PREVENTION'S

YOUR
PERFECT
WEIGHT

The Diet-Free Weight-Loss Method Developed by the World's Leading Health Magazine

Mark Bricklin, Editor, *PREVENTION* Magazine and Linda Konner

Rodale Press, Emmaus, Pennsylvania

Copyright © 1995 by Rodale Press, Inc.
Cover photograph copyright © 1995 by Burk Uzzle

Prevention is a registered trademark of Rodale Press, Inc.

Printed in the United States of America on acid-free ∞ ,
recycled paper containing a minimum of 20% post-consumer waste ♻

"Fight Fat!" table on page 49 is reprinted with permission, *Tufts University Diet and Nutrition Letter*, New York, New York.

Library of Congress Cataloging-in-Publication Data

Bricklin, Mark.
　　Prevention's your perfect weight : the diet-free weight-loss
method developed by the world's leading health magazine / by Mark Bricklin
and Linda Konner.
　　　　p.　　cm.
　　Includes index.
　　ISBN 0–87596–229–7 hardcover
　　1. Reducing. I. Konner, Linda. II. Prevention (Emmaus, Pa.) III. Title.
RM222.2.B777 1995
613.2′5—dc20　　　　　　　　　　　　　　　　　　　　　　　94–5318
　　　　　　　　　　　　　　　　　　　　　　　　　　　　　　　CIP

Distributed in the book trade by St. Martin's Press

2　4　6　8　10　9　7　5　3　1　hardcover

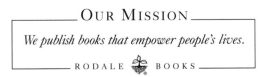

──────── OUR MISSION ────────
We publish books that empower people's lives.
──── RODALE 🌱 BOOKS ────

PREVENTION'S YOUR PERFECT WEIGHT EDITORIAL AND DESIGN STAFF

EDITOR: Alice Feinstein

CONTRIBUTING WRITERS: Lisa Delaney, Greg Gutfeld, Jeff Meade, Marty Munson, Cathy Perlmutter, Linda Rao, Maggie Spilner, Michele Toth

INTERIOR AND COVER DESIGNER: Acey Lee

COVER PHOTOGRAPHER: Burk Uzzle

STUDIO MANAGER: Joe Golden

LAYOUT DESIGNER: Publication Design

TECHNICAL ARTISTS: Kristen Page Morgan, David Q. Pryor

COPY EDITOR: Durrae Johanek

RESEARCH EDITOR: Bernadette Sukley

RESEARCH ASSOCIATE: Sally A. Reith

OFFICE STAFF: Roberta Mulliner, Julie Kehs, Mary Lou Stephen

PREVENTION MAGAZINE HEALTH BOOKS

EDITOR-IN-CHIEF, RODALE BOOKS: Bill Gottlieb

EXECUTIVE EDITOR: Debora A. Tkac

ART DIRECTOR: Jane Colby Knutila

RESEARCH MANAGER: Ann Gossy Yermish

COPY MANAGER: Lisa D. Andruscavage

Jack W. McAninch, M.D.
Chief of urology at San Francisco General Hospital and professor and vice-chairman of the Department of Urology at the University of California, San Francisco

Morris B. Mellion, M.D.
Clinical associate professor of family practice and orthopaedic surgery at the University of Nebraska Medical Center and medical director of the Sports Medicine Center, both in Omaha

Susan Olson, Ph.D.
Clinical psychologist and former director of psychological services at the Southwest Bariatric Nutrition Center in Tempe, Arizona

Thomas Platts-Mills, M.D., Ph.D.
Professor of medicine and head of the Division of Allergy and Clinical Immunology at the University of Virginia Medical Center in Charlottesville

David P. Rose, M.D., Ph.D, D.Sc.
Chief of the Division of Nutrition and Endocrinology at Naylor Dana Institute, part of the American Health Foundation in Valhalla, New York

William B. Ruderman, M.D.
Chairperson of the Department of Gastroenterology at Cleveland Clinic Florida in Fort Lauderdale

Yvonne S. Thornton, M.D.
Professor of clinical obstetrics and gynecology at Columbia University College of Physicians and Surgeons in New York City and director of the Perinatal Diagnostic Testing Center at Morristown Memorial Hospital in Morristown, New Jersey

Lila A. Wallis, M.D.
Clinical professor of medicine and director of "Update Your Medicine," a continuing medical education program for physicians, at Cornell University Medical College in New York City

Andrew T. Weil, M.D.
Associate director of the Division of Social Perspectives in Medicine at the University of Arizona College of Medicine in Tucson

CONTENTS

INTRODUCTION
WHAT YOU GAIN WITH WEIGHT LOSS xi

PART ONE: THE KEYS TO YOUR PERFECT WEIGHT

THE HEALTH BENEFITS OF WEIGHT LOSS 3
Ever feel like giving up the endless struggle to drop those extra pounds? Don't!
Extra weight hurts far more than your appearance.

SETTING YOUR GOAL WEIGHT 12
You want to be beautifully thin. How many pounds should you lose to improve
both your health and your appearance? Here's how to get a handle on the perfect
weight for *you*.

A BEGINNER'S GUIDE TO CUTTING FAT.....................................19
It's not exactly a secret that keeping fat out of your mouth is the best way to get the
fat out of your body. Here's the latest on getting fat out of your life for good.

CREATING THE LOW-FAT KITCHEN 35
Using the right kind of equipment and laying in the right kind of supplies make it a
whole lot easier to prepare scrumptiously slimming meals for the whole family.

SHOP TALK: DEVELOPING YOUR SUPERMARKET SAVVY 41
Don't let your new way of eating get sabotaged in the supermarket aisles. It helps to
have an action plan *before* you find yourself knee deep in chocolate chip cookies.

LOW-FAT COOKING TRICKS 46
There are dozens of ways to eliminate fat in the kitchen without sacrificing taste.
Take advantage of these strategies . . . and your waistline will thank you.

NUTRITION: GETTING THE RIGHT STUFF 51
It's one thing to cut fat grams and calories and quite another to inadvertently
eliminate important nutrients from your diet. Learn to make wise choices without
putting your health at risk.

EXERCISE: YOUR SECRET WEAPON 58
Guess what? You don't have to sweat. A modest amount of comfortably paced
exercise is all it takes to get those pounds off and keep them off forever.

RESISTANCE TRAINING: PUMP UP YOUR WEIGHT-LOSS POWER. 71
Muscle doesn't just look good—it performs weight-loss wonders. Get your muscles
in the right shape, and they'll burn calories for you even while you're just sitting in
front of the TV.

TAMING YOUR STRESS WHILE YOU SHED POUNDS 79
If you nibble whenever you're stressed out, you're not alone. Here are ways to cope
without relying on the soothing, tranquilizing effects of food.

PART TWO: SPECIAL STRATEGIES FOR STAYING THIN FOREVER

CHANGE YOUR WAYS, CHANGE YOUR WEIGHT. 89
You eat when you're bored. You eat for something to do. Sometimes you eat
without even noticing it. . . . If you want to achieve your perfect weight, you'll have
to turn on some healthy eating habits.

JUMP-STARTING YOUR MOTIVATION. 99
Almost everyone gets off to a great start on a new "diet." But what do you do when
your new way of eating is forever . . . and your enthusiasm for the program has
bottomed out at zero?

READER SURVEY RESULTS: THE BEST WAYS TO GET THIN FOREVER 102
Who best knows how to lose weight and keep it off? People who have done it, of
course. Here are the top secrets from those who have walked the walk.

CALLING ALL MEN! 107
For most men, "diet" is a four-letter word. And once they decide to lose weight,
they face their own special challenges. Arming yourself with the right information
makes the battle easier.

FOR WOMEN ONLY. 114
Pregnancy and menopause are the two times in a woman's life during which she's
most likely to put on extra pounds. Knowing what to do ahead of time is a big plus.

HIS/HER GUIDE TO WEIGHT LOSS. 119
There are no two ways about it. Men and women lose weight differently. Here's the
scoop on foods, attitude boosters and exercises most likely to work for each gender.

KEEPING YOUR KIDS SLIM 128
You think adults carrying extra weight have problems? Try being an overweight kid.
With the right program . . . and a lot of understanding . . . you can turn a child's life
around.

DINING-OUT GUIDE 137
It's frustrating: You spend weeks eating right, then cancel out all your progress with
one weekend of celebration. When you know what to order, however, restaurants
are no longer a problem.

SPECIAL SITUATIONS 144
Holidays . . . buffets . . . Caribbean cruises—sometimes it seems like life is one
gigantic dietary obstacle course. Head into these dietary minefields with a field
guide for preserving your low-fat lifestyle.

TIPS FROM TOP SPAS 147
Celebs pay thousands for the spa treatment. But what goes on behind those
exclusive doors is no secret. You can put their tricks of the trade to work in your
own life.

20 UNEXPECTED REASONS WHY WEIGHT LOSS FAILS 153
You thought you were doing everything right. Suddenly, the scale stalls in place
and refuses to budge, or jumps up for no good reason that you can think of. Is it
something you ate? Maybe.

MAKEOVERS TO LAST A LIFETIME 158
There's nothing like someone else's success to motivate you in your own low-fat
living program. Five people share their personal triumphs over major health-risking
weight problems.

KEEPING IT OFF FOREVER 168
You've probably heard it before—losing weight is only part of the challenge. The
really tough part is keeping it off . . . unless you're willing to change the way you
live. Here's what it takes.

PART THREE: ONE YEAR TO YOUR PERFECT WEIGHT

YOUR PERFECT WEIGHT 52-WEEK PLAN 177
You don't have to go it alone. Following this day-by-day, week-by-week program
will help you take all the necessary steps to losing those extra pounds and being
slim for the rest of your life.

YOUR PERFECT WEIGHT SUCCESS DIARY 275
You win a few; you lose a few. You're *always* a winner if you use your slip-ups and
mistakes to prevent future problems, and what better way to do that than by
keeping close track of your progress?

PART FOUR: RECIPES FOR LOW-FAT LIVING

QUICK AND EASY LOW-FAT RECIPES......................................293
Who says low-fat has to mean low satisfaction? These recipes are so scrumptious
you'll think you're eating to indulge yourself. And guess what? You are!

PART FIVE: FOOD GUIDES FOR LOW-FAT LIVING

NEVER SAY NEVER...325
No matter how well you follow your new low-fat lifestyle, sometimes you simply
can't say no to a food craving. This list helps you know what you're getting into, so
you can plan your bounce-back strategy immediately.

TRAINING YOURSELF TO MAKE BETTER CHOICES 328
With all the great new low-fat products on the market these days, you can often
minimize the damage from all those high-fat goodies you sometimes get a yen for.

SLIMMER SELECTIONS FROM FAST-FOOD RESTAURANTS 334
Don't let fast-food fans sabotage your low-fat lifestyle. Yes, you can eat out with
your friends without undermining all the progress you've made.

SURPRISE! FOODS CAN FOOL YOU 342
You think you have a pretty good handle on what's fat and what's not? If you go by
first impressions, you could be fooling yourself. Here are the foods that dieters most
commonly misconstrue.

ONE HUNDRED 100-CALORIE SNACKS 346
In the mood for a little nibble that will hardly count in the long run? Just turn to
this list and choose a quick snack that you can be sure is low in fat and calories.

TERMS FOR PERFECT WEIGHT 351

INDEX...355

INTRODUCTION

What You Gain with Weight Loss

Perhaps you're wondering if this book can really help you lose weight.

Well, it can. But it can do a lot more, too.

Following our program and tips may well deliver major health benefits that you never dreamed were associated with weight loss.

As Linda and I were working on this book, many people in the scientific community had the same idea: It's time for some fresh looks and new approaches to a problem that seems to be becoming worse almost year by year.

Discoveries in the past few years have put a whole new light on the wisdom and benefits of weight control.

Osteoarthritis of the hands is a good example. Now, you may already know that there's a link between osteoarthritis of the knees and being overweight. It's quite easy to imagine how being fat can foul up your knee joints. As Peter D. Wood, D.Sc., Ph.D., of Stanford University puts it, "Imagine carrying around a 50-pound sack of flour all day."

But now there's research from the University of Michigan showing that overweight is also linked to arthritis of the hands. A study that followed about 1,300 adults of Tecumseh, Michigan, found that people who, on first measurement, were 20 percent or more overweight were three times more likely to have osteoarthritis of the hands when checked again 23 years later, compared with slimmer people of the same age. Plus, their arthritis was more severe.

Chief author Wendy Carman of the Department of Epidemiology at the University of Michigan School of Public Health in Ann Arbor and colleagues aren't sure how overweight may lead to arthritis of the hands. While it could involve some mechanical stress, there's the clear possibility that too much fat in our bodies may cause certain chemical or hormonal changes, which in turn damage joints.

And here is something even more surprising: Overweight may also be a major contributing factor to a nerve-conduction problem in the hand known commonly as carpal tunnel syndrome, or CTS. Usually, we think of this problem as being caused by physical stress on the wrist area. But a group from Portland, Oregon, says: "Not so fast!"

Their analysis shows that degree of overweight was the strongest single predictor of carpal tunnel syndrome, being twice as influential as age. Oddly, the kind of work people did had virtually no bearing on whether they'd develop the problem. Occupation might worsen the problem, but it seems that "health habits and lifestyle" are most associated with appearance of CTS, suggests the team from the Portland Hand Surgery and Rehabilitation Center.

Weight Down, Immunity Up

From Japan comes an intriguing study that implicates obesity as a dangerous weakener of the immune system. This could be why obesity has been linked with greater vulnerability to infection and even some forms of cancer. But doctors at the School of Medicine at Yokohama City University took the research a step further.

They took 34 obese people (yes, there are a few in Japan!), measured their blood for strength of immune function and then put them on pretty strict diets for periods ranging from about three to eight months. Then their blood was reanalyzed.

Finding: Immune reaction of the T lymphocytes—key body defenders—nearly doubled after the subjects peeled off an average of about 50 pounds.

More recently, there is research pointing to the fact that women who are extremely (not just moderately) obese have about twice the risk of giving birth to a baby with a neural tube defect—a very serious condition. (However, researchers do not recommend dieting while trying to conceive, since inadequate nutrient intake can also increase the risk of birth defects.)

Although all this new research is still somewhat tentative, we do know for sure that overweight encourages high blood pressure, heart disease and diabetes. So it could be that the biochemical disruptions caused by overweight are more complex than we thought. Perhaps it is best to think of excess body fat not just as something that may hasten problem A or problem B but rather as a kind of toxic condition that may harm virtually every system and organ.

Besides the ones we've mentioned, obesity also has been linked with gallstones, back pain, sleep apnea, heartburn, stroke, gout, varicose veins and even cancer. Rachel Ballard-Barbash, M.D., at the National Cancer Institute, told us the link is strongest with endometrial cancer. And, she adds, it appears that women who carry fat around their middle (as opposed to on the hips and thighs) have a higher risk of developing breast cancer after the age of menopause.

Now here's the weird part. The benefit that's most immediate and often most dramatic with weight loss is just about entirely ignored by medical researchers. Yet we know from interviewing hundreds of people that it's real.

Have you guessed?

It's simple: You feel better!

The word we hear most frequently is "energy." Often, it's coupled with phrases like "unbelievable . . . what a difference! . . . it's changed my life."

When, in effect, you've turned down the force of gravity by 10, 20 even 30 percent, it's only natural to feel incredibly lighter on your feet. You breathe easier, and there's less strain on you back. A whole new, more active and happier lifestyle becomes available.

So, while most people view losing weight as just that—"How much did I lose?"—we look upon it as powerfully positive: "Look what I gained!"

Mark Bricklin
Editor
Prevention Magazine

Part One

THE KEYS
TO YOUR
PERFECT WEIGHT

THE HEALTH BENEFITS
OF WEIGHT LOSS

Excess weight is bad for you. You already know that besides making you look less than svelte in your bathing suit, being overweight is just plain unhealthy. But exactly how unhealthy is it to carry around extra pounds? The answer, in a word, is *very*.

If you've ever needed to boost your motivation to eat better, exercise more and peel away that excess poundage, read on.

First and foremost, you should know that being overweight has been directly linked to the leading causes of death in this country today: heart disease, certain types of cancer, stroke and diabetes. In addition, excess weight is tied to a host of other conditions of varying degrees of severity, ranging from varicose veins to sleeplessness.

In short, the statistics are staggeringly in favor of achieving and maintaining your ideal weight if you want to live a long, healthy life.

And while the most significant health problems crop up when a person is clinically obese—that is, 20 percent or more above her ideal weight—it doesn't take a big weight loss to effect substantial health improvements. If you have high blood pressure, for example, losing just ten pounds can help reduce it, say health officials at the Michigan Department of Public Health.

"Look," you may well be saying, "I just want to drop a few pounds because I want to fit into that size-eight dress I have my eye on." That's fine. But just in case you need further incentive to launch a serious weight-loss and maintenance program, here are some of the main health benefits you'll reap almost immediately after you start to slim down.

Smoke-Free . . . and Chubby?

People quit smoking for the same reasons they lose weight: to look better and improve their health. Problem is, some people who would like to quit keep on smoking because they're afraid that if they toss the butts they'll put on extra pounds.

In fact, many ex-smokers do put on some pounds when they give up their cigarettes, for a number of reasons. First off, nicotine increases the metabolic rate, the rate at which you burn up calories. So as soon as you stop smoking, your metabolism is likely to slow, and the calories you normally consume won't be burned as efficiently.

Second, to give their mouths and fingers something to do, many ex-smokers become nibblers, often unconsciously. So suddenly they're taking in more calories, whether they're aware of it or not. The result? Extra pounds.

And third, nicotine suppresses the body's insulin levels. Insulin is the hormone that helps your body use sugar and keep your sweet tooth at bay. When smokers quit, they may find that they now crave cakes and cookies—not to mention more food in general, which suddenly tastes great because without tobacco their taste buds have sprung to life.

So an ex-smoker's fear of gaining weight is very real. Yet it is possible to quit smoking and keep those extra pounds at bay.

Here's what you can do.

Eat a healthy, balanced diet. If you feel the urge to snack, have cut-up veggies, a handful of thin pretzel sticks, some sugar-free iced tea or mineral water.

Satisfy your sweet tooth. Try low- or nonfat frozen yogurt, nonfat frozen fruit bars or sugar-free versions of kids' fruit drinks.

Having a Healthier Heart

Each year, more than 900,000 Americans die of heart disease. Almost half of these victims are women. Every year an additional 1.25 million have a nonfatal heart attack. And nearly one-third of adults suffer from high blood pressure, which can, among other things, lead to heart disease and stroke. A major cause of all of the above problems is overweight. Think about it: The more you exceed your ideal weight, the more your heart has to keep pumping to do its job and the greater the pressure you're placing on it.

But lose weight and high blood pressure almost inevitably drops. In one

Keep your mouth busy. Chew on sugarless gum or "smoke" a plastic cigarette. Keep your hands occupied with needlework or gardening or by taking a computer class.

Drink plenty of water. It will aid in digestion and help relieve the bloated feeling ex-smokers sometimes get.

Use a food diary. "Your Perfect Weight Success Diary," on page 273, will help you focus on any changes in your eating behaviors.

Exercise. Especially if you tend to be inactive, you'll need to launch a workout schedule—even a modest one—to counteract your now-slower metabolism. Some ex-smokers report that beginning an exercise program a month or two before they plan to quit smoking is easier and ultimately more long-lasting than attempting both simultaneously.

Weigh yourself once a week. The moment you notice a pound or two you didn't notice before, increase your exercise by an extra 30 to 60 minutes a week.

Find a distraction. Start focusing on things other than smoking and eating. Clean out the garage, join a community project, take a workshop in a subject you've always wanted to explore.

Check out a smoking-cessation clinic. Not only will these sessions help you kick your tobacco addiction but also they'll give you support for dealing with your food cravings.

Give yourself a break. Maybe now's not the time to think about quitting smoking *and* maintaining your weight. After all, kicking the cigarette habit is an achievement in and of itself. If you find yourself gaining five or ten pounds and can't handle the thought of dieting, too, perhaps the smartest thing is to wait until you've been smoke-free for a while and then begin "Your Perfect Weight 52-Week Plan," on page 177.

study done at the University of Pennsylvania's Obesity Research Group, people with high blood pressure experienced dramatic reductions in pressure even in the early stages of their weight-loss diet.

The kinds of foods you're eating will also affect your heart, determining whether your arteries are open and free-flowing or as clogged as a drain begging for Drāno. A diet high in fat, particularly the saturated fat that comes from animal sources, causes arteries to plug up with a gooey substance called plaque. Blood has a harder time circulating through plaque-filled arteries. But a diet in which no more than 25 percent of calories come from fat keeps blood flowing smoothly and dramatically cuts your chances of having a heart attack.

Boosting Good Cholesterol

By now you probably know that LDL, or "bad," artery-clogging choles-terol is affected by the foods we eat—especially the amounts and types of fat. But did you know that you can also increase your HDL, or "good," artery-cleaning cholesterol, by being at or near your ideal weight? Regular exercise also helps.

"The younger you are and the less fat you carry, the better your chances of reducing your cholesterol levels to well within the desirable range—say, 175 to 195 milligrams total cholesterol per deciliter of blood," reports Louis J. Aronne, M.D., associate professor of clinical medicine at New York Hospital–Cornell University Medical College in New York City. (An HDL level of 60 milligrams per deciliter of blood or greater is considered good; at less than 35, it's a risk factor for heart disease. And an LDL reading of under 130 is desirable; it's risky when it hits 160 or above.)

Happily, you needn't wait until you reach your goal weight to see good HDL results. "Even rather small weight losses—10 percent of initial weight or so—will result in increased HDL levels," says F. Xavier Pi-Sunyer, M.D., director of the Obesity Research Center at St. Luke's–Roosevelt Hospital Center in New York City.

Your cholesterol may rise as you get older, and while you can't do much to avoid birthdays, you certainly can start to lower your cholesterol readings by lowering your weight.

Decreasing the Risk of Diabetes

Of all the major diseases, diabetes is the one most clearly linked to over-weight. Of the 11 million Americans suffering from the disease, 90 percent have non-insulin-dependent (Type II) diabetes—precisely the type most closely associated with excess weight.

"There's no question that obesity is a major contributor to the develop-ment of diabetes," says Susan Zelitch Yanovski, M.D., an obesity expert at the National Institute of Diabetes and Digestive and Kidney Diseases in Bethesda, Maryland. But here again, the news is good. "Even a modest weight loss," she says, "can significantly reduce risk for the development of diabetes, as well as improve the blood sugar of those who already have it."

Adds Dr. Pi-Sunyer, "In people with non-insulin-dependent diabetes, blood sugar levels improve within days after starting a weight-loss program, and in some cases medication can be greatly reduced or eliminated."

Preventing Cancer

While there's some debate over whether overweight is a factor in breast cancer, there is a distinct relationship between breast cancer and a high-fat

---

What's Up, Doc? (maybe it's your weight)

Want to launch a weight-loss program? Consulting your physician for help and advice is a good idea, but don't assume that he necessarily practices what he might preach to you about a healthy diet.

One survey revealed that more than half (55 percent) of U.S. doctors are overweight. And while they may know the value of eating five daily servings of fruits and vegetables, a scant 20 percent do so. A whopping 66 percent confessed that they ate some candy "in the past week." The survey was conducted in 1993 by Sudler and Hennessey, the health care and pharmaceuticals advertising division of Young and Rubicam.

"I was surprised that so many physicians said they were overweight," says John Chervokas, the Sudler and Hennessey executive vice president who headed up the survey. "We received a much larger response from doctors than we had originally anticipated, which proved to us that the doctors are interested in the subjects of diet and nutrition. Or, maybe they're just interested in food!"

---

diet, which generally leads to overweight as well. In Japan, where until recently fat intake was far lower than ours, the incidence of breast cancer was also far lower.

However, things are changing. As the Japanese eat more fat and their diet begins to resemble the typical high-fat American diet, they are experiencing more breast cancer.

Many experts now believe that limiting dietary fat to no more than 20 percent of calories consumed—a figure substantially lower than the government's recommended ceiling of 30 percent—is the ideal way to ward off breast cancer. But even if you lean more toward the higher percentage, you're still dramatically cutting your chances of getting breast cancer, which strikes one in every nine American women.

In addition to breast cancer, overweight women experience greater incidence of other types of cancer, including ovarian and cervical. "Studies have shown that obesity leads to increased levels of estrone, a cancer-promoting hormone," says Dr. Yanovski. "While not all of the evidence for this is clear right now, it is likely that being at a healthy body weight would help give protection from these forms of cancer."

In men, high-fat diets have been associated with prostate cancer, and so they, like women, would be wise to limit their dietary fat intake to no more than 25 or 30 percent of calories from fat.

Weight Down, Sex Up

Want yet another good reason to lose weight? It'll give a boost to your sex drive!

Ronette Kolotkin, Ph.D., director of the behavioral program at the Duke University Diet and Fitness Center in Durham, North Carolina, conducted a pair of studies examining the relationship between weight and quality of life. Sixty-four overweight people entering a typical one-month weight-loss program at Duke were asked to respond to statements about how weight affects their quality of life, including six about sexual life.

- "I do not feel sexually attractive."

- "I have little or no sexual desire."

- "I don't want anyone to see me undressed."

- "I have difficulty with sexual performance."

- "I avoid sexual encounters whenever possible."

- "I do not enjoy sexual activity."

A month later, after completing a program of eating right, exercising and losing weight—on average 8 to 30 pounds—they were asked about the same six statements. To a man (and woman!), they answered quite positively.

"They reported that now they felt more sexual desire and more sexually attractive," reveals Dr. Kolotkin. "What's interesting to note is that someone answering the questions might have lost 20 pounds and still have had 20 or 50 to go. So the point is, you don't need to lose all your excess weight in order to have a quality-of-life improvement—including your sex life."

Living Longer

Again, the Japanese seem to have many of the answers. Despite their unfortunate, and growing, fondness for our own beloved high-fat fast foods, the traditionally low-fat Asian lifestyle generally means a longer life: Japanese men and women have the longest life expectancy in the world.

A new study has also shown that you'll function better as you age if you keep body fat down. Larry Wier, Ed.D., director of the health-related fitness program at the NASA Johnson Space Center in Houston, Texas, studied 300 women and their ability to use oxygen during exercise. Although it had always been believed that your exercise efficiency inevitably declines with age, Dr. Wier learned otherwise. "We found that the more body fat a person accumulates over the years, the more of a decline he or she will see," he says. "Some folks over 75 are more functional than others who are much younger. As you grow older, it pays to keep your body fat low and your exercise high."

Building Better Backs and Joints

Extra pounds up front also invariably lead to extra stress on your back. It's believed that just 10 too many pounds around your abdomen, centered ten inches in front of your spine, means your back muscles have to exert a force of 50 pounds to counterbalance your gut.

"Over half of all Americans will eventually develop some back problems, and almost every physician will advise overweight patients with back trouble to reduce their body weight," says Dr. Yanovski.

Doctors also suspect that keeping your weight down will help prevent osteoarthritis by taking a load off your already-overworked joints, particularly knee joints. Nearly 10 percent of folks over 65—and more women than men—suffer from this wear-and-tear knee problem, and obesity is a major risk factor. But if, for example, a 5'4" woman who weighs 165 pounds loses 11 pounds and keeps it off, she can reduce her chances of developing this condition by one-third.

Your hip joints will also thank you if you keep your weight down.

Easing through Pregnancy and Childbirth

The closer you are to your ideal weight, the simpler your pregnancy and delivery will be, says registered dietitian Joann Heslin, author of 16 books and co-author of The Pregnancy Nutrition Counter. "If you're physically fit, you'll be able to endure labor more easily," she says. "But if you're heavier, you may complicate it, and you'll put yourself at greater risk should you require surgery—the doctor may have to cut through three inches of fat before she can get to the baby."

There's no real mystery about delivering a baby, Heslin points out—your body knows how to do it naturally. "But if you're in good shape to start out with, you'll help your body do its job nicely," she says.

Dr. Yanovski adds that an overweight new mom is more likely to develop such complications as pregnancy-induced diabetes and high blood pressure.

"Even though the diabetes usually disappears after delivery, a woman who's had diabetes during her pregnancy must work long and hard to prevent the development of diabetes later in life," she says. "A large number of these women do go on to develop Type II diabetes."

Fat: It Hurts More Than Your Looks

Think a steady diet of fattening foods will just make your belly bulge? Nope. It can take its toll on almost every part of your body, and in ways that won't make you too happy. Here's how obesity can affect every part of your body.

Body Part	Problem or Condition
Brain	Stroke
Windpipe	Intensified snoring
Armpits	Excess sweating
Heart	Enlargement, erratic beat, other types of heart disease
Breasts	Cancer
Liver	Cirrhosis
Gallbladder	Gallstones, cancer
Kidneys	Kidney stones, kidney failure due to high blood pressure
Pancreas	Diabetes
Ovaries	Sterility, cancer
Uterus	Cancer
Cervix	Cancer
Hip, knee and ankle bones	Arthritis
Legs	Varicose veins

Getting Well and Staying Well

Any surgery you might need becomes far more difficult and dangerous the heavier you are. But, says Dr. Pi-Sunyer, "just a 10 percent reduction in body weight can reduce the duration of hospitalization and the incidence of postoperative complications."

When you lose weight by cutting fat, you're also giving a big boost to your immune system. That's what scientists at the USDA's Human Nutrition Research Center in San Francisco discovered after monitoring the changes in seven women they studied. Their diets had been reduced from about 41 percent to approximately 30 percent of calories from fat. While this is admittedly a modest study, it suggests that you can only do your immune system good by keeping your weight at a desirable level.

Boosting Energy Levels

Think of how perky you feel when you're lugging home 25 pounds of groceries. Not very? Then you'll have a good idea how an extra 25 pounds (or more) of body weight can drag you down and make you feel more tired and sluggish than necessary. One of the first things dieters report is how much extra energy they have after they've lost even 5 or 10 pounds. They also sleep better.

Many overweight people have a condition known as sleep apnea, and many of those who have it go undiagnosed. Not only do people with apnea snore but also their breathing passages become blocked. Typically, they wake up again and again or sleep fitfully, never getting adequate rest. "They get drowsy during the day and may start to fall asleep during meetings or while driving their car," explains Dr. Yanovski.

Dieting can help tremendously, she says, adding, "Sleep apnea is very responsive to weight loss."

SETTING YOUR GOAL WEIGHT

You're ready to embark on a sensible eating-and-exercise program. And you realize that there's probably something to *Prevention's Your Perfect Weight* philosophy: Instead of dieting, you're going to be making some healthy lifestyle changes that you will follow for the rest of your life.

Fine. But what about all that . . . uh . . . fat? What happens when you know you have some pounds to shed before you're at a healthy weight that's attractive and comfortable for you?

The question then becomes how *many* pounds. Ah, that's the $64,000 question.

Only you can decide on the goal weight you'll be shooting for over the next weeks and months. And just how do you go about determining your goal weight?

It's an important question, because the wrong choice could create health problems. In fact, selecting the wrong goal for yourself may very well have been responsible for diet failures in the past.

If you're choosing your target number based on a picture of bikini-clad Cindy Crawford taped to your refrigerator door, or on a yellowing photograph of yourself in your wedding dress from three decades ago, your goal-weight expectations might be unrealistic. Times, and "ideal weight" guidelines, have definitely changed.

Depending on whom you talk to, you'll get a different opinion about the best weight for you and how to achieve and maintain it.

These suggestions should help you decide on a goal weight that makes sense for you.

Standard Tables Are Not So Standard

Are you one of those people who swears by those standard government height-weight tables? Then you should know that they have been dramatically updated over the past few years. What's more, even the people who put those numbers together insist that you can't just focus on one number. Rather, they insist, you must understand how the numbers were determined. Only then will the goal weight you set for yourself be the best one for you.

Doing It by the Numbers: Suggested Weights for Adults

When picking a weight for yourself, checking the federal government's standard guidelines for adults can be helpful. Don't just land on one number; choose a range of three to five pounds. After all, body weights naturally fluctuate, especially among women, and it's unlikely that your weight will stay exactly the same day after day, no matter how diligent you are about your diet and exercise program. There's no point in setting yourself up for psychological disappointment, and if you allow yourself a range of a few pounds, you'll still be able to monitor how you're doing, *and* catch yourself in plenty of time if your weight starts creeping up past that acceptable limit.

Note that the ranges are for both men and women, with the higher numbers in the range intended for men. Also note that the heights are measured without shoes on and the weights taken without clothes on.

Height	Weight		Height	Weight	
	19 to 34 years	35 and older		19 to 34 years	35 and older
5'0"	97–128	108–138	5'10"	132–174	146–188
5'1"	101–132	111–143	5'11"	136–179	151–194
5'2"	104–137	115–148	6'0"	140–184	155–199
5'3"	107–141	119–152	6'1"	144–189	159–205
5'4"	111–146	122–157	6'2"	148–195	164–210
5'5"	114–150	126–162	6'3"	152–200	168–216
5'6"	118–155	130–167	6'4"	156–205	173–222
5'7"	121–160	134–172	6'5"	160–211	177–228
5'8"	125–164	138–178	6'6"	164–216	182–234
5'9"	129–169	142–183			

Why were those tried-and-true tables changed, anyway? Well . . . because they weren't so true after all. "Originally, the Dietary Guidelines for Americans were based on the 1959 and 1983 Metropolitan Life Insurance tables, using nonrepresentative populations—that is, only people who were applying for life insurance. But the tables were changed in 1990 because we wanted a more representative sampling of the population," explains Jay Green, a registered dietitian with the U.S. Department of Agriculture (USDA).

Up until 1990, the criteria used to create the tables were essentially an insurance applicant's height, frame and gender—that's it. So, if you were a 5'5", medium-framed woman wearing three pounds of clothes and one-inch heels, you should have weighed anywhere from 127 to 141, period. Those early tables assumed that all women who were 5'5" were exactly alike.

But then things changed, for the logical. For the first time, such crucial factors as one's other health problems, such as high blood pressure and elevated blood sugar; a family history of obesity-related problems, including diabetes; and the location of fat in the body were taken into account, explains C. Wayne Callaway, M.D. Dr. Callaway was a member of the nine-person Dietary Guidelines Advisory Committee to the USDA and the Department of Health and Human Services, the government institutions that drafted the proposed changes to the earlier tables. The committee's aim? To encourage people to shift their thinking away from the ambiguous "desirable weight" to "healthy weight."

Suddenly, says Dr. Callaway, the old height-weight charts seemed outmoded. "The notion that ideal body weight is independent of how much body fat you have is foolish," he says. "The amount of body fat is much more important than actual weight as well as where the fat is located and whether you have other health conditions. If all you used was the weight table to determine your healthy weight, it would give you false reassurance if, for example, you had spindly legs but also a potbelly. And healthy pear-shaped women, on the basis of the table, might feel they had to lose weight, even though there's no evidence that fat in the thighs causes harm."

Also added to the new tables were separate sets of weights for folks above and below age 35. The reason? "Our data showed that overweight is much more hazardous in terms of your future health if you're 20 than if you're 60," Dr. Callaway explains. "The adverse health consequences of excess body weight seem to be greater the younger you are."

Which is *not*, he quickly points out, license for older people to pack on the pounds, even though a quick glance at the tables might seem to indicate that. It simply means that no appreciable health risk has been found for slightly heavier weights among older folks.

What Kind of Fruit Are You?

Apples are great to eat, but it's not so great when you look like one.

Most overweight women tend to be pear-shaped, with the excess weight concentrated in their hips and thighs. Most overweight men, on the other hand, are apple-shaped, with their extra pounds packed around their bellies.

A report based on a five-year Iowa Women's Health Study—involving more than 40,000 older women—revealed that the rounder or more apple-shaped a body is, the higher the risk of health complications and even death. Why? Researchers think they have the answer. Any belly fat that's actually within the abdominal cavity can easily enter the bloodstream and deposit it-self onto the liver, leading to higher levels of blood cholesterol, they believe. They also have evidence that excess abdominal fat might cause elevated blood pressure and blood sugar levels.

To determine whether your body shape puts you at health risk, first measure your waist at the narrowest point between the bottom of your rib cage and the top of your pelvis. Then divide that number by the size of your hips at the widest protrusion of your buttocks. The number you get is your waist-hip ratio. If you're a woman and the number you get is larger than 0.8 (or if you're a man and your number is 1.0 or higher), you're carrying more abdominal fat than is good for you. A weight-loss diet will probably help reduce your belly fat—along with your health risks.

So, Dr. Callaway concludes that if all three of the following statements describe you, then there's no health reason for you to lose weight.

1. I have no health problems that would be eased or eliminated through weight loss.

2. My waist-to-hip ratio is acceptable. (To determine your hip-waist ratio, see "What Kind of Fruit Are You?")

3. My current weight falls within the U.S. Dietary Guidelines. (See "Doing It by the Numbers: Suggested Weights for Adults," on page 13.)

Letting Go of False Ideals

If, after all this talk about setting a healthy goal weight, you're still clinging to the dream of someday returning to your college or wedding-day weight, you need to recognize that it just may not be possible—or worth it. After all, as you age your metabolism naturally slows down—and the weight you could easily maintain in your teens or twenties might not be doable today without a considerable decrease in the number of calories you take in or without stepping up your exercise program to superhuman levels.

If your notion of what your body size should be is based on what you see on the TV screen or in the pages of fashion magazines, you may be dooming yourself to failure. The fact is, most of us don't look like actresses or models, and to attempt to make our bodies match theirs is unnecessarily punishing, if not impossible. Obesity expert Kelly D. Brownell, Ph.D., of Yale University's psychology department, estimates that most actresses and models probably have a body-fat composition of just 10 to 15 percent. Normal body fat for healthy women is about twice that much—22 to 26 percent. To try to get your body down to such levels may seriously jeopardize your health.

Getting Real

Rather than forcing your body to conform to some unrealistic ideal, consider what is healthy for you, Dr. Brownell advises.

Dr. Brownell says that for people with relatively small amounts to lose— say, 10 or 20 pounds—shooting for the numbers in the government health tables is fine and probably realistic. "But if you have much more weight to lose, the tables can be an obstacle," he insists. "It presses people to try to achieve weights that, for biological or psychological reasons, may not be attainable for them. They may fixate on the tables, push themselves to try to reach a certain weight, dismiss the value of anything short of that, and then become high risks for relapse."

So rather than aim for an "ideal weight," Dr. Brownell believes that goal weights should be highly personalized and renamed "reasonable weights," attained through reasonable changes in one's diet and exercise. He believes, for instance, that your starting weight and the length of time you've been overweight are key factors in establishing your goal weight. Thus, a 5'4" woman who has weighed 175 pounds for the past ten years, would have a very different target weight compared with a 5'4" woman who weighed 135 for most of her adult life and then suddenly shot up to 150 over the past year. The woman who maintained 135 most of her life might realistically expect to get back to her original, comfortable weight of 135. But the woman who has weighed 175 for the past ten years might be satisfied if she reaches and maintains a weight of 150.

Dr. Brownell knows his theory is controversial. "Many people believe that ideal weight taken from a health perspective is the only weight, and that anyone who is above that mark should lose," he says. "But I think that ignores reality. It would be great if people didn't drink too much or smoke either, but that's not the way it is."

The Bathroom Scale—Friend or Foe?

Are you the sort of person who wakes up, staggers into the bathroom half-asleep, climbs onto the scale . . . and becomes depressed for the rest of the day if you don't see a number you like? You've got lots of company: all those diet fanatics who let the numbers on the scale rule their lives.

Don't misunderstand. Just like standardized height-weight charts, scales are useful tools for gauging your weight-loss or maintenance patterns, and you should buy the best, most accurate model you can afford to help you attain and maintain your goals.

But remember: Your scale is your assistant, not your boss, your mother or your guru. If the number your see today happens to be higher than the number you noticed the last time—regardless of your sensible eating and exercise in the interim—it may be because you drank more water than usual, or because you consumed more water-retaining salt or monosodium glutamate or because your menstrual period is here (or fast approaching). And let's face it, there will be times when your weight goes up for no discernible reason at all.

The real questions to ask yourself as you hop on and off the scale are: How am I eating? How often am I exercising? How do I look? How do I feel? The more you come up with answers you like, the more you'll realize that the number on the scale is just a number.

You might want to determine your goal weight by aiming for the lowest weight you've comfortably maintained as an adult for one year. The thinking is that once you're back at that weight, via a sensible diet and exercise program such as the one outlined in this book, it shouldn't be too difficult to stay there.

Doing What Comes Naturally

Other weight-loss experts recommend aiming for what they call your natural weight. Your natural weight is the weight you will maintain when you eat normally (approximately 1,800 calories per day for a woman, and 2,200 per day for a man) and exercise regularly, doing the equivalent of a one-hour brisk walk daily. Eat right and get the right amount of exercise, many pros say, and you should eventually get down to an easily maintained weight you're happy with. And that weight may well be something other than what you find on any height-weight chart.

Firming Up Rather Than Slimming Down

Another point to consider when establishing your goal weight: You may not love what you see when you look in the mirror, but your spreading bottom or your flabby middle may not automatically mean a weight-reducing diet is in order. Perhaps what you really need is to start a regular program of resistance training to reshape and strengthen your body without weight loss. (To learn how to start a resistance-training program, see "Resistance Training: Pump Up Your Weight-Loss Power," on page 71.)

When it comes to choosing the best weight for you, there are clearly many factors to consider. Don't hesitate to get your doctor's input, *if* she's at a reasonable weight herself! The bottom line, however, is that the number you shoot for should be one you can comfortably live with—now and forever.

A BEGINNER'S GUIDE TO CUTTING FAT

Count fat, not calories. It seems so obvious, so sensible now, and yet it's a relatively new concept in the world of weight loss. It is a concept well worth paying attention to, however. That's because science has shown conclusively that to shed pounds and, incidentally, to prevent diseases of many kinds, fat is what you need to cut, not calories.

Ounce for ounce, dietary fat contains more than twice the calories and is more readily converted to body fat than either protein or carbohydrates. So when you count fat, you're automatically counting lots and lots of calories.

"One of the main benefits of a low-fat diet is the spontaneous reduction of caloric intake and weight loss," says registered dietitian James Kenney, Ph.D., nutrition research specialist at the Pritikin Longevity Center in Santa Monica, California.

Carbohydrates and proteins each have just four calories per gram, compared with nine calories per gram of fat. You don't have to be a mathematician to realize what this means to you, namely, that you can eat twice as many carbs and proteins as fat and still take in fewer calories. That, in combination with daily exercise, is the not-so-magic formula for lifelong weight-loss success.

You probably already know from firsthand experience that, unlike low-fat diets, low-calorie diets are not only potentially dangerous but simply don't work long-term. "That's because when you eat less, your body interprets this as starvation," explains Dean Ornish, M.D., who heads up the Pre-

Figuring Out the Fat

Before you can begin to cut fat, you should have a fairly good idea of how much you're already consuming day to day. Take this quick quiz to find out.

1. How many ounces of meat, fish or poultry do you usually eat per day? (A 3-ounce serving includes one regular hamburger, ½ chicken breast, one pork chop, and so forth.)
    a. None
    b. 3 ounces or less
    c. 4 to 6 ounces
    d. 7 ounces or more

2. How much cheese do you eat per week?
    a. None
    b. Only low-fat cheese, such as low-fat ricotta or cottage cheese
    c. Whole-milk cheese 1 or 2 times a week
    d. Whole-milk cheese 3 or more times a week

3. What type of milk do you use?
    a. Only skim or 1 percent milk
    b. Skim or 1 percent milk, but others occasionally
    c. 2 percent or whole milk

4. How many egg yolks do you use per week?
    a. None and/or egg substitute
    b. 2
    c. 3 or more

5. How often do you eat lunch meat, hot dogs, corned beef, spareribs, sausage, bacon or liver?
    a. Never
    b. About once a week
    c. 2 to 4 times a week
    d. 4 or more times a week

ventive Medicine Research Institute in Sausalito, California, and wrote *Eat More, Weigh Less*. "So your body goes into a survival mode, which means your metabolism slows down and you burn calories less easily. It helps you survive if you are starving to death, but if you're trying to lose weight, that's the last thing you want to have happen," he says. "You'll lose weight at first, but as your metabolism slows more and more, you'll gradually stop losing."

Which is why switching to a low-fat diet means you can shed pounds without starving yourself. "If you change the type of food you eat—from

6. How often do you usually eat foods such as baked goods (cake, cookies, doughnuts, etc.) and ice cream?
   a. None
   b. Once a week
   c. 2 to 4 times a week
   d. 4 or more times a week
7. What's the main type of fat you use for cooking?
   a. None
   b. Safflower, sunflower, corn or soybean oil
   c. Olive or peanut oil, or margarine
   d. Shortening, butter or bacon drippings
8. How often do you eat snack foods such as chips, fries or party crackers?
   a. Never
   b. Once a week
   c. 2 to 4 times a week
   d. 4 or more times a week
9. What spread do you usually use on bread, vegetables and the like?
   a. None
   b. Soft (tub) or diet margarine
   c. Stick margarine
   d. Butter

TO SCORE

For each time you answered (*a*), give yourself 1 point. Each (*b*) gets 2 points, each (*c*) 3 points and each (*d*) 4 points. Now add up the numbers from each of your answers. If you score 15 or less, good for you! You're already following a low-fat diet. Anything higher than 18 can be considered high-fat, and the first step in your quest to cut fat from your diet is to switch as many of your (*c*) and (*d*) answers to (*a*) and (*b*).

high-fat meats, dairy products and processed foods, to low-fat carbohydrates and proteins, such as fruits and vegetables, grains and legumes—you don't really have to worry about the amount," notes Dr. Ornish. "Your metabolism won't slow down; in fact, it may even increase because it can burn protein and carbohydrate calories much more efficiently than fat calories."

The rewards of a low-fat diet are many, the experts agree. The best news of all: They can be yours pretty painlessly. "You do have to change your eating pattern permanently if you're going to keep your weight off," insists Steven Jonas, M.D., professor of preventive medicine at the School of Medicine, State University of New York at Stony Brook, and author of *Take Control of Your Weight*. "But lowering the fat in your diet is the easiest way to do it."

Getting Started

Now that you've determined that counting and trimming fat are tops on your weight-loss agenda, the question is: How exactly do you count fat? And how do you figure out how much is too much for you?

A good place to start is by taking a cold, hard look at just how much fat you're currently eating. And a good way to do that is by taking the simple quiz, "Figuring Out the Fat," on page 20.

If you're already eating a low-fat diet, congratulations! If you're like most Americans, however, you face a few alterations in your daily diet. Perhaps the word *diet* in this context requires a little explanation. We're not taking about something you do short-term to drop a few unwanted pounds. This "diet" is something you're going to embrace and live with for the rest of your life (which, incidentally, should be considerably longer once you make these changes).

So, how much fat cutting are we talking about here? Several nutritional authorities recommend that you lower your fat intake so that it accounts for no more than 30 percent of the total calories you take in each day. We advise, for the sake of your weight-loss program and your health, even lower intakes—a maximum of 25 percent. But is there an easy way to tell when your fat intake is within the guidelines?

The Easy Way to Keep Your Diet Lean

The old standard method was to get out your calculator to figure percentage of calories from fat for individual foods or your entire daily diet. For foods, you'd check the labels for total grams of fat per serving, then multiply that number by 9, divide by the total calories per serving, and multiply by 100. Whew! That's a lot of work when all you wanted was a handful of potato chips. But we have an easier way.

First, check the "Fat Budget" table, on page 23, for your magic number. That's the maximum number of grams of fat you should be eating daily to get no more than 25 percent of your calories from fat while you lose weight. Then, just count the grams of fat you eat each day and make sure the total doesn't exceed your magic number.

Let's take the example of a 140-pound woman who wants to get down to 120 pounds. The chart indicates that to maintain her weight, she's probably eating about 47 grams of fat (and about 1,700 calories) every day. But to re-

Fat Budget

How much fat is too much fat? Frustrated diet cynics would probably snap, "Any fat at all is too much." The fact of the matter is that you need some fat in your daily diet. (Anyway, it's just about impossible to eliminate all the fat.) This chart will help you figure out how much fat you can safely eat in order to reach and maintain your perfect weight.

To use the chart, find your current weight in the first column. The second column shows the number of calories you're probably eating every day to maintain that weight. What you want to memorize is the number in the third column that corresponds to your target weight in the first column.

Weight	Calorie Intake	Fat Limit (g.)	Weight	Calorie Intake	Fat Limit (g.)
WOMEN			MEN		
110	1,300	36	130	1,800	50
120	1,400	39	140	2,000	56
130	1,600	44	150	2,100	58
140	1,700	47	160	2,200	61
150	1,800	50	170	2,400	67
160	1,900	53	180	2,500	69
170	2,000	56	190	2,700	75
180	2,200	61	200	2,800	78

duce her weight to 120 pounds, she should bring her fat intake to no more than 40 grams of fat per day.

Keep in mind that these fat limits are approximate and that the chart is for sedentary people. If you exercise regularly and vigorously, you can afford a few more grams of fat (three grams for every extra 100 calories you burn). The chart doesn't account for age, either, and metabolism slows down with age. So it's particularly important for older people to step up their exercise and keep fat calories within these recommended ranges.

As for identifying the fat grams in a given serving, those numbers appear on just about all packaged foods. For fresh produce, meats, fish, and the like, you can refer to any fat-gram counter. (See the "Fat Finder's Guide," on page 28, to help you get started.)

This approach to counting fat has a way of encouraging some very healthy attitudes toward low-fat eating. For one thing, it correctly implies that it's more important to limit total fat intake than to fret about particular

Bad Fat, Good Fat

Fat, fat, fat. All this talk about cutting fat might lead you to believe that a zero-fat diet is the healthiest one of all. Not really. Dietary fat serves several useful purposes. Dieters and nondieters alike need a minimum of 2 to 5 percent of their calories from fat for energy, to process vitamins A, D, E and K, and to avoid certain skin and liver disorders.

Fat also provides that nice feeling of satiety that keeps you from overeating. So we're not saying you should shun fat altogether, just eat less of it. And stay away as much as possible from the most harmful varieties. The list below will help you separate the good guys from the baddies.

Good: Monounsaturated oils (such as olive and canola) protect against heart disease. Polyunsaturated fats (corn and other vegetable oils) tend to reduce blood cholesterol levels.

Bad: Hydrogenated fats (margarine, shortening and other solid and semi-solid vegetable oils treated with hydrogen) clog coronary arteries.

Worst of all: Saturated fats (butter and other animal fats, which are solid at room temperature) put you at high risk for heart disease and some types of cancers. Both the National Institutes of Health and the American Heart Association recommend that you limit saturated fat to under 10 percent of total calories.

---

foods that contribute to that total. (Dieters often try to forbid themselves from having any high-fat fare, but if you're eating small amounts—an occasional pat of butter, a few slices of lean meat—it'll cost you just a few grams of fat.) And indulging in those once-in-a-while treats can help you avoid that poor-deprived-me mentality that can scuttle your diet.

Also, since high-fat foods can so quickly put you over your daily fat-gram quota, this approach automatically encourages you to choose more delicious low-fat alternatives. As a result, you'll inevitably end up eating extra fruits, vegetables, whole grains and other complex carbohydrates while keeping fat intake (and weight) down.

Take It Easy, Take It Slow

We've talked about how to reduce dietary fat in terms of numbers. But eating habits and food preferences can't be dictated by fat-gram charts and nutrition labels. We're human, after all, and we love the taste of chocolate bars and corn chips, cookie-dough ice cream and thick, juicy steaks. Can we realistically expect to swear off our favorites, no matter how strong our desire to be thin?

No, say the experts, nor do you need to. The key is to make dietary adjustments in stages. "I say it over and over again: When it comes to food and exercise, gradual change leads to permanent changes," says Dr. Jonas. "Cognitively, I may understand that reducing fat is a good idea, but I like the taste, and I know I can't do it instantly. Fine—you don't have to. Eating is a lifetime activity, and you have a better chance of making a permanent change if you don't try to do it all at once. Instead, make food substitutions on a gradual basis."

Let's say you've decided to eat less red meat. "Sit down and make a chart for the past week, counting up how many meat meals you ate out of 21,"

Breakfast (lunch and dinner) of Champions

What do you serve a beefy football player to get the best game out of him? Would you believe . . . bagels? Orange juice? Apples? Yes, insists Dean Kleinschmidt, president of the Professional Athletic Trainers Society and head athletic trainer for the New Orleans Saints professional football team, who's been on a mission to gradually switch players from a high-fat to a high-carbohydrate diet. And it's been working.

The majority of NFL teams are now getting most of their calories from pasta, grains, fruits and veggies rather than fatty foods.

Before, explains Kleinschmidt, "players thought they had to eat pounds and pounds of meat." But now a typical pregame meal includes a choice of fresh fruits and fruit juices; pasta and a couple of low-fat, meatless sauces; pancakes; wheat toast; scrambled eggs; and bagels. What's more, he adds, "every day a produce man delivers crates of fresh fruit, like apples, oranges and bananas, to the practice field, all free for the players."

He was understandably delighted when a 1993 survey of NFL athletic trainers by the Produce for Better Health Foundation revealed that a pro football player eats, on average, six servings of fruit and vegetables a day, compared with the typical American, who consumes just half that number (five a day is considered ideal). "So," says Kleinschmidt, "here's the couch potato, watching football on TV on Sunday, eating only three servings of produce a day and looking at these guys who eat six!"

Kleinschmidt hopes that now that football players know the value of a carbohydrate-rich, low-fat diet, the rest of us will soon follow suit.

suggests Dr. Jonas. "Say that seven had meat as the main component. First, try cutting back to six meat meals a week, substituting chicken or fish or just vegetables for that seventh meal. Then go down to five, then four, then three. Remember, you don't have to be perfect. In fact, aim to not be perfect, because trying to be perfect just leads to guilt and frustration and quitting. But if you manage to drop from seven meat meals a week to three, you've already eliminated a large amount of fat."

Dr. Jonas knows this method works: He's done it successfully himself. "Fifteen years ago, I couldn't contemplate the idea of meatless meals," he confesses. "Now, many of mine are, but I got there gradually."

Making relatively simple adjustments in your food choices, then, is the way to go. It's also the way to stay at a weight you're happy with. "When you talk to people who've successfully lost weight and kept it off, this is how most of them did it," adds Dr. Jonas. "They didn't count calories, and they didn't walk around with diet menus. They simply learned what the high- and low-fat foods are and they significantly reduced the high-fat foods they ate. People lose weight and stay slim by making qualitative changes in their life."

Losing Your Fat Tooth

All this talk about cutting fat still give you the willies? ("I love the way fat tastes! I'll never be able to give it up!") Then you may be surprised to hear that lots of people just like you have happily and painlessly lost their fat tooth. A four-year study of more than 2,000 women at the Fred Hutchinson Cancer Research Center at the University of Washington in Seattle reveals that women who limited their fat intake to around 25 percent of calories lost their taste for fat in six months or less. By the end of the study, say the women, they actually found fatty foods unpleasant to eat.

Dr. Jonas has a similar story to tell, and an explanation. "Now I find that although I still like the taste of chocolate, I can't eat too much of it at one sitting, because later that evening or the next morning I'll wake up with an uncomfortable feeling," he says. "And while I still enjoy the flavor of steak, I know what a large portion of fatty meat does to me. I feel uncomfortable a few hours later, probably due to all the fat lying undigested in my stomach. As a result, it's actually caused my taste for fat to change."

Dr. Ornish, whose very low fat program has produced in his patients actual reversal of heart disease and long-term weight loss, takes what is probably the most radical approach of all to taming your fat tooth. He believes that until you stop eating high-fat foods, your craving for them will never go away.

"Ironically," says Dr. Ornish, "it's easier to make big changes than small ones. If you continue eating some meat or other fatty foods, you never really

The 80-Calorie Lotto

Need proof that fat calories don't fill you up nearly as much as calories that come from carbohydrates or protein? There are approximately 80 calories in just 2 teaspoons of margarine or oil—pure fat. Check out the list below to see what else 80 calories can buy you.

6 ounces skim milk	3 ounces lobster
2 cups snap beans	2 pieces gefilte fish
½ cup oatmeal	½ cup three-bean salad
15 ounces tomato juice	3 tomatoes
1 slice of light bread	1 cup blackberries
4 egg whites	6 dill pickles
3 ounces striped bass	1½ cups watermelon
1½ cups air-popped popcorn	½ cup wild rice
2 cups broccoli	4 ounces frogs' legs
1 medium apple	4 cups iceberg lettuce with 1 tablespoon fat-free salad dressing
½ cup corn grits	
4 prunes	

lose your taste for them—you feel more deprived eating smaller portions of them than if you didn't eat them at all. But if you gave them up completely, your palate would adjust accordingly. For example, if you stop putting salt on your food, initially it will seem like it needs more salt, but then after a few weeks it'll taste fine and eventually the salted foods you used to eat will seem too salty."

No one here is insisting that you slash your dietary fat to the 10 percent level that Dr. Ornish recommends for his heart-disease patients, nor that you quit all of your high-fat favorites cold turkey. Simply retrain your taste buds to love fat less. How? Try substituting low- and nonfat foods, like nonfat frozen yogurt, low-fat salad dressings and leaner meats for your old fatty favorites. That way, you'll feel less deprived, and it's likelier your new eating habits will stick.

Fat Finder's Guide

To find out how many grams of fat are in the specific foods you eat every day, check the labels, or pick up one of the many handy paperback books listing fat-gram counts. This handy guide will get you started.

Food	Portion	Fat (g.)
BREADS AND BREAD PRODUCTS		
Breads		
Italian	1 slice	0
Pita	1	0.6
Cracked-wheat	1 slice	0.9
Mixed-grain	1 slice	0.9
Rye	1 slice	0.9
White	1 slice	1.0
Pumpernickel	1 slice	1.1
Whole-wheat	1 slice	1.1
Oat bran	1 slice	1.2
French	1 slice	1.4
Crackers		
Rye wafer	1	0
Whole-wheat, low-sodium	1	0
Rye snack	1	0.4
Wheat snack	1	0.4
Graham	1	1.3
French toast		
Frozen	1 slice	5.0
Homemade	1 slice	6.7
Muffins		
English	1	1.1
Oat bran, with raisins	1 small	3.0
Blueberry	1 small	4.0
Corn	1 small	4.0
Bran	1 small	5.1

Food	Portion	Fat (g.)
Pancakes and waffles		
Waffles, frozen	2 (2.5 oz. each)	7.0
Plain pancakes	4 (4")	7.6
Buckwheat pancakes	4 small	8.0
Rolls and biscuits		
Brown-and-serve roll	1	2.0
Hard roll	1	2.0
Hamburger/ hot dog bun	1	2.1
Biscuit	1 small	5.1
Others		
Melba toast	1 piece	0
Matzo	1 piece	0.3
Rice cake	1	0.3
Corn tortilla	1	1.1
Bagel	1	1.4
Taco shell	1	2.2
CEREALS		
Wheat flakes	1 cup	0
Corn squares	1 cup	0.1
Puffed rice	1 cup	0.1
Puffed wheat	1 cup	0.1
Farina	1 cup	0.2
Shredded wheat	1 biscuit	0.3
Bran flakes	1 cup	0.7
Cornflakes	1 cup	0.7
Wheat germ, toasted	1 Tbsp.	0.8
Raisin bran	1 cup	1.0

Food	Portion	Fat (g.)
Bran squares	1 cup	1.4
Oat rings	1 cup	1.5
Oatmeal, instant	1 pkg.	1.7
Oatmeal, cooked	1 cup	2.4
Wheat germ, toasted	½ cup	6.1
Granola	1 cup	33.1

CONDIMENTS

Food	Portion	Fat (g.)
Horseradish	1 Tbsp.	0
Soy sauce, low-sodium	1 Tbsp.	0
Teriyaki sauce	1 Tbsp.	0
Worcestershire sauce	1 Tbsp.	0
Cranberry sauce	¼ cup	0.1
Dill pickle	1 med.	0.1
Ketchup	1 Tbsp.	0.1
Sweet pickle	1 small	0.1
Sweet relish	1 Tbsp.	0.1
Tamari	1 Tbsp.	0.1
Yellow mustard	1 Tbsp.	0.6
Brown mustard	1 Tbsp.	1.0
Green olives	5	2.9
Tartar sauce	1 Tbsp.	8.0

DAIRY PRODUCTS AND EGGS

Cheeses

Food	Portion	Fat (g.)
Yogurt cheese	1 oz.	0.6
Cottage cheese, 1% fat	½ cup	1.2
Parmesan, grated	1 Tbsp.	1.5
American, singles	1 oz.	2.0
Swiss, diet	1 oz.	2.0
Mozzarella, skim-milk	1 oz.	4.5
Cottage cheese, 4% fat	½ cup	4.7
Blue cheese	1 oz.	4.9

Food	Portion	Fat (g.)
Ricotta, part-skim	¼ cup	4.9
Feta	1 oz.	6.0
Monterey Jack, light	1 oz.	6.0
Mozzarella, whole-milk	1 oz.	6.1
Swiss	1 oz.	7.8
Brie	1 oz.	7.9
Ricotta, whole-milk	¼ cup	8.0
Monterey Jack	1 oz.	8.6
American, processed	1 oz.	8.8
Colby	1 oz.	9.1
Cheddar	1 oz.	9.4
Cream cheese, regular	1 oz.	9.9

Eggs

Food	Portion	Fat (g.)
White only, raw, large	1	0
Whole, raw, large	1	5.0

Milk and cream

Food	Portion	Fat (g.)
Evaporated skim	½ cup	0.3
Skim	1 cup	0.4
Nondairy whipped topping, frozen	1 Tbsp.	0.9
Nondairy creamer	1 Tbsp.	1.0
Half-and-half	1 Tbsp.	1.7
Buttermilk	1 cup	2.2
Low-fat, 1%	1 cup	2.6
Sour cream, imitation	1 Tbsp.	2.6
Cream, light	1 Tbsp.	2.9
Sour cream, cultured	1 Tbsp.	3.0
Low-fat, 2%	1 cup	4.7
Cream, heavy, whipping	1 Tbsp.	5.5
Whole, 3.3%	1 cup	8.2
Evaporated whole	½ cup	9.6

(continued)

Fat Finder's Guide—Continued

Food	Portion	Fat (g.)	Food	Portion	Fat (g.)
DAIRY PRODUCTS—CONTINUED			**Doughnuts**		
Yogurt			Plain	1 (2 oz.)	10.8
Plain, nonfat	1 cup	0.4	**Frozen desserts**		
Plain, low-fat	1 cup	3.5	Fruit-flavored frozen yogurt	½ cup	1.0
Plain, whole	1 cup	7.4	Orange sherbet	½ cup	1.9
DESSERTS AND SNACKS			Vanilla ice milk	½ cup	2.8
Cakes			Vanilla ice cream	½ cup	7.2
Angel food	1 slice (2 oz.)	0.1	Vanilla ice cream, premium	½ cup	11.9
Sponge	1 slice	3.1	**Pastries**		
Strawberry shortcake	1 slice	8.9	Apple turnover	1 oz.	4.7
Pound	1 slice (1 oz.)	9.0	Eclair, with custard and icing	1	13.6
White, with chocolate icing	1 slice	11.0	Cheesecake	1 slice	16.3
Candies			**Pies**		
Chocolate fudge, plain	1 oz.	2.9	Apple	1 slice	13.1
Milk chocolate, with almonds	1 oz.	10.1	Custard	1 slice	14.0
Milk chocolate, with peanuts	1 oz.	10.8	Blueberry	1 slice	15.0
			Chocolate cream	1 slice	15.1
Cookies and brownies			Pecan	1 slice	27.0
Gingersnap	1	0.6	**Pudding and gelatin**		
Vanilla wafer	1	0.9	Gelatin	½ cup	0
Fig bar	1	1.0	Vanilla pudding, sugar-free, 2% milk	½ cup	1.2
Chocolate chip	1	2.2			
Chocolate/vanilla sandwich	1	2.3	Chocolate pudding, sugar-free, 2% milk	½ cup	1.9
Brownie, with chocolate icing	1	5.0			
			Chocolate pudding	½ cup	4.0
Cupcakes			Tapioca pudding	½ cup	4.0
No icing	1	3.0	Rice pudding, with raisins	½ cup	4.1
Devil's food, with icing	1	4.0	Vanilla pudding	½ cup	5.0
Chocolate, with icing	1	5.0	Custard, baked	½ cup	7.5

Food	Portion	Fat (g.)
DIPS AND DRESSINGS		
Dips		
Clam, garlic or French onion	1 Tbsp.	2.0
Guacamole	1 Tbsp.	2.0
Jalapeño or green onion	1 Tbsp.	2.0
Bacon and horseradish	1 Tbsp.	2.5
Dressings		
Italian, no oil	1 Tbsp.	0
Sweet-and-sour	1 Tbsp.	0.3
Blue cheese, low-fat	1 Tbsp.	0.9
French, low-calorie	1 Tbsp.	0.9
Italian, low-calorie	1 Tbsp.	1.5
Mayonnaise-style	1 Tbsp.	5.2
French	1 Tbsp.	6.0
Ranch-style	1 Tbsp.	6.0
Italian, regular	1 Tbsp.	7.1
Blue cheese	1 Tbsp.	7.6
Russian	1 Tbsp.	7.6
Vinegar and oil	1 Tbsp.	8.0
Thousand Island	1 Tbsp.	8.1
FATS AND OILS		
Butter		
Whipped	1 tsp.	2.4
Regular	1 tsp.	3.8
Margarine		
Corn oil, diet	1 tsp.	1.9
Whipped	1 tsp.	2.7
Corn oil, stick	1 tsp.	3.8
Corn or safflower oil, soft	1 tsp.	3.8
Mayonnaise		
Low-calorie	1 tsp.	1.3
Regular	1 tsp.	3.7

Food	Portion	Fat (g.)
Oils		
Olive	1 tsp.	4.5
Vegetable	1 tsp.	4.5
FRUITS AND JUICES		
Dried fruits		
Dates	½ cup	0.4
Prunes	½ cup	0.4
Raisins	½ cup	0.4
Figs	½ cup	1.2
Fresh fruits		
Grapefruit	½ med.	0.1
Grapes	10	0.1
Peach	1 med.	0.1
Casaba melon, cubed	1 cup	0.2
Figs	2 small	0.2
Honeydew melon, cubed	1 cup	0.2
Orange, all varieties	1 med.	0.2
Papaya, cubed	1 cup	0.2
Kiwifruit	1 med.	0.3
Apricots	3 med.	0.4
Cantaloupe, cubed	1 cup	0.4
Apple, with peel	1 med.	0.5
Banana	1 med.	0.6
Blueberries	1 cup	0.6
Mango	1 med.	0.6
Nectarine	1 med.	0.6
Strawberries	1 cup	0.6
Bartlett pear	1 med.	0.7
Pineapple, cubed	1 cup	0.7
Raspberries	1 cup	0.7
Sweet cherries	10	0.7
Watermelon, cubed	1 cup	0.7
Plums	2 med.	0.8
Florida avocado	1 med.	15.4
California avocado	1 med.	30.0

(continued)

Fat Finder's Guide—Continued

Food	Portion	Fat (g.)
FRUITS AND JUICES—CONTINUED		
Juices		
Cranberry	1 cup	0.1
Prune	1 cup	0.1
Grape	1 cup	0.2
Apple	1 cup	0.3
Orange	1 cup	0.5
GRAVIES AND SAUCES		
Gravies		
Beef, canned	¼ cup	1.2
Turkey, canned	¼ cup	1.2
Mushroom	¼ cup	1.6
Chicken, canned	¼ cup	3.6
Sauces		
Chili	¼ cup	0
Tomato, canned	¼ cup	0.1
Barbecue	¼ cup	1.2
Taco, canned	¼ cup	1.4
Marinara, canned	¼ cup	2.1
Spaghetti, canned	¼ cup	3.0
White, thin	¼ cup	4.9
White, medium	¼ cup	7.8
White, thick	¼ cup	10.6
White, very thick	¼ cup	13.5
LEGUMES		
Beans		
Mung, sprouted	1 cup	0.2
Lima, boiled	1 cup	0.5
Navy, cooked	1 cup	1.0
Red kidney, canned	1 cup	1.0
White, small, boiled	1 cup	1.2
Refried	1 cup	2.7
Garbanzo, canned	1 cup	4.6
Others		
Lentils, boiled	1 cup	0.7

Food	Portion	Fat (g.)
Peas, split, dried, cooked	1 cup	1.0
MEATS		
Beef		
Bottom roast, lean	3.5 oz.	9.6
Arm pot roast	3.5 oz.	9.9
Rib roast, lean	3.5 oz.	13.7
Blade pot roast	3.5 oz.	15.2
Hamburger, extra lean	3.5 oz.	16.0
Hamburger, lean	3.5 oz.	18.4
Salami	3.5 oz.	19.9
Lamb		
Rib chop, lean, broiled	1	7.4
Leg, lean, roasted	3.5 oz.	7.7
Shoulder, lean, roasted	3.5 oz.	10.7
Pork		
Canadian bacon	1 slice	2.0
Tenderloin roast, lean	3.5 oz.	4.8
Ham, extra lean	3.5 oz.	5.5
Ham roast	3.5 oz.	8.9
Loin roast, lean	3.5 oz.	13.5
Shoulder roast	3.5 oz.	14.9
Chop, lean, broiled	3.5 oz.	15.2
Italian sausage links	1½ (3.5 oz.)	17.2
Bologna	4 slices (3.5 oz.)	19.7
Loin roast, lean and fat	3.5 oz.	21.5
Chop, lean and fat, broiled	3.5 oz.	27.0
Sausage patties	4 (3.5 oz.)	30.9
Sausage links	8 (3.5 oz.)	32.4

Food	Portion	Fat (g.)	Food	Portion	Fat (g.)
Veal			**Duck**		
Shoulder and arm roast, lean	3.5 oz.	5.8	No skin, roasted	3.5 oz.	11.1
Rib, lean, braised	3.5 oz.	7.8	With skin, roasted	3.5 oz.	28.2
PASTAS AND GRAINS			**Goose**		
			No skin, roasted	3.5 oz.	12.6
Pastas			With skin, roasted	3.5 oz.	21.7
Whole-wheat macaroni, cooked	1 cup	0.8	**Turkey**		
Spaghetti, cooked	1 cup	1.0	Breast, no skin, roasted	3.5 oz.	0.7
Spinach pasta, cooked	1 cup	1.3	Turkey loaf, from breast	3.5 oz.	1.6
Egg noodles, cooked	1 cup	2.0	Smoked	3.5 oz.	3.9
Chow mein noodles	1 cup	11.0	Turkey ham, from thigh	3.5 oz.	5.0
Grains			Dark meat, no skin	3 oz.	7.2
White rice, cooked	1 cup	0	Turkey pastrami	3.5 oz.	7.2
Bulgur, cooked	1 cup	0.4	Turkey roll, light meat	3.5 oz.	7.2
Brown rice, cooked	1 cup	1.8	**NUTS AND SEEDS**		
Spanish rice, cooked	1 cup	4.2	Chestnuts, roasted	½ cup	0.9
POULTRY			Sesame seeds, roasted	1 Tbsp.	4.3
Chicken			Pumpkin/squash seeds, roasted	½ cup	6.0
Breast, no skin, roasted	3.5 oz.	3.5	Cashews, oil-roasted	½ cup	31.4
Thigh, no skin, roasted	1 small	5.7	Cashews, dry-roasted	½ cup	31.8
Chicken roll, light meat	3.5 oz.	7.3	Pistachios, dry-roasted	½ cup	33.8
Breast, with skin, roasted	3.5 oz.	7.8	Almonds, dry-roasted, whole	½ cup	35.6
Leg, no skin, roasted	3.5 oz.	8.0	Peanuts, oil-roasted	½ cup	35.7
Leg, no skin, stewed	3.5 oz.	8.1	Sunflower seeds, dried	½ cup	35.7
Breast, floured, fried	3.5 oz.	8.8	Spanish peanuts, dried	½ cup	35.9
Thigh, floured, fried	1 small	9.2	Filberts (hazelnuts)	½ cup	36.0
Breast, batter-fried	3.5 oz.	13.1	Pecans	½ cup	36.6
Leg, roasted	1 small	15.4			*(continued)*
Dark meat, with skin, roasted	3.5 oz.	15.8			
Salad	3.5 oz.	17.5			

Fat Finder's Guide—Continued

Food	Portion	Fat (g.)	Food	Portion	Fat (g.)
NUTS AND SEEDS—CONTINUED			Shrimp, breaded, fried	3.5 oz.	12.1
Persian/English walnuts	½ cup	37.1	**VEGETABLES**		
Brazil nuts	½ cup	46.4	Carrot, raw	1 med.	0.1
Macadamia nuts	½ cup	49.4	Celery	1 stalk	0.1
SEAFOOD			Romaine lettuce	1 cup	0.1
			Sweet potato, baked	1 med.	0.1
Finfish			Zucchini, boiled	1 cup	0.1
Anchovy, fillet, canned	1	0.4	Butternut squash, baked	1 cup	0.2
Tuna, light meat, canned in water	3.5 oz.	0.5	Cauliflower, raw	1 cup	0.2
Cod, cooked	3.5 oz.	0.9	Potato, baked, no peel	1 med.	0.2
Haddock, cooked	3.5 oz.	0.9	Spinach	1 cup	0.2
Flounder, broiled	3.5 oz.	1.5	Acorn squash, baked	1 cup	0.3
Sole, broiled	3.5 oz.	1.5	Mushrooms	1 cup	0.3
Red snapper, cooked	3.5 oz.	1.7	Sweet pepper	1 small	0.3
Halibut, broiled	3.5 oz.	2.9	Tomato	1 med.	0.3
Rainbow trout, cooked	3.5 oz.	4.3	Broccoli, boiled	1 cup	0.4
Swordfish, cooked	3.5 oz.	5.1	Cabbage, boiled	1 cup	0.4
Pink salmon, canned	3.5 oz.	6.0	Green beans, boiled	1 cup	0.4
Bluefin tuna, cooked, dry heat	3.5 oz.	6.2	Asparagus, boiled	1 cup	0.6
Salmon, cooked	3.5 oz.	7.5	Summer squash, boiled	1 cup	0.6
Tuna, canned in oil, drained	3.5 oz.	8.1	Brussels sprouts, boiled	1 cup	0.8
Sardines, canned, in tomato sauce	3.5 oz.	11.9	Corn, fresh, boiled	1 small ear	1.0
Mackerel, cooked	3.5 oz.	17.6	Onion ring, fried	1	3.0
Shellfish			French fries, frozen	10 pieces	4.4
Shrimp, cooked	3.5 oz.	1.1	Hash-brown potatoes, frozen	½ cup	9.0
Scallops, steamed	3.5 oz.	1.4	Potato salad, homemade (eggs and mayonnaise)	½ cup	10.3
Clams, cooked	3.5 oz.	5.8			
Scallops, breaded, fried	3.5 oz.	11.4			

CREATING THE LOW-FAT KITCHEN

If you've got a weight problem—and a growing family—then chances are you've got a kitchen bulging with the kinds of foods designed to keep all of you overweight. Cupboards crammed with creamed soups and cookies . . . freezers filled with fatty cuts of meat and ice cream . . . pantries packed with potato chips and sugary breakfast cereals. If that sounds like your kitchen, join the club.

"The typical American kitchen tends to have foods that are high in fat and high in calories, with too little fresh produce and whole-grain products," says registered dietitian Gayle Shockey Hoxter, a Murrieta, California–based nutritionist. "To have a balanced diet, we need a balanced kitchen, with items from all five food groups—fruits and vegetables; milk, yogurt and cheese; meat, poultry, fish, eggs and beans; bread, cereal, rice and pasta; and fats and oils. To accomplish this in the average kitchen, it usually means adding more produce and whole-grain products and cutting back on high-fat items."

Okay—we hear you out there. "How can I *not* keep chips and cheese and ice cream in the house? They're what my husband and my kids enjoy! And, frankly . . . so do I!" We understand. No one's saying you have to toss all your favorite foods into a Dumpster. What we're suggesting is making slow, gradual changes in the contents of your fridge and cupboards. The basic idea is to keep the kinds of foods you and your family love on hand but, wherever possible, swapping them for low-fat, low-cal versions.

Make one food swap per month—more, if you're ambitious. You'll still

(continued on page 38)

A Kitchen Makeover

You've heard of beauty makeovers? Well, here's a makeover you can do on your kitchen. By adding a bit of this and subtracting a smidgen of that, says Murrieta, California–based nutritionist Gayle Shockey Hoxter, R.D., you can turn your fat-making kitchen into a low-fat haven for you and your whole family. Here's how.

Swap . . .	For . . .
IN YOUR FRIDGE	
Whole-milk dairy products (including 1% or 2% milk)	Low-fat or nonfat dairy products
Regular yogurt	Low-fat or nonfat yogurt
High-fat cheeses	Low-fat or nonfat cheeses
Eggs	Egg substitute or egg whites
Butter; regular margarine	Reduced-calorie margarine
High-fat deli meats, hot dogs or bacon	98% fat-free deli meats; 80% fat-free hot dogs; 90% fat-free turkey bacon
High-fat salad dressings or mayonnaise	Low-fat or nonfat salad dressings or mayonnaise

(Always have on hand: a variety of fresh fruits and vegetables.)

Swap . . .	For . . .
IN YOUR FREEZER	
Regular frozen waffles	Low-fat frozen waffles
Regular frozen entrées (including pizza)	Low-fat frozen entrées; pizza
Regular breaded fish and other breaded products	Light breaded fish, etc.
High-fat meats and poultry	Lean cuts of meat; skinless poultry; 90% fat-free ground turkey or beef
Regular frozen cakes	Fat-free frozen cakes
Regular ice cream	Low-fat or nonfat frozen yogurt, frozen dessert or ice milk
Fruit juice concentrates with added sugar	100% fruit juice concentrates

Swap . . .	For . . .
Frozen fruit in sugar	Unsweetened frozen fruit
Creamed and buttered frozen vegetables	Frozen vegetables without sauces

(Always have on hand: whole-grain breads, bagels, English muffins.)

IN YOUR PANTRY

Shortening and oils such as vegetable oil and peanut oil	No-stick vegetable oil spray; alternative healthy oils—olive oil, canola oil and light oils
Tuna, salmon and other fish or meat packed in oil	Water-packed tuna and salmon
Baked beans refried in sauce	Canned, dried or frozen beans (no salt added) such as kidney, lima, garbanzo, fat-free refried beans
Regular or chunky peanut butter	Natural peanut butter without salt or sugar (drain off excess oil); use sparingly
Canned spaghetti; pasta and rice mixes	Plain pasta; rice and grains; low-fat seasoned pasta
Sugared breakfast cereals	High-fiber, sugar-free cereals
Granola	Low-fat granola
High-fat cookies	Low-fat cookies (including graham crackers and whole-wheat fruit bars)
High-fat snacks (including high-fat microwave popcorn)	Pretzels; air-popped popcorn; low-fat microwave popcorn; raisins; fat-free chips
Canned fruit in syrup	Canned fruit packed in water or juice
Commercially prepared muffins	Low-fat muffin mixes
Jams and jellies with added sugar	100% fruit preserves
Cake mixes	94% fat-free cake mixes; 97% fat-free frostings
Creamed and high-sodium soups	99% fat-free and low-sodium soups

(continued)

A Kitchen Makeover—Continued

Swap . . .	For . . .
IN YOUR PANTRY—CONTINUED	
High-fat crackers	Low-fat crackers; rice cakes
Gelatin and puddings	Sugar-free gelatin and fat-free or sugar-free puddings
Hot chocolate mixes and beverage mixes with sugar	Sugar-free hot chocolate and sugar-free beverage mixes
Cooking sherry	Red or white table wine (for cooking)

(Always have on hand: canned tomatoes, tomato paste, salsa, horse-radish, ketchup, Dijon mustard, pickle relish.)

IN YOUR SPICE RACK	
Salt; seasoned salt	Reduced-sodium salt; seasoned salt
Soy sauce	Reduced-sodium soy sauce
Bouillon cubes	Reduced-sodium bouillon cubes

(Always have on hand: a variety of spices, dried and fresh herbs.)

NOTE: You'll notice that some of the changes we've made are for low-sodium versions of various products. While sodium per se isn't fattening, it can affect your weight loss. Sodium may cause your body to retain water, which means that even if you've been eating carefully, you might still register a weight gain on the scale.

reap lots of low-fat benefits. Take milk, for example. "Not everyone likes the taste of skim milk, but you'll still be better off if you switch from whole milk to 1 or 2 percent milk," says Hoxter. "Or if you don't like fat-free or low-fat mayonnaise, mix a bit of it with regular mayonnaise. You'll be cutting some fat and calories and still be keeping most of the taste."

For the lowdown on other switches you can make, see "A Kitchen Makeover," on page 36. And in a year's time there'll be a lot less lard in your larder—and on you.

Tools of the Low-Fat Brigade

Losing weight isn't just a matter of what you're cooking—it's also a matter of what you're cooking with. Thanks to the vast array of kitchen gadgets and gizmos available today, cutting fat and calories from your home-cooked meals is easier than ever. Follow this checklist to see what you may be missing.

No-stick skillet. Toss a tablespoon of butter or oil into a regular pan and you're adding 110 needless calories and 12 grams of fat to your meal. Instead, you can fry or sauté your favorite dish the low-fat way using a no-stick skillet and a squirt of no-stick vegetable oil spray. Buy the best skillet you can afford—you'll be using it a lot. You'll also need a set of plastic or wooden utensils so you won't scratch the skillet's surface.

Steamer. Steamers have been around for some time, and cooks who use them know how great they are for steaming veggies, rice and other foods without cooking away their taste and nutrients. Now you can also get stackable steamers so you can prepare several items at the same time.

Blender. Another all-around favorite in the kitchen, the blender's calorie-cutting potential is tremendous. Blenders help retain the creamy consistency that's often lost when the fat in food is eliminated, and, as you know, blenders are tops for whipping up frothy drinks, creamy soups, dips and desserts. Besides the traditional countertop models, there are newer, handheld immersible ones that can be used right in the pot or bowl.

Plastic or metal strainer. Strainers are terrific for skimming fat from soups and stews.

Microwave oven. "Your microwave is a great aid to low-fat cooking because it lets you cook without added fat," says registered dietitian Nancy Clark, director of Nutrition Services at SportsMedicine Brookline in Brookline, Massachusetts, and author of *Nancy Clark's Sports Nutrition Guidebook.* It also helps you jazz up simple foods. "Plain old boring fruit cooked in the microwave is very appetizing," adds Clark.

Double meat loaf pan. Traditional meat loaf is an American favorite—but it also packs on about 18 grams of fat per four-ounce serving when prepared the usual way. Now, thanks to this nifty device—which allows the fat to drip out of the inner, perforated pan into the outer pan—you can cut fat by as much as 75 percent.

Popcorn popper. If you automatically think of popcorn as a healthy, fiber-rich snack food, hold on: Some ready-to-eat and microwave brands may contain a whopping ten grams of fat per three-cup serving, reports registered dietitian Judy E. Marshel, director of Health Resources of Great Neck, New York. But you can have your popcorn and eat it, too—guiltlessly—if you prepare it in an electric or microwave air popper. (You can buy low-fat microwave popcorn.)

Salad spinner. This gadget isn't just for drying wet lettuce. "A salad spinner is great for keeping salad items crisp and ready," says Marie Simmons, syndicated columnist and author of *The Light Touch* and several other cookbooks.

Plastic freezer bags. "One reason people don't eat more vegetables is that they have to stop, clean and peel them," says Simmons. "So after you bring your veggies home from the store, trim them, cut them up and store them in resealable bags so they're ready whenever you want a quick hit. They're especially good for kids, so they can help themselves." Keep enough plastic bags handy for cutting up and storing (in the fridge or freezer) fresh fruit, too.

SHOP TALK: DEVELOPING YOUR SUPERMARKET SAVVY

Ah, those gleaming aisles filled with shiny eggplants and apples . . . those knee-high boxes of puffed cereal . . . those famous faces smiling on bottles of salad dressing and jars of spaghetti sauce. Where else can you get this close to Paul Newman but in your favorite supermarket—the place where dreams of creating delicious, healthy, low-fat meals are made.

And the trend is indeed toward smarter-than-ever food-buying habits. A survey done by the Atlanta, Georgia–based Calorie Control Council (CCC) revealed that the demand for "light" products is still growing, with nine out of ten American adults 18 years and older enjoying low-calorie and sugar-free foods and beverages, as well as reduced-fat foods. We're talking about 171 million fans of these products, one-third of whom are actively dieting to maintain and lose weight, says CCC spokesperson Russ Lemieux.

"Long-term weight control requires changes in eating behavior, and these products can give the dieter many of the foods she enjoyed all along without the unnecessary fat and calories," says Lemieux.

A survey conducted by the Food Marketing Institute in Washington, D.C., in connection with *Prevention* magazine, has equally good news to report. According to Tom Dybdahl, director of Market Research for *Prevention*, 47 percent of the supermarket shoppers interviewed were committed to good nutrition and said they consistently made healthful food choices.

But as heartening as these statistics are, there's no question that many waist watchers continue to find the supermarket a scary place. Why? Because it's all too easy to go astray, despite our best intentions.

Supermarket Shopping: It Isn't Kid Stuff

How often have you been at the supermarket and watched a mother—her cranky, crying child in tow—grow so exasperated that she finally snaps, "Here! Eat this!" ripping open the first bag she can lay her hands on.

Hmmm . . . maybe *you've* played that scene once or twice yourself. It's tough. How can you go shopping with your children and avoid feeding them or bringing home foods you wish they wouldn't eat? "Leave the kids at home!" laughs Judsen Culbreth, editor-in-chief of *Working Mother* magazine and the mom of two. But if you simply can't, she's got some savvy strategies for dealing with children who might try to lure you into feeding them the entire candy section or thwart your efforts to stick to your sensible shopping list.

Feed 'em first. If you think it's bad for you to go to shopping when you're hungry, it's twice as bad if your kids are starving—they'll want to eat anything and everything they see on the shelves. Take the edge off their appetites by giving them a healthy snack—a piece of fruit, a frozen fruit bar, even a bowl of cereal—before you leave the house.

Bring low-fat munchies. "Why not keep some things in your pocketbook for your kids to snack on if they get hungry in the supermarket?" Culbreth suggests. Pack up some pretzels, air-popped popcorn or breadsticks in case they get a snack attack while you're cruising the supermarket aisles.

Involve your child. If your youngster is a preschooler, create a simple supermarket game by asking him to help you locate some healthy foods you plan to buy. For example, tell him, "Now we need to get some apples. Can you find the apples?" If it's an older child, make it more challenging. Turn your supermarket expedition into a scavenger hunt, and ask her to bring back to your shopping cart several items at a time. In both cases, your kids will learn to associate going to the market with selecting healthy foods.

Don't say no all the time. If something your child wants is off your shopping list, you can simply and firmly say, "No, we're not buying that today." But, adds Culbreth, "there's a new way of thinking—that certain foods shouldn't be completely off-limits. There are really no bad foods, just some that we shouldn't have as much of. It's okay to let your child occasionally have that candy bar. Don't make food a bigger issue than you have to."

But we *have* to eat, and we *have* to buy food. How do we make our weekly outings to the market a more pleasant experience and be sure we come home with precisely those items that will do our diet good? Weight-loss and nutrition experts offer these tips.

Never shop when you're hungry. "It's dangerous, because your willpower is down and you might want everything in sight!" warns Jim Fobel, the author of *Jim Fobel's Diet Feasts*. "Sometimes just a glass of water and a carrot before leaving the house will curb your appetite."

Always shop alone. Doing your marketing with friends might be more fun, but you might also be inclined to take home the same high-fat, high-calorie foods that look so tempting in your friend's shopping cart.

Use a list, but be flexible. A well-thought-out shopping list is always a good idea. But, says Fobel, who has lost more than 100 pounds, "you might see something at the store that's lean and wonderful, like some fresh fish or a lean cut of meat. Something might be so perfect that you may want to deviate from your list sometimes."

Buy the makings for a one-pot meal. "I love soups," says Nancy Clark, director of Nutrition Services at SportsMedicine Brookline in Brookline, Massachusetts, and author of *Nancy Clark's Sports Nutrition Guidebook*. "So once a week I might make a big pot of soup and add different vegetables to it each day—lentils one day, cabbage the next—it varies according to my mood. Or I'll make a week's worth of chili and eat it plain one day, add some ground turkey another day, make it into a taco salad the third day or serve it with rice the fourth day."

Fobel does something similar with his "perpetual pot of chicken stock," to which he adds veggies, tiny meatballs or egg noodles, depending on how he feels that day. Stocking up at the market for the various ingredients you'll need for this meal in a pot means less work once you get home.

Shun the free samples. You don't need to eat that wedge of Swiss cheese to know how it tastes. Passing up that one-ounce chunk means saving a whopping 105 calories and eight grams of fat.

Check out the fresh herbs and spices. "There are so many more of them to choose from now and they're found in so many supermarkets," notes Marie Simmons, author of *The Light Touch*. "The more fresh ingredients you use, the less you miss the fat."

Go easy on the additives. Fobel is a fresh-food fan and an avid label reader. "If the ingredient list is too long, I'm automatically suspicious! I tend to put the package right down. My favorite cereal is shredded wheat, and the only ingredient listed is wheat!" Low-cal and low-fat products are certainly a boon to dieters, but don't omit "real" things—fresh fruits and veggies and other unprocessed foods—from your daily diet.

Buy foods in season. "During asparagus season," says Fobel, "I eat

The Food Label Lowdown

"Low-fat." "Low-calorie." "Light." "Lite." It was enough to make anyone light-headed. How were you supposed to make smart supermarket selections when food product descriptions were so downright confusing?

The Food and Drug Administration (FDA) agreed that there was a dizzying array of misleading terms being tossed around grocery stores everywhere. And so as of May 1994—courtesy of the Nutrition Labeling and Education Act of 1990—a uniform system for labeling just about every type of processed food has been making life a lot easier for weight-conscious consumers.

Says FDA spokesperson Brad Stone: "Congress passed this law in response to concerns that it was hard for consumers to figure out what a lot of the terms really meant. It was also hard for people to compare different foods because many products did not have nutrition information at all. In other cases the serving sizes varied from one brand to another. The aim is to give people a clearer, more reliable way to understand the nutritional values of the foods they eat."

As a result, every serving size for some 140 food categories is now uniform, product for product. It therefore makes it far simpler for you to compare the fat and caloric breakdowns of everything from pudding to peanut butter. Suddenly, deciding whether Heinz tomato soup, Progresso minestrone or Campbell's chicken with rice is the best bet for your diet is a cinch.

In addition, all health-oriented claims found on food packaging must now be fully substantiated. "For instance," says Stone, "a container of milk may carry the message that the calcium in the milk may help reduce the risk of osteoporosis only if the milk meets FDA requirements—that is, if it has the required level of calcium per serving."

Perhaps the best news of all for confused dieters: Any diet-oriented product description must conform to standardized FDA definitions. They include:

- *Calorie-free:* up to five calories per serving

- *Sugar-free:* up to 0.5 gram of sugar per serving

- *Fat-free:* up to 0.5 gram of fat per serving

- *Low-fat:* up to 3 grams of fat per serving or per 100 grams of the food

- *Light or "lite":* products containing one-third fewer calories than usual

asparagus almost every day—it's wonderful. You can never go wrong buying fresh produce in season." If you live near a greenmarket where farm-fresh fruits and vegetables are available, better yet.

Buy the best. Select the highest-quality foods you can afford, insist the experts, and your taste buds won't miss some of the fattening items you're trying to avoid.

Don't buy things "just in case." The words "just in case"—just in case company drops by, or just in case the kids want something sweet—have scuttled many a weight-loss program. Choose only those items you know are tasty yet low-fat and low-calorie, and shop with you and your immediate family in mind, not some phantom guests who may or may not show up. Even if they do, you can serve them the same delicious, low-fat foods you have on hand.

LOW-FAT
COOKING TRICKS

True or false: Healthy, low-fat meals take too long and are too complicated to make on a regular basis. False! And the clever cooking tips that follow prove it. Sure, brown rice and dried beans, for instance, do take their own sweet time to cook, and certain calorie-conscious recipes involve lengthy ingredient lists. But there are still plenty of quick-'n'-lean dishes (dozens of which can be found in this book) that can save you prep time and skim fat from your favorite meals.

And we are talking about skimming fat, not eliminating it altogether. After all, as Marie Simmons, author of several cookbooks, including *The Light Touch*, points out, "You can't just leave out the fat completely, because fat tastes really good! But you can compensate. If a recipe, say, calls for ¼ cup of olive oil, instead of leaving out the oil, use just 1 tablespooon during cooking and then maybe add another ½ tablespoon at the end, so you still have that good taste."

Rodale Press nutritionist and registered dietitian Anita Hirsch, who teaches healthy-cooking classes, says that her students are always worried that recipes won't turn out well if they cut back on fat. "But then," she says, "they'll make a dish with half the usual oil, and later they'll tell me their husbands ate it and didn't know the difference! That's the ultimate test."

Here are some easy, fat-trimming ideas that can help you create fabulous food at home any night of the week.

Get ready for super soups. In preparation for whipping up easy soups or quick sauces, stock your fridge with canned broth—it adds instant flavor to almost any dish. And by keeping your cans chilled, you can scoop off the solidified fat at a moment's notice.

Take stock. For a near-instant, completely fat-free stock, pour boiling water over porcini, shiitake or other dried mushrooms. Soak for about 15 minutes. Strain the broth, which has a surprisingly meaty flavor, and use it as the liquid ingredient in pilafs or to add depth of flavor to stews or sauces.

Fry not. Poaching fish instead of frying saves fat grams galore. To poach a fish fillet without a recipe or an endless list of ingredients, just grab that can of crab boil that's probably hiding in the back of your spice cabinet. Shake this savory blend of spices into a frying pan half full of water, add your fish and simmer until done—less than ten minutes for thin fillets.

Or, if you're cooking your fish in the oven, skip the butter and baste with a little lemon juice, orange juice or spicy vegetable-cocktail juice for tangy taste appeal.

Sauté sans oil. Sautéing is fine, says Hirsch—as long as you monitor the oil you use. "Use a no-stick pan, and start out with as little oil as possible." You can always add a bit more later or fat-free chicken broth.

Alternatively, "sauté" your food in a few tablespoons of a tasty, nonfat liquid such as wine, tomato juice or fat-free chicken or beef broth.

Think juicy. If you're used to sautéing your veggies in a pan coated with a half inch of oil, here's a better way. Bring out their natural flavor by cooking them in a no-stick pan over a low flame in a mixture of a little oil plus water, advises Simmons. "Some vegetables are already about 90 percent water," she says, "and at low temperatures you can easily coax out those juices."

Serve special spuds. Who needs fat-packed french fries when you can make delicious, nutrient-rich yam or sweet potato "fries." Cut the unpeeled potatoes into thick slabs (about ½ inch), then dredge them in a mixture of low-sodium soy sauce and a few drops of sesame oil. Grill or broil until crisp and golden.

Fix low-fat pizza, pronto. "If I'm in the mood for pizza, I simply take some crushed canned tomatoes—*not* prepared pasta or pizza sauce—and put a little of that on a pita, top it with part-skim mozzarella cheese, some sliced raw mushrooms, a sprinkle of oregano and a pinch of grated Parmesan, and pop it in the oven for a couple minutes. It's very satisfying and sensible," says cookbook author Jim Fobel, author of *The Whole Chicken Cookbook.*

Don't wait for rice. When you haven't got 45 minutes to watch a pot of brown rice boil, try one of these quick-cooking, superhealthy grains instead. Each of these should cook to perfection within 5 to 12 minutes after your water boils: quick-cook brown rice (10 minutes), quick-cook barley (12 minutes), bulgur (7 minutes), couscous (5 minutes).

Spray it again, Sam. No-stick vegetable oil sprays, including flavorful butter and olive oil varieties, are a boon to waist-conscious cooks. Use them for whipping up everything from frittatas to stir-fries for impressive fat savings.

Think virgin. If you're going to use oil, suggests Simmons, opt for the extra-virgin kind. "It costs more," she concedes, "but the flavor goes further, so you'll use less."

Get in tune with tuna. To whip up a terrific luncheon salad in no time, toss a can of beans with a can of water-packed tuna (both rinsed under cold water to remove the sodium and canning liquid). Add chopped peppers and onions, minced parsley and any other fresh herbs you like. Dress with vinegar and a bare splash of oil. For extra zip, sprinkle on some capers or cherry tomatoes. Voilà! A low-fat, warm-weather salad.

Veg out. Everybody always says to steam vegetables until they're al dente, but Fobel has another opinion: "When they're slightly well cooked—a little more tender than al dente—they'll be moister and juicier, and you won't miss the butter on them."

Mind your milk. Drink or cook with two glasses of whole milk every day for a year and you'll be saddled with a whopping 12 pounds of dietary fat. Switch to the same amount of 1 percent milk and you cut your fat intake by a third. Better yet, skim milk, which, at two glasses daily, adds up to a mere 0.1 pound of fat by year's end.

Trim down meat. Simplify the task of trimming visible fat and skin from meat. First stick the raw beef, pork or chicken in the freezer for 15 to 20 minutes. When blasted with cold air, fat quickly hardens and slices off easily.

Shed the skin. "Some people will remove the skin from chicken before they cook it, but then they're not happy because the chicken tastes dry," acknowledges Hirsch. "If you want to cook it with the skin on, just be sure to peel it off before you eat it."

Be a little saucy. You can pare fat calories from muffins, cakes and other home-baked goods by swapping the cooking fat for applesauce. This trick works best in recipes with other wet ingredients, like skim milk or fruit. Just exchange one part oil, butter or margarine for one part applesauce. For example, instead of using ⅓ cup of oil and two whole eggs when preparing lemon cake from a mix, substitute ⅓ cup applesauce and three egg whites and save 4.5 grams of fat and 40 calories per slice.

Fix fat-busting burgers. Dieters don't have to give up hamburgers, says Hirsch, but you can prepare the beef a lower-fat way. "I use shredded vegetables such as carrots, onions and green peppers to replace some of the meat." Better yet, try ground turkey or ground chicken for your burgers, or any other recipes that call for ground beef.

Skinny up your potato salad. Rather than make your favorite potato salad recipe with mayonnaise—or even with yogurt, which is too watery—make it with yogurt cheese, advises Simmons. "Put the yogurt in a fine strainer over a bowl overnight—all the whey comes out, so what remains is much thicker."

Achieve pasta perfection. Pasta dishes don't have to be loaded down with oil or cream to taste great. For a delicious instant pasta primavera, toss some dried pasta into boiling water. About three minutes before it's done, throw in a bag of frozen mixed vegetables—they'll take just a short time to thaw in the boiling water. Drain well and toss with a smidgen of olive oil and a dusting of grated Parmesan.

Fight Fat!

Want to save loads of fat and calories from your everyday meals? No sweat! Here are the quick-'n'-easy ways to lop off fat and calories. Just follow the guidelines below.

Instead of ...	Use ...	Savings
1 cup whole milk	1 cup skim milk	8 g. fat, 64 cal.
	or	
	1 cup 1% milk	5 g. fat, 48 cal.
1 cup cream	1 cup evaporated skim milk	60 g. fat, 392 cal.
1 cup sour cream	1 cup nonfat sour cream	39 g. fat, 256 cal.
	or	
	1 cup nonfat yogurt[*]	40 g. fat, 289 cal.
	or	
	1 cup low-fat yogurt[*]	37 g. fat, 272 cal.
	or	
	1 cup 1% fat cottage cheese whirled in blender with 1 Tbsp. fresh lemon juice	38 g. fat, 249 cal.
1 whole egg	2 egg whites	5 g. fat, 47 cal.
	or	
	¼ cup egg substitute	6 g. fat, 54 cal.
1 oz. unsweetened baking chocolate	3 Tbsp. cocoa powder + 2 tsp. vegetable oil	4 g. fat, 63 cal.
1 cup cream cheese	1 cup pot cheese	72 g. fat, 672 cal.
1 cup whole-milk ricotta cheese	1 cup 1% fat cottage cheese	30 g. fat, 268 cal.

[*]In recipes where a yogurt sauce is to be cooked, stir in 1 tablespoon cornstarch for every cup of yogurt to prevent separation.

Prepare fruit in a flash. Keep peeled and sliced fruit in your freezer, to whip up a yummy, fat-free fruit dessert at a moment's notice. Store the fruit in plastic bags, and then puree the pieces in a food processor until smooth. All different kinds of fruit work tremendously well this way—berries, peaches, plums, bananas, mangoes, papayas and kiwis, just to name a few.

Be spicier. You won't miss the taste of butter or oil on your veggies, fish or meats if you learn to cook with herbs and spices. To simplify your spice rack, buy seasoning blends. Supermarkets carry everything from authentic (preblended) curries to multiherb seasonings and pumpkin pie spice. There are even blends targeted to fish, chicken, meat and vegetables. With these premixed spices on hand, you can spice up your meal in a flash—and keep it low in fat.

Another tasty idea for salads or recipes calling for vinegar: Add a splash of fruit- or herb-flavored vinegar.

NUTRITION: GETTING THE RIGHT STUFF

Today's simple rules for good nutrition are a lot easier to follow and a lot more sensible than those of even a few years ago. And they've probably changed a lot since you were in school.

Remember those brightly colored pictures of cholesterol-choked red meat, glasses of whole milk and hunks of high-fat Swiss cheese that cheerfully adorned our grade-school classrooms? The Basic Four food groups were around for decades. They are the dietary guidelines we grew up—and grew fat—with.

Today all that advice to eat four-plus servings a day of whole-milk products (ice cream? cheese? sugar-packed puddings?) and two or more servings a day of meat (which could conceivably mean a 12-ounce porterhouse steak) seems laughable. In fact, it's downright frightening in light of what we currently know about eating right.

Back in those days, dietitians were mainly concerned about people getting all the nutrients their bodies needed, according to Dianne Odland, acting director of the Office of Government Affairs and Public Information for the Human Nutrition Information Service at the United States Department of Agriculture (USDA).

"It wasn't until the '70s that we began to realize that there's more to food than getting nutrients, that there are some components of food we shouldn't get too much of," she explains. "There is now a greater awareness of the diet-disease connection."

Using the Food Guide Pyramid

Finally, in April 1992, after about $1 million worth of research and a good deal of tinkering, the USDA finally unveiled what we now know as the Food Guide Pyramid.

The pyramid isn't perfect. It doesn't, for example, make mention of low-fat or low-sodium versions of foods within each category, or take health restrictions such as diabetes into account. But it has brought Americans into a new and healthier age. With its emphasis on grains and breads, fruits and veggies, and its deemphasis of fats and oils, sugar and alcohol, the pyramid comes quite close to ensuring those who follow it a sound and varied diet.

"The Food Guide Pyramid emphasizes the fact that a healthy diet is a balancing act, that no one food group can stand alone," says registered dietitian Gayle Shockey Hoxter, a nutritionist from Murrieta, California. "Suddenly, looking at the Food Guide Pyramid, it becomes painfully clear that if you've ever been on an all-fruit diet or a protein-only diet, you were playing fast and loose with your health."

You can make especially good use of the Food Guide Pyramid if you're trying to eat right and lose weight at the same time, says Hoxter. Use it as a basic guideline, she suggests, with these additional guidelines.

Think condiments. It's time to stop thinking of meat and dairy products as the main course. Instead, treat them like condiments, serving smaller portions along with complex carbohydrates—grains and breads, fruits and vegetables.

Think thin. Within each category, select reduced-calorie, low-fat or sugar-free versions. Within the Meat/Poultry/Fish/Dry Beans/Eggs and Nuts category, choose the very leanest cuts of meat and poultry, and use eggs in moderation, egg substitutes or the whites of the egg only.

Watch those servings. Lean toward the low end of the recommended number of daily servings, for instance, women who are trying to drop a few pounds should have two daily servings of dairy products and six servings from the Bread/Cereal/Rice/Pasta category.

Love those veggies. Do not go below the recommended five servings of fruit and vegetables a day. (Remember vegetables are lower in calories than fruit.)

Get the Nutrients You Need

Whatever dietary guideline you choose to follow as you strive to shed pounds, keep in mind that losing weight without maintaining basic nutrition is foolish and potentially harmful. As registered dietitian Jayne Hurley, associate nutritionist at the Center for Science in the Public Interest in Washington, D.C., says, "You can lose weight on any diet, but you must first follow a healthy way of eating."

To ensure maximum health while dieting, heed the following precautions.

Be safe, not sorry. "I really believe in taking one daily vitamin/mineral supplement as a margin of safety, because people have such erratic eating patterns," says Donna Dispas-Gebert, director of nutrition services at the

Getting Your Fair Share

When you're trying to lose weight, you have to be especially careful that you're getting enough nutrients. But exactly how much is enough? Following are the most current U.S. RDI (Reference Daily Intake) standards for the major vitamins and minerals that your body needs.

Nutrient	Daily Value
VITAMINS	
Vitamin A	5,000 IU
Thiamin	1.5 mg.
Riboflavin	1.7 mg.
Niacin	20 mg.
Vitamin B_6	2 mg.
Vitamin B_{12}	6 mcg.
Biotin	0.3 mg.
Folic acid	0.4 mg.
Pantothenic acid	10 mg.
Vitamin C	60 mg.
Vitamin D	400 IU
Vitamin E	30 IU
MINERALS	
Calcium	1 g.
Copper	2 mg.
Iodine	150 mcg.
Iron	18 mg.
Magnesium	400 mg.
Phosphorus	1 g.
Zinc	15 mg.

Benjamin Franklin Weight Management and Metabolism Center in Allentown, Pennsylvania. "And in wintertime, when vegetables and fruits are sitting on a truck for longer periods of time and lose some of their nutrients, a supplement is an especially good idea."

Pay attention to iron. Any woman consuming fewer than 1,800 to

(continued on page 56)

Climbing the Great Pyramid

It looks simple enough—a pyramid with four sections and the major food groups listed as servings. Eat all the servings listed on the pyramid each and every day, and voilà, you've got a road map to good nutrition. But what counts as a serving? Here's an easy guide to serving size for each type of food.

BREAD, CEREAL, RICE AND PASTA GROUP

1 slice bread

½ cup cooked rice or pasta

½ cup cooked cereal

1 ounce ready-to-eat cereal

VEGETABLE GROUP

½ cup chopped raw or cooked vegetables

1 cup leafy raw vegetables

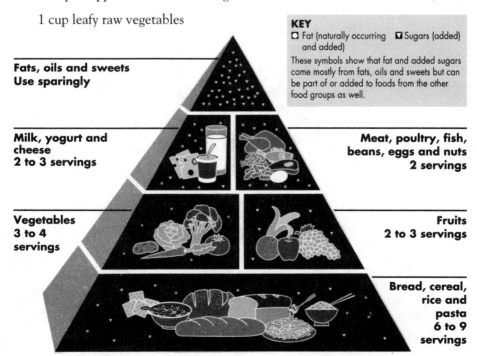

KEY

☐ Fat (naturally occurring and added)   ◼ Sugars (added)

These symbols show that fat and added sugars come mostly from fats, oils and sweets but can be part of or added to foods from the other food groups as well.

**Fats, oils and sweets
Use sparingly**

**Milk, yogurt and cheese
2 to 3 servings**

**Meat, poultry, fish, beans, eggs and nuts
2 servings**

**Vegetables
3 to 4 servings**

**Fruits
2 to 3 servings**

**Bread, cereal, rice and pasta
6 to 9 servings**

SOURCE: U.S. Department of Agriculture, Human Nutrition Information Service, August 1992, leaflet no. 572.

FRUIT GROUP

1 piece fruit or melon wedge

¾ cup juice

½ cup canned fruit

¼ cup dried fruit

MILK, YOGURT AND CHEESE GROUP

1 cup milk or yogurt

1½ to 2 ounces cheese

MEAT, POULTRY, FISH, DRY BEANS, EGGS AND NUTS GROUP

2½ to 3 ounces cooked lean meat, poultry or fish

Count ½ cup cooked beans, or 1 egg, or 2 tablespoons peanut butter as 1 ounce of lean meat

FATS, OILS AND SWEETS

Limit calories from these, especially if you need to lose weight.

How many servings do you need each day?

	Women and Some Older Adults (about 1,600 calories*)	Children, Teen Girls, Active Women and Most Men (about 2,200 calories*)	Teen Boys and Active Men (about 2,800 calories*)
Breads	6	9	11
Vegetables	3	4	5
Fruits	2	3	4
Milk	2–3†	2–3†	2–3†
Meats	2 (5 oz. total)	2 (6 oz. total)	3 (7 oz. total)

*These are the calorie levels if you choose low-fat, lean foods from the five major food groups and use foods from the Fats, Oils and Sweets group sparingly.

†Women who are pregnant or breast-feeding, teenagers and young adults to age 24 need three servings.

2,000 calories a day—and that means most women trying to lose weight—is at risk for an iron deficiency, warns Dispas-Gebert. "Women have a tendency to lose some iron during menstruation anyway, and then if there's a calorie-restricted diet on top of that, they probably won't get their daily 18 milligrams of iron," she says.

You might want to make sure that any vitamin/mineral supplement you take has an extra boost of iron. Better still, work on increasing your dietary iron by eating lean cuts of meat, chicken or fish, as well as iron-enriched cereals.

Make sure you get enough calcium. Another potential nutrient deficiency for all women and particularly dieting women: calcium. Says Dispas-Gebert: "You need about 1,000 milligrams a day. And if you're not consuming about 2,000 calories a day or if you have an allergy to milk products, you probably won't get sufficient amounts of calcium."

Women past the age of menopause in particular, but even women as young as 35, need substantial doses of calcium to head off osteoporosis. As a result, many nutritionists and doctors recommend even higher dosages than found in the Reference Daily Intakes (RDIs)—up to as much as 1,500 milligrams. And since it's virtually impossible for women to get all the calcium they need solely from their diet, supplements are crucial.

Dispas-Gebert feels that "multipreparations" don't contain enough calcium to do the trick, so she suggests taking calcium carbonate, which is calcium in its most absorbable form. "Oscal or Tums are good," she says.

Don't skimp on protein. While focusing on cutting calories, you musn't neglect dietary protein, warns Lila Wallis, M.D., founder and first president of the National Council on Women's Health. If any dieter is at risk for a protein deficiency, it's someone who's on an excessively low-calorie diet—below 1,000 calories or so a day (of course, you don't ever want to go that low). When you eat too little protein, according to Dr. Wallis, you may lose muscle and bone. "A very low protein diet and the resulting potassium deficiency may affect heart muscle contractility," she says. "This condition is the most common cause of fatality in people on a very low caloric diet."

Get the right fats. While the watchword today is low-fat, the danger is that some dieters may attempt to cut all fat from their diet, says registered dietitian Judy E. Marshel, director of Health Resources of Great Neck, New York. This practice can lead to what's called essential fatty acid deficiency, she explains.

"When you see ridges in your fingernails or if your hair starts falling out, those could be signs of essential fatty acid deficiency," she explains. "You need some omega-3 and omega-6 acids, found in fatty fish like salmon and mackerel, and in vegetable oils. If you choose your food wisely, you can still follow a low-fat diet, but you must include some of these foods."

And while we're on the subject of vegetable oils, as an added bonus they can also help lower cholesterol levels and are good sources of vitamin E—a nutrient that experts say can help boost the body's immunity to certain diseases.

Drink lots of water. If have an eye on your waistline, then surely you've been stepping up your exercise routine. This may mean you're at risk for yet another deficiency: water. Luckily, this one's got a simple solution: Drink up!

"Most Americans are pretty dehydrated in general," says Dispas-Gebert. "Water constitutes 55 to 60 percent of total body weight, and the typical American working out 20 to 40 minutes, three times a week, needs about 64 ounces of water a day to maintain that level."

What about sports drinks like Gatorade? Do they have any special benefit plain old water doesn't? Sports drinks contain electrolytes, including potassium, sodium and chloride, that can be depleted during vigorous activity. We're talking *really* vigorous activity that makes you sweat a lot. In that case you might want a sports drink to replace some potassium, says Dispas-Gebert. "For the average person, there are enough electrolytes in water to compensate for what might be lost," she adds.

EXERCISE: YOUR SECRET WEAPON

Why is it so hard to stay slim? Most people would swear they don't eat all that much. Most, in fact, are convinced they eat less than they did years ago, when they were 10, 20 or even 50 pounds lighter than they are today, and perhaps it's true.

So what's the real reason so many of us are overweight? We believe it's found in the title of the classic Charlie Chaplin film *Modern Times*. What these modern times have done is create a huge deficiency—a deficiency of exercise, resulting in a nation struggling with the awful problem of obesity.

Despite all we've heard and read about America's alleged obsession with aerobics, fitness walking and all the rest, the average person today gets much less exercise than her counterpart did a generation or two ago.

Back then, people burned excess calories just by living—that is, living in the 1940s or '50s or even '60s. But the '90s have made us exercise-deficient, and remarkably few people realize the extent of this deficiency even when the result of it is staring at us from the snickering face of a bathroom scale. The tricky part is that the deficiency comes from lots of little things—so little that they're nearly invisible, but still making a big difference in our weight.

Imagine, if you will, a split-screen image, with 1955 on the left side and 1995 on the right, and witness the dramatic effects of an exercise-free lifestyle.

Calorie Burning: 1955 versus 1995

It's morning, and Mrs. 1955 walks a quarter mile to the bus, followed by another quarter-mile walk to her job on the second floor of an elevator-less building. Once ensconced at her desk, she spends the day pounding away on an old Underwood.

Now let's look at Mrs. 1995. She drives to work, then takes the elevator to her fifteenth-floor office, where she spends her day pounding the keyboard of a computer.

The difference doesn't seem so great, does it? After all, Mrs. 1955 wasn't working in a steel mill, and she climbed only one flight of stairs to reach her desk. Yet, in fact, the difference is about 16 pounds. Yes, assuming they're the same size with the same metabolism and eat the same amount of food, just this small part of Mrs. 1995's daily regimen will, in time, make her close to 16 pounds heavier.

That's because Mrs. 1955 burned 100 calories a day walking to and from her bus stop, with about another 100 extra calories using a manual typewriter instead of an electronic keyboard. A few daily trips up and down the stairs at work burn about another 20 calories, for a total of 220. For roughly every 15 calories you stop burning on a daily basis while eating the same amount of food, you will in time get 1 pound heavier, for a total of 16 big ones in Mrs. 1995's case.

Then versus Now

Meanwhile, her husband drives 30 minutes to work, just like his dad did 40 years ago. As a salesman he drives through city traffic for about three hours a day, just like his dad did. The difference? Nearly 12 pounds a year, because Mr. 1995 has an automatic shift, while his dad, using a stick, actually burned an extra 140 calories a day.

And that's just the beginning. Because they're a two-job family, our modern couple eats out three nights a week. Over on the left side of the screen, our '50s couple ate out just once a week. The difference? For whoever does the kitchen work, about another five pounds—the result of not preparing dinner twice a week. And don't forget that our modern couple has a dishwasher!

Come evening, our '50s couple liked to watch their new TV set, though Mr. 1955 used to pop up about 15 times a night to fiddle with the aerial or change the channel. Our modern-times guy just sits there with his thumb resting on the remote.

And while Mrs. 1955 usually did her knitting while she watched TV, our modern woman just sits and watches. The difference: probably about two pounds each. Plus, one more pound can probably be tacked on because, instead of scampering to get the phone (in the kitchen) every time it rings, our contemporaries have a cellular that's always in reach.

Weekends, Mr. 1955 did yardwork. So does his son in 1995. But while Dad spent an hour and a half at a time pushing a mower over the homestead, Junior uses a riding mower and is done in 20 minutes. The difference? At the rate of 20 mows a year, four-plus pounds.

Walking Off the Weight

Perhaps the simplest, most pleasant and most effective form of exercise is walking. After all, what's not to like about it? You can do it anywhere, anytime, with a minimum of equipment—just a good pair of walking shoes and comfortable clothes. You can walk alone and use the time to unwind and contemplate. Or you can walk with others and take that opportunity to catch up with a friend or a family member. Little wonder so many people choose walking as their favorite form of exercise.

The combination of low-fat eating and an hour of brisk walking is nothing short of diet dynamite. But walking is such a powerful weight-loss method that even if you didn't change your present eating routine, just adding two brisk, hourlong walks each week would result in a ten-pound weight loss within a year.

A walking program doesn't have to be intense to be intensely satisfying . . . and effective. Here is a week's worth of tips to get you started.

See the doctor. If you're a sedentary person who is starting to exercise for the first time, tell your doctor that you're planning a walking program, and ask if she has any special advice for you.

Invest in a pair of walking shoes. It's a small price to pay for the weight-loss and health benefits you'll be getting. Comfortable, supportive shoes not only protect you from injury but make walking a more pleasurable experience as well. Walking shoes have heels specifically designed for the angled impact of your foot on the ground, making correct walking motion easier.

And when the snows came to Mr. 1955's hometown in the Northeast, he'd shovel his steps, pathway and sidewalk all by hand—about a 600-calorie job. Junior, like so many moderns, lives in the Sunbelt, and at ten no-snows per year, he's just gained two more pounds.

Back in the '50s, our couple frequently took short walks to the grocery store, fish market, butcher shop, library, drugstore and dry cleaner. Today, it's one-stop shopping via a drive to the mall. Carry a bag of groceries two or three blocks? Ha! Who does that anymore? You can probably slap on another six pounds.

By now, it's likely that, together, our modern couple is a good 50 pounds heavier than their '50s counterparts, even if they eat considerably less food. As for our modern houses, their very design makes us fatter. Many of us who were raised in vertical homes now live in ranches—no more up and down the stairs ten times a day. And appliances! Who kneads dough by hand or

Start slow. Eventually, your goal is to walk at least 30 to 40 minutes, three times a week, but for now try 5 or 10 minutes every day. It takes time to condition your muscles and your feet to walking, and sore muscles and blisters may weaken your resolve. You can take several 5-minute walks a day to help build your sense of commitment to an active lifestyle. You'll be less likely to get sore muscles or blisters than if you take one long walk. In the long run, walking every day won't hurt you and will increase your fitness level.

Watch your posture. Stand tall, relax your shoulders and let your arms swing naturally. Have a friend check your posture. The straighter you stand, the less strain you put on your neck or back. Try to keep your pelvis tucked forward, keeping the lower back as straight as possible. As your abdominal muscles get stronger, you'll be less likely to experience lower-back pain.

Find a favorite route. In the beginning, it's best to establish your walking habit by walking at the same time and place, if possible. Later you can change your route for variety. Walk facing traffic if you live in an area where there are no sidewalks.

Don't worry about stretching. Unlike other exercises, you don't really need a formal warm-up and cooldown period. Just start out each day by walking slowly, giving your legs a chance to limber up and get used to the idea. Cool down the same way.

Keep a log. Jot down how much you've walked each day so you can look back over the week and chart your progress. Writing it down helps you keep track and increases your sense of commitment.

stirs a thick batter by spoon anymore when there are automated ways of doing just about everything short of peeling a banana?

And we haven't even mentioned the VCR, the PC, the CD-ROM and the don't-get-up-and-change-the-record-you-might-burn-a-calorie multidisc CD player.

Curing Virtual Immobility

We used to hear that modern lifestyles were becoming sedentary. Well, we're way past that. Today we're into virtual immobility. And we're paying the price, with our weight and even with our lives: A sedentary lifestyle has now officially been designated as one of the major risk factors for heart disease.

All the normal, everyday, no-big-deal things we unconsciously did to burn calories and keep slim are gone, never to return. Which is why creating an exercise program for yourself is crucial. It's the best way to prevail over an environment destined to keep you overweight, no matter how diligently you may watch your diet. And, the weight-loss experts agree, it's the only way to stay thin forever.

Sure, you can lose weight just by going on a reduced-calorie diet. But why do it that way when adding exercise to your eating plan is like adding a booster to your weight-loss rocket? Study after study has proven beyond any doubt that dieting without an accompanying exercise program makes weight loss much more difficult and weight maintenance nearly impossible.

"Exercise is an important part of a weight-control program," says Steven N. Blair, P.E.D. (doctorate in physical education), director of epidemiology and clinical applications at the Cooper Institute for Aerobics Research in Dallas. "The addition of exercise to diet produces more weight loss than does dieting alone. Exercise has a favorable effect on body-fat distribution, and it's especially important in maintaining weight."

In fact, a survey done by researchers at the University of California,

---

Time Out for Working Out

Too busy to exercise, you insist? Remember, exercise doesn't take time as much as it creates time.

How's that?

After the first week or so of beginning a regular exercise program, many people report that their levels of energy and stamina surge to the point where they feel like they've actually gained extra productive hours in each day.

Exercise also helps you gain time in the most literal sense: By reducing your risk of heart disease, osteoporosis and other life-threatening diseases through regular aerobic workouts, you can add days and even years to your life.

Still wondering how to shoehorn an hour of exercise into an already-snug schedule? Try these ideas.

Be active in the morning. Borrow an hour of early-morning snooze time. Before your day begins, little can come between you and your workout. That may explain why morning exercisers tend to stick with their fitness programs better, says obesity expert Susan Zelitch Yanovski, M.D., at the National Institute of Diabetes and Digestive and Kidney Diseases in Bethesda, Maryland.

"When patients come to me and say they're always tired, I say, 'Get up early and take a brisk walk!' Inevitably, they come back and say, 'I feel great and have much more energy,'" adds cardiologist Debra Judelson,

Davis, showed conclusively that exercise is an important key to successful long-term weight loss. A whopping 90 percent of the successful dieters surveyed—people who had kept off 20 pounds for at least one year—said they did aerobic exercise at least 30 minutes, three times a week.

The word is definitely in: If you're interested in keeping those pounds off once you get them off, you need to put together an exercise program that you can live with on a long-term basis. And just how do you go about doing that?

Exercise: No Sweat

If until recently your idea of exercise has been confined to reaching for a can of mixed nuts from a top shelf, you may be worried that launching an exercise program means plenty of pain and exertion. Not at all. Forget heart monitors, forget pedometers, forget finding your pulse.

The latest research shows that working out at a moderate pace is best

M.D., chair of the American Medical Women's Association's subcommittee on cardiovascular disease.

Walk 'n' talk. Time usually spent chatting on the telephone, over lunch or across a desk may provide an opportunity for fitness. Whether it's an intimate tête-à-tête with a good friend or a brainstorming session for an annual fund-raiser, consider carrying on the conversation while you fitness-walk.

Improve your mind. Do what Morton H. Shaevitz, Ph.D., a weight-loss expert and director of the Institute for Family and Work Relationships in La Jolla, California, does: Get fit while you get the news. Each day he rides his stationary bike while reading the paper or watching CNN.

Shop for fitness. If you leave the car at home, you can turn hauling home the groceries into an effective workout. Make sure your groceries are fairly evenly divided between two handled bags when you leave the store. Grab one in each hand and, as you walk, raise and lower your bags by bending your elbows—one at a time or, better yet, at the same time. When your arms get tired, simply carry the bags normally for a block or two. Repeat until you get home!

Exercise on the go. Is traveling a big part of your job? Make those pockets of time work for you and your fitness regime. Plan on getting to your destination 30 or 60 minutes early so you can use the hotel gym or jogging path. Stuck at the airport between planes? Check your carry-on luggage in a locker, tie on your sneakers and do a couple of brisk laps around the terminal.

for weight control—and that your most important piece of equipment is your watch.

"It's not intensity that leads to better health, it's the time you spend exercising," says John Duncan, Ph.D., exercise physiologist at the Cooper Institute for Aerobics Research.

Experts used to believe that you had to exercise quite vigorously to reap all the benefits of exercise, explains Dr. Duncan. "But we now know that metabolic changes occur at very moderate exercise intensities," he says, "and that those metabolic changes confer health benefits. We found that women who walked at a moderate pace lost more weight than women who walked the same distance at a fast pace. The difference is that the slower walkers spent more time walking."

In fact, you should only worry about how hard you're working if you think you're working too hard. If you find you're gasping for breath or can't carry on a conversation, then you're not exercising for weight loss, you're just wearing yourself out. The faster you go, especially when you're out of shape, the sooner you're going to want to call it quits *and* the longer it'll be before you want to get moving again. The number-one rule of exercise: Enjoy it so you spend more time doing it!

The Bonus Plan

You know that exercise helps promote weight loss, which is precisely why you're reading this book. But the benefits of exercise go far, far beyond helping to shed pounds. Here's what exercise will do for you in addition to peeling off unwanted pounds.

- Increase lung and heart efficiency

- Improve cholesterol levels

- Lower blood pressure

- Build stronger bones

- Improve sleep

- Enhance mental ability

- Improve self-esteem and create a more positive attitude

- Reduce anxiety and depression

- Improve sex

Creative Calorie Burning

Hate to sweat? You know moving your body on a regular basis is an oh-so-necessary part of your lifestyle if you're going to maintain your perfect weight, but you're tired of aerobic dance, bored to oblivion by the stationary bike and running hurts your knees. Is there anything you can do besides going for a nice brisk walk? Yes!

Here are some other fun activities, and the number of calories they burn per hour (for a 130-pound person).

Activity	Calories Burned per Hour
Fast dancing	500
Roller skating/in-line skating	500
Square dancing	480
Gardening	330
Playing with your kids in the park	270
Slow swimming	250
Bowling	218
Shopping (including carrying heavy packages)	180
Kissing and hugging	135

The Joy of Exercise

Once you discover a sport or activity you truly love—whether it's running on the beach, playing racquetball or tap dancing—it'll be all you can do to not do it every day.

Here are a few more ideas that underscore the "pleasure principle" of exercise.

Play to your preferences. Think about an activity you enjoy—any activity, not necessarily fitness-oriented. Then get creative, combining fun with a physical challenge.

Love to shop? Forget the home shopping channel! Instead, fitness-walk along your favorite shopping district before the stores open and preview the window displays. Got the travel bug? Sign up for a fitness-oriented vacation. Are you crafty by nature? Then take a nature walk and collect pine cones, twigs and other found objects for your next project.

Have it your way. If you have an aversion to exercise, a fresh perspec-

Exercise Lite

You've heard of light beer, light margarine and light crackers. How about light exercise?

It's a concept whose time has come, say experts armed with compelling evidence to prove that some physical activity—even as little as 30 minutes' worth spread out during the day, a few times a week—is far better than none at all.

"We made a mistake by insisting early on that exercise must be sustained, aerobic activity," says Steven N. Blair, P.E.D., director of epidemiology and clinical applications at the Cooper Institute for Aerobics Research in Dallas. And, he suspects, that's probably why so many of us (20 to 30 percent of the U.S. population) are totally sedentary, at high risk for heart disease, and probably battling a weight problem to boot.

Chances are a lot of us have been intimidated by the mere thought of running or playing singles tennis or swimming laps for hours each week. But now, says Dr. Blair, short bursts of calorie-burning activities—including 10 to 20 minutes here and there of stair-climbing, lawn mowing and Frisbee playing with the family pooch—can provide many of the same health and weight-loss benefits of sweating it out on the jogging trail for 45 straight minutes.

Has "Exercise Lite"—as it's being called by the American College of Sports Medicine (ACSM) and the U.S. Centers for Disease Control and Prevention—reduced national fitness goals to the lowest common denominator? Not at all, says Dr. Blair, the program's biggest booster.

"If you look at the energy expenditure resulting from the traditional exercise prescriptions over a one-week period and compare it with the energy expenditure from our new recommendations, you'll see they're in the same ballpark," says Dr. Blair. "It's not a lowering of standards. We're simply presenting an alternative to getting the same energy expenditure, which should give comparable results."

"I see this as very good news for the public," says Russell Pate, Ph.D., president of the ACSM and chairman of the Department of Exercise Science at the University of South Carolina in Columbia. "What it does is demystify this whole exercise thing. If you're not the kind of person who's attracted to vigorous exercise, public exercise or rigid approaches to exercise, there are still lots of ways to lead a physically active life. Find a few and incorporate them into your lifestyle."

So put down that TV remote, get off your duff . . . and get moving!

tive may help, says obesity expert Susan Zelitch Yanovski, M.D., of the National Institute of Diabetes and Digestive and Kidney Diseases in Bethesda, Maryland. "In our field, we're getting away from prescribing specific exercises," she says. "Instead we encourage our patients to develop an active lifestyle."

Add variety. Try all kinds of activities—bird-watching, gardening, Ping-Pong, horseback riding, social dancing. The best workouts aren't necessarily the ones that deliver the greatest calorie burn; rather, they're the activities you're more likely to do because you honestly enjoy them.

Make fitness friendly. Instead of a sit-down dinner party, throw a backyard badminton bash, serving light finger foods and fresh fruits or vegetable cocktails between sets. Or invite a few buddies over to join you on a nature hike and share a picnic lunch. Don't miss a step at holidays, either. Take part in active celebrations with others. In some cities, for instance, there are organized runs on December 31 to help ring in the new year with friends old and new. For additional ways to burn calories that you won't find on any traditional exercise lists, see "Creative Calorie Burning," on page 65.

Getting Started on Getting Fit

How do you begin a new exercise program? Whatever you do, it shouldn't be like trying to muscle a square peg into a round hole. Your workouts should accommodate your tastes, your time constraints and your level of physical ability.

"If they don't and you miss a couple of days, you may feel you've fallen off the exercise wagon," says Thomas A. Wadden, Ph.D., director of the weight and eating disorders program at the University of Pennsylvania in Philadelphia. "Then you feel so bad that you have trouble getting back on."

Weight-loss experts suggest you aim for an exercise-induced calorie burn of about 300 a day. Then, if you also work on cutting back the fatty foods in your diet, you'll end up with a daily 500-or-so calorie deficit—and a loss of about a pound a week. But because doing too much too soon could burn you out or sideline you with an injury, set your sights lower at the beginning. That means you may have to cut back a little more on food to make up the difference—one less snack or treat a day should do the trick.

To find out where your starting point is, see "Your Exercise Quota," on page 68. The 300-calorie figure has been converted into activity points, to make it easier for you to keep track. "Your Exercise Quota" lists exercise options and the number of points you can earn per 20 minutes. (If you're out of shape or have been sedentary for a while, it's probably a good idea to see your physician before you embark on a new exercise regimen.)

Your Exercise Quota

How much exercise do you need to do in order to achieve your perfect weight and stay there for the rest of your life? Probably less than you think.

This handy activity point system will tell you exactly what you need to do to attain your goals.

All you need to do to burn off one pound a week is earn 210 points a week, or 30 points a day. Half your weekly goal of 210 points should come from list 1 on the opposite page—the more exercise-oriented activities. You can rack up the rest by choosing from the everyday activities in list 2.

You may not be able to jump into this much activity right away, however, especially if you're not used to it. No problem. To gain a little more insight into your personal exercise requirements, read the assessment under the statement that best describes you.

I am not currently physically active. That puts you on an eight-week track to your 210-point goal. The first week, your total quota is a mere 30 points. That increases to 45 points in Week 2 and 60 points in Week 3. Then you progress in 30-point increments for the remaining five weeks (90 points for Week 4 up to 210 points for Week 8).

I exercise no more than 20 minutes twice a week. You're an intermediate. You've got six weeks to work up to the 210-point goal. Your first week's quota is 60 points, then add 30 points each week until you reach 210 points in Week 6.

I exercise three or more times a week for at least 20 minutes at a time. You're in the advanced category. That means you can reach the 210-point goal within four weeks. Start your fitness program by earning 120 points the first week, increasing your quota by 30 points until you reach 210 points in Week 4.

The figures are based on 20 minutes of activity for a woman weighing 130 pounds or a man weighing 180 pounds. If you weigh more, you'll earn slightly more points for every 20 minutes; if you weigh less, you'll earn a fraction fewer.

Choosing Your Activity

Now you'll also need to figure out what kinds of activities suit you best. That's fairly easy to do. For starters, decide where you'd like to work out. If you're a nature lover, try some outdoor sports. If music motivates you and

Activity	Points Earned per 20 Minutes	
	130-lb. Woman	180-lb. Man
RECREATIONAL ACTIVITIES		
Badminton	11	16
Cross-country skiing	16	22
Cycling (10 mph)	12	16
Golf (walking)	10	14
Hiking (hilly)	16	22
Jogging (10-min. mile)	18	25
Jumping rope	16	23
Resistance training	8	11
Rowing machine	13	19
Scuba diving	16	23
Swimming (slow crawl)	15	21
Table tennis	8	11
Tennis (doubles)	8	11
Tennis (singles)	13	17
Volleyball	10	13
Walking	10	14
HOUSEHOLD CHORES		
Cleaning windows	7	10
Gardening (digging, hoeing)	14	19
Mopping floors	7	10
Mowing lawn	12	16
Painting (outside)	9	13
Raking	7	9
Scrubbing floors	13	17
Shoveling snow	17	23
Trimming hedges	9	13
Trimming trees	15	21
Washing car	7	9
Weeding	9	12

you like working out with other people, join a gym. If you like your privacy, choose solo activities like walking, cycling and swimming. Or, work out at home with an exercise video or handheld weights.

You don't have to schedule two-a-day sweat sessions in a gym to earn your activity points, either. Walking takes little or no athletic prowess (unless you're a competitive speed- or racewalker). And according to our system, you can earn activity points for everything from hoeing a few new rows in the vegetable garden to putting a good gloss on the old Chevy. Just being more active in your everyday life can take a big bite out of your daily calorie total.

"But to get the optimum fitness and weight-loss benefits, you have to work out a little harder," says Wayne L. Westcott, Ph.D., YMCA national strength-training consultant and strength-training consultant to the National Academy of Sports Medicine and the American Council on Exercise. "So try to earn at least half of your weekly total with more traditional workouts, like walking, resistance training, swimming or cycling." And make sure you're always ready to go by keeping a well-stocked gym bag handy.

If you prefer to work hard in short spurts, you'd probably respond best to high-intensity, strength-based exercise that involves most of your major muscle groups. That probably means something like circuit training. Circuit training consists of a series of resistance-training exercises with bouts of aerobic exercise, like brisk walking, jogging, cycling or stair-climbing in between. A stationary cycle, with handles that you push and pull as you ride, is also an option. Cross-country skiing and rowing—or their indoor incarnations—may hold some appeal for you, as well.

If you like to exercise at a slower pace for a longer period of time, consider exercise involving continuous, repetitive movement—walking, jogging, swimming and cycling on a standard stationary bike are good options for you.

If you find that you become easily bored, try cross-training, an array of aerobic exercises you can mix and match. Come up with a set of workouts for the week equal to your point quota: Each day's workout could consist of several different types of exercise. Or you could devise a couple of standard workouts and rotate among them. Cross-training also reduces your risk of injury. "If you work the same muscles every day, they get stronger while the others get weaker," Dr. Westcott says. "That sets up an imbalance that almost always leads to injury."

RESISTANCE TRAINING: PUMP UP YOUR WEIGHT-LOSS POWER

Not so long ago, resistance training—also known as strength training or weight training—was only for the likes of Arnold Schwarzenegger or for the 97-pound weakling hoping to avoid getting sand kicked in his face by bigger guys at the beach. The average man simply didn't pump iron. And what woman wanted biceps like Rocky Balboa?

But those days are over. Today, health clubs and home gyms (even if that means no more than a corner of the bedroom or basement) are beehives of muscle-making activity. And we're all a lot savvier about resistance training and how it works: You provide a challenge to your muscles, and your muscles react by growing and getting stronger. When you challenge the muscles on a regular basis, you create a better, firmer, more attractive body, without becoming muscle-bound.

In fact, many people are beginning to realize that a complete program of health and fitness is . . . well, incomplete without some resistance training built into it. Resistance training helps increase your body's power and endurance, and it reduces the risk of injury to muscles, ligaments and tendons during everyday activities and especially while doing sports. The nice part is, you see results very quickly.

"The gratification is immediate," says William J. Evans, Ph.D., who heads the Laboratory for Human Performance Research at Penn State University and is the co-author of *Biomarkers: The 10 Determinants of Aging You Can Control.* "You get stronger by the second week, and in just 12 weeks you can double or triple your strength." Little wonder, then, that strength training can even boost your self-confidence. In addition, strength training has been found to help boost HDL (or "good") cholesterol and lower your risk of developing diabetes.

Creating the Look You Want

As if all that weren't enough, resistance training is also a key ingredient in any weight-loss plan. How? Since resistance training helps the body burn fat and build muscle, you'll look firmer and more toned. Remember that resistance training by itself isn't likely to produce weight loss—after all, muscle weighs more than fat. But once you start a regular program of resistance training, your body shape will definitely improve. In fact, don't be surprised if you notice you've dropped a dress size even without a change on the bathroom scale.

And because muscles burn calories at a faster rate than stored body fat does, sticking to your resistance-training regimen after you reach your goal will make weight maintenance much easier.

This is more important than you might think. When people lose weight by diet alone, a futile cycle can develop. They lose weight so quickly that their body shifts into starvation mode—that is, it tries to conserve as much energy as it can. The rate at which you burn calories then slows to a crawl, so you have to cut calories even more to continue losing weight. And once you start eating normally again, your body conserves each one of those precious calories in the form of fat. But with resistance training, "we're trying to maintain the metabolic rate so people can have a much easier time losing weight," says Miriam Nelson, Ph.D., a Tufts University research scientist at the U.S. Department of Agriculture's Human Nutrition Research Center on Aging.

Resistance training is particularly helpful for older people who want to stay trim. "Metabolism and muscle mass definitely decline as we age, which makes it tougher to keep off excess weight," explains Dr. Nelson. Resistance training helps the aging body hold on to its muscle, says Dr. Evans.

Get Your Questions Answered

If you think launching a resistance-training program means enrolling in a pricey health club filled with scary-looking hardware and Sylvester Stallone clones, think again. While it is a good idea to learn the basics from a fitness pro—to avoid possible injury and to see how to get the greatest benefit from your workout—you can easily continue your regimen using some simple gear at home, or at your local Y or community center.

Be sure to talk to your doctor or physical therapist before starting a

Women, Don't Resist Resistance Training!

Resistance training may offer the most benefit of all to women past the age of menopause. Ironically, that's precisely the group that seems to be the most reluctant to work out with weights.

You won't end up looking like the Terminator, but you will notice a dramatic improvement in your mobility and flexibility by performing a few simple exercises three times a week for eight weeks. In one study with a group of people over 90, a couple of them even ended up throwing away their canes!

Resistance training is particularly important for older dieters. That's because it can help ward off crippling osteoporosis by strengthening and maintaining bone so often lost during dieting. "When a woman loses 20 or 30 pounds, she loses not only fat but also muscle and bone, which may compromise her health," says Miriam Nelson, Ph.D., Tufts University research scientist at the U.S. Department of Agriculture's Human Nutrition Research Center on Aging. Dr. Nelson is conducting studies at Tufts to test the effect of resistance training on bone mass, and she hopes to prove that adding strength training to a weight-loss program will mean the end of dangerous muscle and bone loss. "The results aren't in yet," she says, "but we speculate that the only thing these exercising women will lose is fat."

So, get pumping! Invest in a pair of one- or two-pound weights and a resistance band, and get directions for a basic upper-body workout from a resistance-training pro. If you've got a stationary bike, it will provide you with resistance exercise that benefits the crucial hip area. "Just increase the resistance against which you're pedaling," says osteoporosis expert Sydney Lou Bonnick, M.D., research professor at the Center for Research on Women's Health, Texas Women's University, Denton, Texas. "This strengthens the muscles of the upper hips and thighs so they pull on the bone, which is a good stimulus to bone growth." You can get the same effect on a bicycle outdoors by going uphill.

resistance-training program. This advice is particularly important if your doctor has told you that you may be at risk for osteoporosis or muscle tearing. When you start your program, stick to very light weights, follow instructions closely, go slowly and pay attention to form to avoid sprains or strains.

Here are answers to the most common questions that beginners ask.

Boost Your Muscles and Your Ego!

While you're losing weight, how would you like to lose all those bad feelings about yourself that accumulated along with the extra pounds? Pumping iron can help pump up your self-esteem as well.

"Exercise has a powerful impact on the way we view ourselves," says Robert Motta, Ph.D., director of the doctoral program in school community psychology at Hofstra University, in Hempstead, New York. "It offers one way to attain mastery over a task, while in life's other activities we might not be so successful." Mastery—becoming successful in a given area—is key for self-esteem, whether it occurs in your work, a hobby or a recreational sport. "In addition, resistance training compounds the benefits of mastery by offering almost immediate, powerful feedback in the shape of increased muscle and a trimmer body," says Dr. Motta.

Self-esteem then benefits from a double dose of physical medicine: You've mastered something real, with the tangible rewards seen clearly in the mirror. "That's something you may not be able to do with other kinds of programs," says Dr. Motta.

What's more, to attain mastery of resistance training, you don't need to be a master. "You can reap all these physical and psychological benefits without necessarily being an athlete or expert. Improvement is generally a function of effort and motivation," says Dr. Merrill J. Melnick, the State University of New York sports sociologist. You don't need a Ph.D. in quantum physics to load up a barbell, lie on your back and push up a weight, but it does take discipline, enthusiasm and drive. And it also makes you feel better about yourself.

Q. How much time must I spend on resistance training? (I already do aerobics for 30 minutes, three times a week.)

A. You can get the greatest benefit from your resistance-training program if you do it for about the same amount of time you do your aerobics, around 30 minutes, three times a week. It's best to space out your workouts, giving yourself a day off in between.

Q. How many repetitions do I need to do of each exercise?

A. Each activity—arm curls, knee extensions, whatever—should be done in sets of two or three, 8 to 12 repetitions per set. Give yourself a couple minutes' rest between each set before continuing.

Q. Are warming up and cooling down as important in resistance training as they are in aerobics?

A. Yes! You need to get your muscles, ligaments and tendons loose and supple before starting your workout. A five- or ten-minute warm-up—in which you walk around or do some easy stretches—is a good idea. Then cool down after your workout with a slow five-minute walk.

Q. What kind of equipment do I need to buy?

A. Little, if any. Sure, you can invest in barbells or hand weights, but beginners might want to start by using clean, plastic milk or detergent bottles (with handles), filled with water or sand. Ideally, each should have the capacity to be filled to two or three times the weight you can comfortably lift now. (So, if you can easily lift 10 pounds, after ten or so weeks of training, you might progress to 20 or 30 pounds of weight per bottle.) But don't overdo it; it's best to start very slowly and easily and work up from there.

Q. How do I know when I've reached a muscle-building plateau?

A. You've plateaued when you can do more than 8 to 12 repetitions (reps) of an exercise with practically no rest time in between them and when your muscles don't feel fairly exhausted afterward. When that's the case, you should either add more weight to the barbells or hand or leg weights or try a new exercise aimed at building that muscle (or muscle group).

Q. When can I quit my resistance-training routine?

A. Uh . . . we were afraid you'd ask that question. The answer is: never, not if you want to maintain the benefits you've achieved. Unfortunately, as soon as you stop resistance training, your body will return to its prefitness levels within a couple of weeks—although Dr. Evans has some evidence that you might be able to reduce your regimen to just once a week following a ten week, three-day-a-week program and maintain your fitness level. But stop completely? Once you start, you're going to look and feel so terrific, why would you even think of it?

On Your Mark, Get Set . . . Pump!

Here's a simple strategy to ensure and maintain success.
Personalize your program. If you want to succeed at resistance training,

take the workout offered below and create your own version of it. "The key is to construct an individualized program that meets your needs and has realizable goals rather than a general one-size-fits-all program with goals that are not attainable," says Merrill J. Melnick, Ph.D., a sports sociologist at the State University of New York, College at Brockport.

Write it down! Plan your exercise routine, then keep a log of your efforts. "Keeping track of your workouts shows your accomplishments on paper, which accentuates the ones reflected on your body, providing even more motivation," says Leo Totten, head coach for the 1987 U.S. Weightlifting Team for the Pan-Am Games, and assistant coach for the United States in the 1989, 1990 and 1991 World Games. Establish a baseline weight for each exercise you do, and enter it in "Your Perfect Weight Success Diary," on page 275. After you run out of pages, you can simply continue your record-keeping in another notebook. Keep track, workout by workout, as you get stronger.

Set realistic goals. Start at a low-enough level to allow you to work your way up. Underestimate your strength in the beginning and step up the ladder slowly—a pound on this machine, a pound on that. By improving slowly, you're less likely to burn out or plateau.

Reward yourself. Keep the momentum at a peak. Periodically give yourself gifts—say, some new clothes and a night out in them, or perhaps just a new T-shirt—to reward your efforts and your success at meeting new challenges.

Change your routine. For instance, you can increase the repetitions instead of the weight and work on endurance. You may even want to drop some weight and increase the number of repetitions in order to concentrate on form and work on defining and toning muscle. Use a variety of exercises for the same muscles and muscle groups. By switching exercises, you help maintain the momentum that may be stymied by a plateau in your workout. "With the lifters I coach, I stress a great deal of variety," says Totten. "The body needs a 'shock' to the system to jolt it out of the doldrums."

Go slow. Avoid jerky, fast movements. If you do your exercises sloppily, you just open yourself up for injury. A sore shoulder or pulled muscle will definitely put a dent in your momentum.

Recruit a workout partner. It can be a spouse, a friend or a neighbor, who can offer moral support as well as safety-helping you (spotting) while you do an exercise. And having someone else around is just more fun, and more likely to keep you going.

Getting Started

Here's a beginner's resistance-training workout with two purposes: to give you a sense of momentum, and to produce results you can see. These

The Total-Body Battleground

Besides helping you lose weight and stay trim, how else can resistance training help you? Let us count the ways! (If you're unfamiliar with some of these exercises, have a fitness pro explain what they are and how to perform them properly.)

- Neck exercise: reduces strain; improves posture

- Bench press: builds upper-body strength; improves posture

- Lateral raise: protects rotator cuff; boosts upper-body strength

- Dumbbell row: improves posture and back flexibility; may build bone mass

- Arm curl: boosts forearm and biceps strength; targets wrist bone

- Stomach curl: builds abdominal muscle; tones belly; adds stability for back

- Hip flexor: may build up bone supply at hip

- Hamstring curl: builds thigh muscle; improves mobility

- Quadriceps extension: adds to knee stability and overall mobility

- Calf raise: boosts calf strength; may guard against shin-splints

two purposes combined offer the best motivation for you to continue exercising for the rest of your life. Each exercise hits major muscle groups to ensure fast, noticeable results. For instance, we've included the bench press because it builds the chest, shoulders and back, while in turn making your midsection appear slimmer.

Begin with one set of 8 to 12 repetitions, working up to two or three sets if you feel up to it.

Bench press. Lie on your back on an exercise bench with your knees bent so your feet are flat on the floor. Grasp the barbell from the rack (or have it handed to you) with your hands slightly more than shoulder-width apart. Slowly lower it to your chest. Press the barbell up until your arms are almost fully extended, with elbows almost, but not quite, locked.

Arm curl. Stand with your back straight. Hold the barbell with both hands, palms up, with the bar at arm's length against your upper thighs. Curl the bar up in a semicircular motion until your forearms touch your biceps. Keep your upper arms close to your sides. Lower the bar slowly to starting position, using the same path.

Squat. In a standing position, with feet about 16 inches apart, and using a comfortable grip, place the barbell (with light weights) across your shoulders, behind your head. With your back straight and head up, squat slowly until upper thighs are parallel to the floor. Return to the original position and then repeat. (Note: Start with a light weight or none at all—this exercise is a toughie, but it offers a lot in return. If it's too difficult to go all the way down, try a partial squat instead, returning up before your thighs become parallel to the floor.)

Lat pull-down. Grasp the bar at the lat pull-down station of a weight machine with your hands about 36 inches apart. Then sit down, allowing your arms to extend overhead. Pull the bar down slowly until it touches the back of your neck right above your shoulders. Then return to starting position. (Note: For variation, bring the bar down in front of you.)

Military press. Grasp the barbell and sit at the end of a bench or chair, with your feet firmly on the floor. Lift the weight over your head and rest it on the back of your shoulders. Push the bar up until your arms are almost extended, then lower it to starting position and repeat. (Note: This can be done with a straight barbell or separate dumbbells, or on a weight machine. Also, if you find this movement too difficult, try raising and lowering the weight in front of your shoulders.)

TAMING YOUR STRESS WHILE YOU SHED POUNDS

Are you overworked, overwhelmed . . . and, as a result, overweight?

Join the crowd. There's a raging epidemic these days of too much to do and never enough time to do it. To cope, some people unleash their energies in all directions at once, always starting but never finishing anything. Others procrastinate, so today is always spilling over into tomorrow, and they're always late. Many, already burdened past endurance, choose to make their lives impossible by taking on even more.

Something has to give, and usually does—quality time with your family gets scarce, your health suffers and weight control is out of control.

While most of us can't stop working or dealing with family responsibilities, we can work smarter, learn to set saner priorities and adopt strategies to minimize stress. And while we can't expect to be at the perfect weight all the time, we can avoid the self-defeating cycle of weight gain that all too often accompanies stress. Here are some realistic ways to do it.

Take a walk! Regular walking is one strategy that can attack all your symptoms at once: It can help you lose weight, give you the perfect opportunity to sort out goals and priorities and reduce stress in a big way. (See "Strolling Off Your Stress," on page 80.)

Just say no. "Stressed-out people often can't assert themselves," says Joan Lerner, Ph.D., a counseling psychologist in private practice in Philadelphia and a psychologist at the University of Pennsylvania Counseling Service. "So they swallow things. Instead of saying, 'I don't want to do this,' or 'I need some help,' they do it all themselves. Then they have even more to do."

Asking for help seems obvious, but for many of us, it's not. Many over-

Strolling Off Your Stress

By now you've surely heard that one brisk 20- to 30-minute walk can have the same calming effect as a mild tranquilizer. And you probably know that, over time, a regular exercise program can enhance self-esteem and reduce depression. But now there's research suggesting that a comfortable stroll can leave you feeling less anxious and more positive. By adding simple mental techniques, strollers get the same positive mental benefits that brisk walkers enjoy.

How, you may be asking, can an overworked, overwhelmed person find the time for regular walks in the first place? Simple: Regular exercise such as walking helps you create time by increasing your stamina and energy, which can enable you to get more done in less time. Investing 20 to 30 minutes a day in walking, then, may actually save you more time than that.

So what's the lowdown on this special destressing stroll? Recently, researchers explored how cognitive or "mindful" exercises might enhance the effect of exercise on the body and mind. The study was conducted by Ruth Stricker, director of the Marsh: A Center for Balance, in Minnetonka, Minnesota, and James M. Rippe, M.D., director of the Exercise, Physiology and Nutrition Laboratory at the University of Massachusetts Medical School in Worcester.

This research, called the Ruth Stricker Mind/Body Study, studied 135 people divided into five groups of walkers for 16 weeks. Group one walked at a brisk pace, and group two at a low-intensity pace.

Group three walked at a low-intensity pace but added an extra ele-

whelmed people keep their resentment and their enormous load of responsibilities all to themselves, explains Sally Ann Greer, Ph.D., a Virginia psychologist who specializes in stress management and weight reduction. Asking for help and learning how to say no are skills that the overworked must practice.

What's more, you can learn to say no tactfully, insists Merrill Douglass, D.B.A., president of the Time Management Center in Marietta, Georgia, and co-author with his wife, Donna, of *Manage Your Time, Manage Your Work, Manage Yourself.* Often, saying no while on the job is a matter of giving your supervisor choices, Douglass says. "Say, 'I'd really like to take this on, but I can't do that without giving up something else. Which of these things would you like me to do?' " Douglass advises. Most bosses, he adds, can take the hint.

ment: They practiced a mental technique to bring about the "relaxation response" developed by Herbert Benson, M.D., president of New England Deaconess Hospital's Mind/Body Medical Institute, in an attempt to see how the mind and body work together. (The relaxation response is a physiological response characterized by decreased heart rate and blood pressure, and feelings of tranquillity.)

Group three was asked to pay attention to their footsteps, counting one, two, one, two. They were also instructed to visualize the numbers in their minds. If they found their thoughts drifting, they were to say "Oh, well," and come back to counting their footsteps. Group four practiced "mindful exercise," a Westernized application of t'ai chi ch'uan developed by Stricker, and group five served as controls—they asked not to change anything about their lives.

The results were "dramatic," according to Dr. Rippe. Group three showed decreases in anxiety and had fewer negative and more positive feelings about themselves—equal to the stress-reducing effect that the brisk walkers gained. These effects were evident after just one exercise session and were maintained over the duration of the study. Group two—the low-intensity walkers who did not use the cognitive approach—showed no improvements until the 14th week, and then the improvements were not as extensive. And group four experienced similar results to group three.

"For people who have difficulty with brisk walking or other moderately intense exercise, this is an encouraging study," says Dr. Rippe. "They can be encouraged to exercise knowing that with a simple mental technique they can get the same psychological benefits as a person who can exercise at a higher intensity."

Also, he suggests, examine the reasons behind your inability to say no. Some people don't want to turn down a request from a spouse, a child or a co-worker because it makes them feel guilty. "It might create a conflict," he says. "But often the people who keep asking you to do more don't see it as a conflict. It becomes a vicious circle, and *you* have to slow it down."

Get your signals straight. Overwork often triggers stress. But instead of finding a way to reduce their anxiety, some people respond inappropriately, often seeking solace—or maybe just distraction—by eating.

"People who are stressed may get their signals confused," says Dr. Greer. "Because food is a source of comfort, they might interpret stress as a signal to eat rather than as a signal to reduce the stress."

You may have friends who react in just the opposite way: When they're stressed out they're either too busy or too worried to eat. If you're wondering

Sex, Stress and Pigging Out

Time: the day before final exams.

Place: a college library.

The room is filled with eager-beaver students of both sexes, intently studying their textbooks and taking notes. But something else is going on: While the female students are reading and writing, they're also busily devouring Kit Kat bars, containers of chocolate milk and bags of popcorn, while the guys are . . . just studying. What's this all about? Something that psychologist Richard Straub, M.D., of the University of Michigan, Dearborn, has long suspected, namely, that women under stress tend to overeat, whereas men don't.

A study conducted at the University of Michigan, Dearborn, involved men and women ages 17 to 41, who were shown an anxiety-producing movie and a pleasant one. Snack foods were available while they watched. The men tended to consume 140 fewer calories during the stressful flick compared with the calmer one, while the women ate more during the high-anxiety movie.

It isn't simply that women eat more than men when they're stressed out, says Dr. Straub. He believes that women are usually so much more controlled in their eating habits than men that when given the chance to finally let loose, they do. And what they choose to eat also has a lot to do with stress, researchers say.

When your nerves are fried, do you long for some french fries? When your boss has just bitten your head off, do you feel like biting into a Butterfinger? There's a definite connection between the stress you're feeling and the food you crave.

"Some people who are stressed out go for soft, creamy, comfort foods, such as mashed potatoes with plenty of butter," explains Maria Simonson, Ph.D., Sc.D., professor emeritus and director of the health, weight and stress clinic at Johns Hopkins Medical Institutions. "Or they want baked foods, like a milk and cookies snack. It's the nothing-says-loving-like-something-from-the-oven syndrome."

If you're turning to food in response to stress or bad feelings like depression, loneliness or sadness, it's important to develop a brand-new strategy, urges Dr. Simonson. "Before you eat, ask yourself, 'How am I feeling about myself right now? What happened this week to upset me? Am I eating this because I'm hungry or because I'm upset?'" Anti-stress measures, from counseling to yoga, can help you feel better . . . and eat less.

why that's not *your* problem—and you wish it were!—it's because studies suggest that overweight people tend to overeat in response to stress. Another study done at Cornell University reveals that if you're overweight to begin with, you may use food as a mood elevator, even when you're *not* under stress. (So-called normal-weight people, in contrast, generally eat less when under stress and more when they've had a good day.)

If you tend to eat when you're overwhelmed and overworked, you need to pay more attention to what you're feeling. The next time you feel the urge to eat when it isn't mealtime, ask yourself if you're *really* hungry. If you aren't, Dr. Lerner recommends a nonedible alternative. One of the women she counseled in a weight-and-stress-reduction program at the University of Pennsylvania would, during her work break, buy herself a single red rose instead of a snack. "There are other ways to fill yourself up," says Dr. Lerner.

In one national study called the "Mitchum Report on Stress in the '90s," 75 percent of those polled said they listened to music to help alleviate stress. When stress hits, it's not signaling the need for Raisinets. It is telling you that you need rest or relaxation.

Still other people use food not as a way to cope with stress per se but as a way to avoid dealing with the very thing that's driving them crazy in the first place. "Food is kind of a diversion," explains Dori Winchell, Ph.D., a psychologist in Encinitas, California, who specializes in eating disorders. "It's a way for you to *not* fix what needs to be fixed," she explains. "You hate your job and you hate your boss, so you are miserable and say, 'I might as well be nice to myself and eat some ice cream.'"

The more appropriate response to those signals of distress: Confront what's making you fed up. Easier said than done, Dr. Winchell acknowledges. But, she adds, "If you are living the life you want to be living, I guarantee that stress is not going to make you overeat."

Another option, from Paul J. Rosch, M.D., president of the American Institute of Stress, is progressive muscular relaxation. Alternately tense and relax the muscles of your body, going from one group to the next, shoulders to arms to hands, and so on. "Some people," he adds, "use visual imagery or meditate."

And if you *must* eat, try something that's low-fat—say, some air-popped popcorn or nonfat frozen yogurt.

Put time on your side. Stressed-out people often seem overwhelmed because they're simply disorganized. They're the ones who don't start making the kids' Halloween costumes until the night before. They also tend to apply equal vigor to every task, even though some tasks are more important than others, and so they feel out of control—a leading cause of workplace anxiety, according to Douglass.

If you recognize the symptoms of disorganization in your at-home and on-the-job habits, Douglass recommends coming up with a system to keep track

Best Stress Busters

When you're feeling beat,
And you wanna eat,
Who you gonna call?
Stress Busters!

It may not have quite the same zing as the *Ghostbusters* song, but you get the idea. Next time you feel stress getting the best of you, don't reach for that container of leftover Chinese food in the fridge—reach for this list of great ideas on how to take the edge off your negative emotions. Try a different one each time, and see which gives you the best results.

- Call a friend.
- Read a book or magazine.
- Take a scented bubble bath.
- Go to the gym.
- Write your feelings in a journal.
- Play with your kids or your dog.
- Have a massage.
- Go to a movie.
- Take a 30-minute walk.
- Buy (or pick) some flowers.
- Listen to music.
- Take a catnap.
- Work on your hobby.
- Rent a video.
- Do volunteer work.
- Drop in on a neighbor.
- Take a yoga class.
- Do three total-body stretches.
- Meditate or pray for 15 minutes.
- Do five 1-minute meditations.
- Watch one of your favorite TV shows.
- Spend 15 uninterrupted minutes catching up with your spouse.
- Sit silently for 10 minutes.
- Have a heart-to-heart with a friend.
- Walk around the mall and buy yourself a small present.

of your tasks. You might use a notebook, for example. Make a list of everything you need to do, and check off each item as you go along. Most pressing tasks go at the top, and the least time-sensitive go toward the bottom.

You might also write daily chores on Post-it Notes, and throw each one away as you finish the task written on it. In this way, you can see progress *and* what remains to be done.

Whatever system you use, Douglass notes, it ought to be compatible with your work style. "If it adds too much structure to your life, you're unlikely to use it," he says. "Time-management techniques have to be compatible with who you are and how you're going to use them."

It also helps to establish goals and set deadlines for yourself, he says. Without self-imposed deadlines, your work may expand to fit your time and probably tempt you to put everything off.

"And most people don't have any goals," says Douglass. "But those who do, and are actively pursuing them, probably feel in control of most things and also feel less stressed. They may be working just as hard, but they feel that they're getting somewhere. The feeling of stress has less to do with your workload than with whether you're in *control* of your workload."

Part Two

SPECIAL STRATEGIES FOR STAYING THIN FOREVER

CHANGE YOUR WAYS, CHANGE YOUR WEIGHT

It never fails. Every Friday, Ginny plans a million different activities over the weekend—everything from giving herself a pedicure to checking out the local craft shop. Yet by 3:00 or 4:00 on Saturday afternoon, she always finds herself alone and totally bored and ends up spending what's left of the weekend overeating.

Ellen has had another phone fight with her mom, over yet another trivial issue. And, as usual, Ellen ends the conversation by slamming down the receiver and heading straight for that carton of almond fudge ice cream stashed in the fridge.

Bob wants very much to lose 45 pounds. He'd also like to meet a nice woman and get married. But right now he believes that no woman could possibly like him looking the way he does. So, even though his doctor put him on a low-fat diet and even though he just bought himself a rowing machine, Bob's going out tonight with his buddies for some pepperoni pizza and three or four beers.

These folks aren't doing anything evil or criminal. But what is criminal is the way they've fallen into the habit of mindlessly doing what they've always done, month after month, year after year and, in the process, blocking any chance of getting and staying slim. Food has become an all-purpose pill to help them through life's ups and downs—the fatigue and the boredom, the loneliness and the anxiety, the anger and even the joy. Half the time, they don't even realize how much or what they're eating!

Sound familiar?

What all of them (and perhaps you?) could use is a hearty dose of behavior modification. If that seems like a scary concept, it isn't, really. All it means is modifying your behavior, making an adjustment in the often-unconscious habits that have kept your weight at its current level. And we can help! Our triple-A program involves three keys to positive behavior change.

- Awareness

- Attitude

- Action

Opening Up Your Awareness

Simply being conscious of your behavior is an important first step. Here are some keys to paying attention to the things you eat and do that have an impact on your weight.

Open your eyes to your eating. You can't change your poor habits if you're not even aware of what they are. But, says Dean Ornish, M.D., head of the Preventive Medicine Research Institute in Sausalito, California, "when you learn to eat with awareness, you'll find you won't need the excessive amounts of food that can lead to overweight. Even the *tiniest* amounts become pleasurable—one teaspoon of a rich, chocolate dessert you really focus on can actually be more satisfying than a whole bowl of something you've mindlessly downed while watching TV. Whether it's a spoonful or a bowlful or a half gallon, at some point you finally have enough, and when you pay attention to what you're eating, that point comes much sooner."

"To change unwanted behavior, you must first observe it," says Laura Stein, author of *The Bloomingdale's Eat* Healthy Diet*. Stein has taught behavior modification in her EAT (Effective Appetite Training) Healthy workshops in New York City.

Pay special attention to your feelings. If you've ever tried to drown your sorrow in a bag of cookies or a bowl of ravioli, you know that overeating is ultimately an ineffective way to handle unpleasant feelings. "Many people use food as a way to cope with the loneliness and pain they feel—in a way, the fat 'coats' their nerves and numbs the pain," says Dr. Ornish. Yet you know what always happens: As soon as the food's gone, the problems—along with a few additional pounds around your middle—return.

Dr. Ornish has a better solution: meditation. "If you can quiet down your mind," he says, "you can experience a greater sense of inner peace and well-being. Meditation is really the art of paying attention, and when you pay more attention to your eating behaviors, many good things start to happen." Such as losing the urge to overeat and becoming increasingly aware of how what you're eating affects you, for better or worse.

Says Dr. Ornish: "When you really pay attention to how your body is reacting after having a steak or a cheeseburger, you might find that you're

Cure Those Cravings!

You're walking along, minding your own business, when out of the distance it appears, golden and sparkling in the sun: the bakery. And suddenly you tell yourself that you'll die if you don't go in and buy one or two of those sticky buns right now. Before you know it, an empty bakery bag is in your hand, and the buns are down the hatch.

It doesn't have to be that way. Cravings can be cured, insists Laura Stein, author of *The Bloomingdale's Eat* Healthy Diet*. Stein has taught behavior modification in her EAT (Effective Appetite Training) Healthy workshops in New York City.

"What you want to do," she explains, "is to break up your automatic response to a food craving."

She suggests that you ask yourself four key questions before you go ahead and eat that unplanned-for food.

1. Am I really hungry?

2. Did something just happen to trigger that craving?

3. Would something else, something less fattening perhaps, satisfy me just as well?

4. What do I care about more—the food or having a slimmer, healthier body?

After you have answered all four questions and you're still craving that tempting hot dog or candy bar, delay the action a bit longer by telling yourself:

• First I'll try an alternative activity from my list.

• I can always eat that food later. (And with any luck you'll forget about it or won't want it then.)

• I'll eat it after I exercise today.

The goal, she explains, is not to forbid yourself from ever eating the things you want, but to make certain that you want to eat when and what you think you do. "Choose your food. Don't let the food choose you," she urges.

Perhaps her best advice of all, though, is to gradually wean yourself off those no-no foods that are interfering with your weight-loss plans. "You don't crave what you don't eat," she insists.

feeling sleepy and sluggish, and that your thinking is fuzzy. Once you cut the fat from your diet, though, you'll probably feel so much better right away that the wise food choices will seem obvious to you."

If you're a frequent victim of the oh-my-God-did-I-really-eat-that? syndrome, you might want to tune into your feelings more by giving meditation a whirl. Inexpensive classes are available around the country; check with your local Y or university extension program.

Write on. Another way to start developing your eating awareness is by filling in and regularly reviewing "Your Perfect Weight Success Diary," on page 275.

"Write down any unplanned eating and the circumstances under which it occurred," urges Ronette Kolotkin, Ph.D., director of the behavioral program at the Duke University Diet and Fitness Center in Durham, North Carolina, and co-author of *The Duke University Medical Center Book of Diet and Fitness*. Review your notes so you can start anticipating food triggers and plan smarter ways to deal with them. "Our research at Duke and other research have shown that writing down what you eat is helpful to weight loss," says Dr. Kolotkin.

Hold that thought! Another aspect of awareness means recognizing your impulses—and deliberately not acting on them. "Just because something is in your mind doesn't mean you have to do it," notes Howard Rankin, Ph.D., a psychologist and clinical director at the Hilton Head Health Institute in South Carolina. "It's a powerful notion, that you have the ability to make a decision about how you'll manage an idea. It's impulse control, and eating is a good example of it. Some people always say to themselves, 'When cheesecake is in front of me, it's inevitable that I'll eat it. I want to eat it, I deserve it, and I'll start my diet again tomorrow.' But if you keep thinking that way for five or ten years, you're not likely to lose weight."

So, how do you break the pattern? The answer, again, is through awareness. "You must become very aware—as most people are not—of the long-term consequences of your behavior," says Dr. Rankin. Eat that cheesecake every time the spirit moves you, and it's only a matter of time before your stomach will start to feel like a big, squishy cheesecake. Take your mind off your cravings with some diversionary tactics. (See "20 Alternatives to Eating," on the opposite page, and "Cure Those Cravings!" on page 91.) And practice saying no to yourself a bit more often. "At some point, it's critical to get tough with yourself if you want to see results," says registered dietitian Judy E. Marshel, director of Health Resources of Great Neck, New York.

Adjusting Your Attitude

Simply paying better attention is not enough, however. You have to want to make positive changes in your behavior.

Forget about "dieting." Changing your bad eating habits is essential to

20 Alternatives to Eating

You're bored. You eat. You're depressed. You eat. You're stressed out from your job. You eat. What's wrong here? Nothing, if you like looking at that expando version of yourself in the mirror. If you want to see your slim, trim self, however, this kind of behavior has to stop.

"Most people don't think about managing their eating behavior as they manage other things in their life. But you need to apply the same principles so you can be prepared for those specific situations that cause problems for you," explains Howard Rankin, Ph.D., a psychologist and clinical director at the Hilton Head Health Institute in South Carolina.

Let's say the coffee-and-doughnut wagon at work seems to call out your name every afternoon at 3:00—and you're trying to lose 25 pounds. So, how 'bout dipping into your list of alternative activities instead of diving headfirst into a jelly doughnut? What list of alternative activities? This list, the one you should always have nearby at times like these. Add any other suggestions you think will work for you.

AT HOME

1. Drink a glass of water or two.

2. Brush your teeth and/or gargle with mouthwash. (People report that this kills cravings.)

3. Take a walk.

4. Take a nap.

5. Take a bath.

6. Call or write the person who's making you angry.

7. Go to a movie (but bypass the candy counter!).

8. Buy yourself a nonedible gift for under ten dollars.

9. Have sex.

10. Snack on something with zero or little fat, such as an apple, a rice cake, a carrot.

AT WORK

11. Call a friend.

12. Meditate.

13. Have a piece of fruit at your desk.

14. Leave the building for ten minutes.

15. Play with your computer.

16. Catch up on office gossip with a co-worker.

17. Have a drink from the water cooler.

18. Go to the restroom and splash cool water on your face.

19. Check your appointment book for next week.

20. Walk up a few flights of stairs.

weight loss and maintenance, to be sure. But, says Dr. Kolotkin, "attitude modification is actually more important than behavior modification."

What does she mean? "Most people develop a diet mentality," says Dr. Kolotkin. "They look at what they're doing as a weight-loss program, but they're missing the big picture—that this is a lifestyle-change program forever. It's not just a matter of doing certain things until you lose weight, but rather examining how the way you live your life contributes to your weight. Take a broad view. Don't think of what you're doing as simply dieting, with the typical all-or-nothing perfectionist attitude, because that usually leads to weight yo-yo-ing. The fact is, you won't be perfect—you will overeat and you won't exercise sometimes. What you need is to develop strategies to pick yourself up, to learn how to forgive yourself and keep going."

Stein stresses a similar principle: to think in terms of changing your diet, not dieting. "There's a big difference between the two," she says. "When you change your diet, you focus on progress, not on perfection, the way people do when they're dieting. And when you think in terms of changing your diet, you can view an eating setback as a learning experience. You'll say, 'Why did I have all that pie at my mother's house? How can I avoid doing that the next time I visit her?' instead of saying, 'I've blown it!'—and maybe compounding the problem by eating some more."

Firm up with affirmations. "We believe what we tell ourselves," says Stein. Therefore, the more positive messages you send to yourself, the more you'll want to do what's needed to slim down. Each day, she suggests, write or say aloud these kinds of affirmations.

- I'm losing weight now.

- I'm enjoying how I'm feeling now.

- I love the food that makes me thin.

- I love the feeling of making progress.

- Losing weight is effortless.

- I'm making things easy for myself now.

- My body is getting stronger, slimmer and healthier every day.

It's important, she adds, that all your affirmations be in the present tense to give them a greater sense of power and immediacy. Talk about the ways you hope to be and feel in the future and you'll be less apt to take action today.

Oh, grow up! Think about the way you've dealt with your dieting self in the past. Chances are you've assumed the role of strict parent, telling the little boy or little girl in you, "No! You can't have that!"

"That's how people have typically dieted—'Mustn't eat that chocolate! Bad! Bad!'" says Dr. Rankin. "But after a few hours or days or, if

---

Don't Leave Home without It

It's so easy to skip breakfast—grab a cup of coffee and your car keys and zip out the door. That should save you about 350 calories. Right? Wrong!

"Eat a good breakfast," Mom always said. Turns out she was right, especially if you want to lose weight. At least that's the picture that emerged from a study on the role of breakfast in successful weight loss conducted at Vanderbilt University in Nashville, Tennesee.

Researchers placed 52 moderately obese women on a 12-week diet, in which some ate three meals a day including breakfast while others passed up their morning meal. The women who ate breakfast tended to snack less during the day on high-fat, high-calorie goodies. In other words, they were less inclined to cheat on their diets.

The moral of the story? Get out that cereal bowl and dig in!

---

you're particularly strong-willed, after a few weeks, the child in you rebels and says, 'So, I can't have that candy bar? We'll see!' And then you have three." However, Dr. Rankin says that changing behavior should be viewed as a choice.

"You're responsible for your own behavior," he asserts. "Adults have to realize that every action has a price and a payoff—every action, whether it's eating three candy bars now or eating 1,200 calories a day and exercising five times a week. Act from a position of choice, as opposed to feeling like the parent of an unruly child."

Be a buddy to yourself. "The bottom line is liking yourself—that's a powerful motivator," says Marshel.

Similarly, Stein has taught her workshop clients to assimilate this powerful message: "No matter how I feel, I always treat myself well."

Bad moods and bad days will come and go—that's the reality of life. You'll always have challenges to face, even after you're thin! But once you make the commitment to be your own best friend and treat yourself accordingly, you'll eventually stop looking to food to solve your problems.

Taking Appropriate Action

"You can analyze your weight problem forever, but unless you take action, forget it. Action is critical," says Marshel. "And, your overall goal should be to learn to act and not react, so that you come from a positive place."

What that means is getting in the driver's seat of your own life. It means planning for daily success and therefore minimizing your chances for failure.

Every day you're going to plan on having three low-fat meals, with a healthy snack or two if you want them, and that you'll do some form of pleasant exercise. Whatever surprises crop up, you'll plan on dealing with them, too. So whether it's a sick baby or a less-than-glowing report from your boss or a fender-bender or a check that's lost in the mail, you do not spell relief F-O-O-D. You now have a program for weight-loss success, and this time you're going to see it through.

Make a contract with yourself. Perhaps you work for a company that rewards you for achieving your six-month or yearly goals. You can success- fully apply the same principle to your weight-loss goals. Decide—on paper— what you hope to achieve and when, giving yourself small but meaningful rewards as you reach each minigoal.

"Contracts should be short-term, and should focus on increasing healthful behaviors associated with weight loss, rather than on weight loss itself," say John P. Foreyt, Ph.D., and G. Kent Goodrich, Ph.D., weight-loss experts at Baylor College of Medicine, Houston, Texas, who have studied the effectiveness of various behavior-modification techniques on dieters.

Marshel agrees. "I focus on self-care goals, not weight-loss goals, with my clients," she says. "So if, for example, part of someone's contract is to ex- ercise three times a week and he does it, then he might reward himself by going to the movies on Sunday afternoon."

Why avoid establishing weight goals when, after all, you're trying to lose weight? "Because weight-loss goals are difficult to control and predict," she points out. "And anyway, weight loss is simply a by-product of other positive changes you make. In the long run, it's not the exact number of pounds that counts as much as making adjustments in your behavior and attitude. If you make consistent changes and meet your self-care goals, you will inevitably experience weight loss."

Get the lowdown on high-risk situations. "Different people have dif- ferent vulnerabilities," notes Joyce D. Nash, Ph.D., a clinical psychologist specializing in weight control and author of *Now That You've Lost It: How to Maintain Your Best Weight.* You might, for instance, do fine at an ice-cream stand but lose all control at a buffet table. Someone else might handle buf- fets like a pro but go to pieces at the sight of Reese's Pieces.

"Ask yourself what your high-risk situations are," suggests Dr. Nash. "Is it going out with friends? When you're feeling down and sorry for yourself? When you're in a bakery? Do a personal analysis. Once you know your eating triggers, you can focus your efforts and determine which strategies you can use to cope better."

For some people, this might mean not eating at restaurants, or at least not until they have had some success with their weight-loss program. Other restaurant-coping techniques include not looking at the menu (simply order

---

Midnight Bites

It may not be just what you eat that determines the number on the bathroom scale, but when. A preliminary study indicates that midnight snacking may slow down what in metabolic lingo is called diet-induced thermogenesis (DIT)—the food's natural ability to boost metabolism and burn more energy. This means you'll burn off fewer calories after the meal and you'll pack on more weight.

On three separate days over five weeks, nine men ate either a morning, afternoon or late-evening (1:00 A.M.) snack. Every other aspect of their diet was controlled. Researchers found a big difference between the DIT of the morning and late-evening snack. (The afternoon snack had no significant effect.)

"Eating at night produces less heat and burns fewer calories than eating a snack in the morning," says registered dietitian Judith Stern, Sc.D., professor of nutrition and internal medicine at the University of California, Davis. "Over a period of time, it may mean trouble. By eating the bulk of your food late at night, even in one year there might be a substantial increase in body weight."

The bottom line: Lay off the midnight snacks.

---

the low-fat items you know are available) and asking the waiter to serve your fish or chicken broiled, with the sauce on the side.

The key is to figure out your most effective strategies. "You can't draw up a list of 12 things that will work for everybody. It must be personalized," says Dr. Nash.

Make believe you're motivated. The day's going to come—if it hasn't already—when it's just too cold (or too hot, or too something) to go out for your 30-minute walk. Or there's some leftover pizza hiding out in the back of the refrigerator, and you can't think of a single good reason why you shouldn't eat it at 4:00 A.M.

"Even if you're not motivated to continue your weight-loss plan, act as if you are," says Marshel. "You may not feel like exercising, but don't give yourself the luxury of negotiating the issue with yourself—just do it. What we're talking about here isn't willpower, it's acting *as if*. Simply cut off that negative line of thinking." Marshel guarantees that, within a few minutes, you'll feel better and more motivated.

Don't wait if you deviate! Don't let one binge or a week without exercise lead to a what-the-hell-now-I've-blown-it attitude from which you may never recover. "If you've deviated from your plan, write down what happened and the ways in which you might learn from it," says Dr. Kolotkin. "Identify your destructive thoughts and reactions—for example, exaggerating how bad the eating episode was and the all-or-nothing thinking. You've got to start replacing those destructive thoughts with constructive strategies."

How? Dr. Kolotkin suggests you recall, and pat yourself on the back for, your previous weight-loss successes. Reevaluate and maybe modify your goals—you might be expecting too much, too soon. And create a controlled environment. "What are the things you can change that can put you in greater control of your eating?" she asks. "Maybe it's throwing out the peanut butter and ice cream from the fridge, or keeping more veggies handy, or rearranging your schedule if working late means bad eating habits, or asking the kids to keep their candy in their room."

"Monitor your behavior day to day, but not obsessively," adds Dr. Nash. "If you haven't exercised for the past two days, get yourself out there today. Take action sooner rather than later."

Recruit a diet buddy. Maybe you need more support than you can give yourself. Fine. There's plenty of help available if you just look around. You can try a formal weight-loss support group like Weight Watchers or Overeaters Anonymous (check the phone book for locations), or simply ask your spouse, your teenager or your friend to be your exercise or low-fat-dining buddy. A helping hand does help when it comes to weight loss: One study at Purdue University reveals that dieters with supportive partners lost 30 percent more weight than those who attempted to diet on their own.

"Having someone who knows you and understands what you're going through can be very inspirational," says Ronna Kabatznick, Ph.D., psychologist with Weight Watchers International.

Say goodbye to perfectionism. "When I talk to patients about behavior-changing techniques, I tell them they won't do it right 100 percent of the time, but you don't have to," insists Dr. Rankin. "If, for example, you're now successfully managing your food temptations 20 percent of the time, and then you go up to 60 percent, it will make a huge difference. What you want to aim for is just enough of a change to make a significant improvement. The quickest way to kill off your chances of weight-loss success is to demand perfection of yourself."

JUMP-STARTING YOUR MOTIVATION

You were fired up and raring to go when you first opened the pages of this book. Remember? It wasn't so long ago. Slimming down—and changing your life—was high adventure then, a challenge you rose to immediately. The world was full of new discoveries: that a low-fat lifestyle is much easier and more palatable than you ever thought possible, that sweating through a workout or exploring your neighborhood through daily walks is actually fun!

But now—just maybe—the honeymoon's over. Some days you have to pry yourself out of bed for your prework walk. You have delicious dreams about burgers and fries. You're eating your way through stressful days, and when your mood hits rock-bottom, you seriously consider hanging it all up.

In short, you need a kick in the pants—a little boost.

And here it is! Below is a plan to help you maximize your motivation when you're having a tough time sticking with your weight-loss program. Simply follow the plan, step-by-step, and you should regain your inspiration in no time! What's more, you can use the same plan over and over again, anytime you feel you're in a rut.

Step 1: Do a cost-benefit analysis. Divide a sheet of paper into two vertical columns. In the left column, list all the benefits of sticking to your weight-loss plan. For example: "I've already dropped six pounds"; "I have more energy"; "I deal with stress better." Under those items, jot down the costs of not sticking with the program, like "I'll be out of shape," or "My belly will come back."

In the right column, write the costs of following your program: "I have to give up certain favorite foods that aren't healthy"; "I have to make time

99

for exercise." Then, include the benefits of abandoning the program, such as, "I'll have more time to myself because I won't be walking every day," or "I'll be able to eat and drink whatever I want."

"The things in the left column are the thoughts that will motivate you. When your thoughts start drifting to the right column—to the costs of making the changes and the benefits of not bothering—that undermines your motivation," says clinical psychologist Joyce D. Nash, Ph.D., a weight-loss expert in the San Francisco Bay area and author of *Now That You've Lost It: How to Maintain Your Best Weight*. You should feel free to add to each column as you come up with new pros and cons about sticking with your diet. Be sure to post the list where you can see it every day, as both a visual and mental reminder.

Being honest and open about your negative thoughts can help you figure out why you're starting to feel burned out, Dr. Nash says. Then you know just when to focus on the many good ideas found here in *Prevention's Your Perfect Weight*.

Step 2: Check your records. Look at your weight, body measurements, cholesterol levels and any other vital statistics you noted at the beginning of "Your Perfect Weight Success Diary," on page 275. Where are you now? If you haven't been charting your progress, start now. Record your weekly weight, the amount of time you spend exercising, even your blood pressure and cholesterol readings whenever you have them taken. Avoid thinking about how far you have to go to reach your long-term weight-loss goals. Instead, pat yourself on the back for the progress you've already made!

Step 3: Set daily minigoals. Vow to eat a healthy bowl of whole-grain cereal for breakfast, instead of a short stack floating in butter and syrup. Or to skip your late-night snack, or to walk ten minutes more today than you did yesterday. "Today is your time horizon, not the rest of your life," Dr. Nash says. Looking too far ahead—such as at the 25 pounds you still have to lose—can be overwhelming and self-defeating.

Step 4: Write it down. Having your goals on paper where you can see and update them will make them seem more real—and boost your motivation to achieve them. So, put your minigoals on paper, then give yourself a star once you accomplish them. Or make a formal "contract" with a buddy. Include your goal and the reward for reaching it. You may feel more committed to your goals if you use these techniques.

Step 5: Swap the cookie jar for the "reward jar." Think of at least 20 little rewards for yourself—simple, short-term things you would like to have or do that don't take a lot of time or money. (The more doable they are, the less likely you are to find reasons not to treat yourself, Dr. Nash says.) It could be taking a soothing mineral bath, gathering a bouquet of fresh flowers from your garden, calling a good friend for a long chat or reading a chapter of a novel you never seem to have time to finish. Try to include as many of your favorite (inedible!) treats as possible.

Then, write each one on a separate slip of paper and keep them in an empty cookie jar or canister. Each day, as you accomplish your minigoals, draw from the reward jar—that's your treat for the day. (And replace the slip in the jar, so you'll be able to choose that reward again in the future!)

Step 6: Change your workout routine. Take your act on the road! Instead of stationary cycling, traverse wooded trails on a mountain bike. Walk in a new area—or with a new partner. Try a workout in the morning instead of waiting till afternoon. Take up a new sport, or switch from weight-lifting machines to a free-weight workout. Or experiment with interval training: After a 10- or 15-minute warm-up, step up your pace for about 2 minutes. Slow down to catch your breath, recovering for about 1 minute, then speed up again for another 2. (This works for walking, cycling, running, swimming—even stair-climbing and stationary rowing.) Vary your workouts as much as you like in order to keep them fresh and exciting.

Step 7: Spice up your diet. Give your taste buds a treat: Try a new, exotic fruit or vegetable, or a different type of fish or low- or nonfat product each week. Once each week or so, try one of the yummy, low-fat recipes in this book. Start an herb garden and add fresh sprigs of basil, oregano, cilantro or parsley to your recipes. There are plenty of healthy ways to keep your palate interested and satisfied without straying from your sensible eating plan.

Step 8: Ask for support. Tell a close friend or your spouse that you're having a hard time sticking to your eating-and-exercise plan. Be specific about what that person can do to help you through it. "You may need someone to tell you how much they admire your efforts, or just to show some interest in what you're trying to do," Dr. Nash says.

"Sometimes," she adds, "what you need most may be for your friends and family to say nothing at all. Tell them not to nag you, watch what you're eating or give you that quizzical look when you miss a workout. Let them know if you need to get through this on your own."

Step 9: List your high-risk situations and your defense strategy. Maybe you tend to overeat at restaurants. Or you have an aversion to working out in cold weather. Or you have trouble stopping at just two nonfat oatmeal-raisin cookies (you tend to keep at it until the box is gone). Write each of your most tempting situations on the front of a three- by five-inch index card. Then think of as many counterstrikes as you can and include them on the back of the card. For example, order child-size portions when you eat out. Try mall walking or gym workouts in the winter. Buy individually wrapped snacks, such as nonfat granola and fruit bars, to keep you from going on a granola bar binge. With your defense at the ready, you'll be equipped to handle anything and stay motivated right to the weight-loss finish line.

READER SURVEY RESULTS: THE BEST WAYS TO GET THIN FOREVER

What's the best way to lose weight and keep it off forever? We posed that question to *Prevention* magazine readers—men and women throughout the nation who are committed to keeping themselves healthy, slim and fit. We asked for weight-loss strategies that really work, and more than 6,000 readers answered the call.

The gist of the responses and the basic philosophy of this book is this: If you make small changes in your diet, daily activities and behavior, without drastically overhauling your life, the numbers on your bathroom scale will gradually go down for good. That's terrific news if you've been trying for years to starve off and sweat off those extra pounds.

The fact is, you don't have to quit red meat cold turkey. You can have a sliver of cheesecake once in a blue moon. And you don't have to spend hours in the gym every day. All of that flies in the face of the traditional ways of weight loss, where a main meal might consist of an undressed salad and a naked chicken breast, or worse, a low-cal meal-replacement "shake" with no identifiable flavor whatsoever.

Cutting-edge weight-loss researchers agree: That old approach just doesn't work. "Dieting isn't the way to lose weight, because in people's minds dieting means skipping meals, depriving yourself and designating 'forbidden foods,'" says John Foreyt, Ph.D., professor in the Department of Medicine and director of the Nutrition Research Clinic at Baylor College School of Medicine in Houston, Texas, and co-author of *Living without Dieting.* Sure, you'll probably shed the pounds short-term. But chances are you'll balloon back up in the long run.

Of course, to lose weight you must create a calorie deficit. You can do that by taking in fewer calories, by burning more calories through activity or by doing both at the same time. The *Prevention* reader survey suggests—and the latest weight-loss research confirms—that doing both is the best way to lose weight long-term.

"Most of the data show that people who have lost weight will just not keep it off unless they've made some significant changes in their physical activity," says Steven N. Blair, P.E.D. (doctorate in physical education), director of epidemiology and clinical applications at the Cooper Institute for Aerobics Research in Dallas. But that calorie deficit doesn't have to be big—only about 500 calories a day. And it's amazing how easy that is. Switching to diet soda, walking instead of taking the car—simple substitutions like these can make a big impact on the scale and on your health.

The 20 weight-loss strategies identified by those surveyed add up to a top-notch weight-loss program. This campaign against the scale can help you lose weight the right way and be more likely to keep it off. In fact, if you begin to put these strategies into effect immediately, you can lose a good ten pounds within the next three months.

Fine-Tuning Your Diet

Reducing the amount of fat in your diet was the number 1 successful weight-loss strategy by far: 65 percent of those surveyed gave it top priority. That makes perfect sense, because fat contains more than twice as many calories as carbohydrates or protein. Plus, fat is more readily stored in your body, while those other foods are more easily converted to and burned off as fuel.

What's surprising is that cutting calories—the old-school way of weight loss—ranked only at number 3 and cutting back on sweets (another refrain from previous dieting days) was even farther down the list, at number 5. It's not that reducing calories and sweets isn't important. But if you concentrate on fat, you'll probably make a big dent in the other two as well, because fat and sugar often come together in foods, says F. Xavier Pi-Sunyer, M.D., professor of medicine at Columbia University and director of the Obesity Research Center at St. Luke's–Roosevelt Hospital Center, in New York City.

How do you cut fat and calories? For one thing, you make a practice of reading labels—number 9 on the list of top strategies (on page 104). The fat content of most foods is easy to find, thanks to improvements in product labels. Products that don't pass muster—that have too many grams of fat per serving—

Top 20 Weight-Loss Strategies

Losing weight is not enough. Keeping it off is more than half the game. Here, from more than 6,000 weight loss "experts"—real people who have figured out what works for them—are the techniques that make all the difference.

1. Reduce fat intake.

2. Exercise regularly (any kind of exercise).

3. Reduce total calories.

4. Drink more water.

5. Eat fewer sweets.

6. Keep problem foods out of the house.

7. Walk for fitness.

8. Increase high-fiber foods.

9. Read food labels for fat and calories.

10. Keep a food diary.

11. Eat low-fat or nonfat foods.

12. Cut back on meat intake.

13. Enjoy exercise.

14. Increase your self-esteem.

15. Plan what you'll eat.

16. Eat smaller but frequent meals.

17. Have a support group.

18. Do aerobics.

19. Become more conscious of why you eat at certain times.

20. Eliminate or reduce be-tween-meal snacks.

should never make it from the grocery store shelves to your kitchen. (Keeping problem foods out of the house was number 6 on the list of strategies.)

Eating low-fat or nonfat foods (number 11 of the top 20) is something you can do to substitute for your favorite decadent desserts, creamy salad dressings and spreads. But make sure you swap them portion for portion—otherwise, you could actually gain more calories than you lose. For example, if you swap a piece of raspberry-cheese pastry for a fat-free slice, you cut a whopping 15.9 grams of fat and 65 calories from your meal. But if instead of eating one slice of the skinny version you eat two, you actually add 205 calories to your daily total. So go easy on the serving size.

Number 12 on the list of top successful weight-loss tactics is reducing your intake of meat. Meat is one of the major sources of fat in American diets, especially saturated fat, which also ups your risk of heart disease. "But keeping some meat in your diet isn't bad—you just have to watch the portion size," Dr. Pi-Sunyer says. Once in a while, indulge in a steak if you want, but instead of the 12-ounce T-bone, order the 4-ounce fillet, and cut off the excess fat. Round out your weekly diet with leaner meats, such as baked or broiled turkey and chicken, and fish (many of which contain heart-healthy omega-3 fatty acids).

When you turn your nose up at fat, you tend to fill up on other, more healthy food and drink. Indeed, the number 4 tip was increasing water intake. Experts say that often, when you think you're hungry, you're really thirsty. So first try to douse that urge to eat with a glass of H_2O. (Aim for eight eight-ounce glasses of water a day.)

Eating more high-fiber foods like cereals, vegetables, fruits and beans ranked number 8 on the top 20 list, and filling up on starchy foods like whole-grain breads, pasta and rice is likewise a diet-smart rule to follow. "Those foods tend to be low-fat, so they drive you to a lower-calorie diet," Dr. Pi-Sunyer says. "They're also bulkier, so smaller amounts of them might fill you up more." Research suggests that it takes your body longer to digest fiber-dense foods, so they help keep your blood sugar levels stable. That helps you avoid the severe blood sugar peaks and valleys that may trigger your appetite.

Eating smaller but frequent meals, number 16 of the top 20, may also have the same blood sugar–stabilizing effect. That means snacking can be okay, as long as your idea of a midafternoon treat is low-fat, complex-carbohydrate fare like pretzels, fruits and nonfat or low-fat yogurt. But reducing or eliminating between-meal snacks like handfuls of honey-roasted peanuts or bags of M&M's is a must if you're to lose weight (strategy number 20).

Exercising Your Options

It's no surprise that being more active earned the number 2 spot among weight-loss strategies that work. But activity doesn't necessarily mean exercise in the classic sense—donning a sweat suit and hammering through a daily hourlong walk, run or weight workout at the gym. "These things are fine, but many people have trouble fitting them into their schedules," Dr. Blair says.

It may be more convenient for you to put in 30 minutes of brisk vacuuming, mopping or leaf raking instead of brisk walking—and consider that part of your workout for the day. Although research hasn't shown how such lifestyle workouts compare with more fitness-oriented workouts, anything that gets you moving, no matter how hard you're working, helps you burn calories. "Your muscles don't know whether they're digging in the garden or whether you're on the fanciest weight machine in the gym," Dr. Blair says.

So when walking for fitness (our number 7 strategy) or taking an aerobics class (number 18 on the list) isn't possible, you've got a whole host of options. Take the active way out whenever you can. Use the stairs, wash your dinner dishes by hand or go on a house-cleaning binge. Combine these lifestyle workouts with your favorite fitness activity, whether it's swimming, cycling, hiking or walking. Try to accumulate about one hour of activity daily—it can provide you with about 300 calories of the 500-calorie deficit you're trying to achieve each day.

Perhaps the best thing about having so many exercise options to choose from is that you're more apt to find something you like. Enjoying exercise—number 13 of the top 20—means you're likelier to stick with it, Dr. Blair says.

Psyching Yourself Thin

Increasing your self-esteem ranked number 14 in the top 20. But isn't a higher opinion of yourself a result of losing weight, not a way to lose weight? Not necessarily, explains Dr. Foreyt.

"You do not get true life's joy from focusing on the bathroom scale," he insists. "It's more important to focus on relationships with other people, being more productive at work, being more organized, and viewing life as a series of opportunities and growth experiences." That—along with small steps to change your diet and increase your activity—can help you feel as though you're more in control of your life and your weight problem. And when that happens, weight loss may not seem like such a chore. "The long-term weight-loss successes are people who change their lifestyles for them-selves, not because their high school reunion is coming up or because they want to fit into a pair of size-ten jeans," he says.

You can enhance that feeling of control by using self-monitoring tech-niques, such as keeping a food diary (number 10) and planning what you're going to eat (number 15). When you record what you've eaten, jot down how you were feeling and what you were doing at the time—"Your Perfect Weight Success Diary," on page 275, will show you how. This simple routine will help you become more conscious about why you're eating—number 19 of our weight-loss top 20.

"Often, what drives your eating is not hunger but feelings—boredom, anger, tension, stress or hostility," Dr. Foreyt points out. Handling these feel-ings, instead of feeding them, can not only help you lose weight but also help you create a healthier emotional lifestyle. Whether it's an organized group of fellow dieters, an understanding family or a close friend who's also on the weight-loss track, having a support group—the number 17 weight-loss strategy—can help you stay motivated. What's more, it can enhance your sense of well-being to an even greater extent than the number of pounds you ultimately lose.

"Our weight is such a trivial part of our lives, but so many of us judge ourselves by what the scale says," Dr. Foreyt says. "Being skinny doesn't mean you'll be happy."

CALLING ALL MEN!

Your wife and kids love you. You have a job you like with enough money coming in. You're active in your community, you have a good, solid group of buddies and once or twice a year you and the family take nice vacations. Things are, well . . . just about perfect.

Now, if you could only lose that beer belly!

If, over the years, you've seen your body slowly get out of shape, you're certainly not alone. According to national statistics, 29.6 percent of American men 18 years old and over are considered clinically obese—that is, more than 20 percent above their desirable weight. And millions more, while not quite that overweight, are still heavier than they'd like to be.

For all the talk on TV and in magazines about women's weight woes, there are actually more obese men in the United States than women. Not only is this a problem from an appearance standpoint but it creates a serious health hazard as well. It is now estimated that one out of five men will have a heart attack by age 60, and their excess pounds, poor eating habits and lack of exercise are all contributing factors.

The type of man who typically finds himself overweight is middle-aged and of a higher-than-average socioeconomic status, according to clinical psychologist Morton H. Shaevitz, Ph.D., director of the Institute for Family and Work Relationships in La Jolla, California. President Bill Clinton is a prime example. "President Clinton is an overworked, overstressed, moderately overweight man who makes food choices destined to keep his weight right where it is," notes Dr. Shaevitz, author of *Lean and Mean: The No Hassle, Life-Extending Weight Loss Program for Men.* "He may jog, but it's usually to McDonald's for a cheeseburger."

But whether you're the chief executive living on Pennsylvania Avenue or a construction worker living in Altoona, Pennsylvania, overweight is a very real threat to both your looks and your life span. The reasons men have a hard time eating right and staying slim are many.

Ignorance Is Blubber

The biggest cause of male weight gain is lack of information. "Smart men are nutritionally ignorant," asserts Dr. Shaevitz. "They just don't know what's in the food they're eating and why it can be harmful."

For example, a chef's salad and a diet soda is many men's idea of a healthy lunch. But they couldn't be more wrong. A chef's salad is a 750- to 1,500-calorie, high-fat meal, usually containing cheese and luncheon meat—each approximately 100 calories per ounce and about 80 to 90 percent fat—all smothered in two or three ladles of dressing for an additional 250 to 750 calories. A man will wash the salad down with a diet drink and feel virtuous because the soda has no calories. But in fact he may have just consumed more than half his caloric and fat limit for the entire day.

The What-Me-Worry? Syndrome

Unlike a woman, who focuses much more on her weight and who can probably tell you how many calories she and everyone else at the table just consumed, a man tends not to think about these things very much at all.

This casual—and in some ways healthier—attitude about weight and overall body image is first developed when we're very young. "Differences in how men and women perceive their bodies start real early," says registered dietitian Linda H. Eck, an assistant professor in the psychology department of Memphis State University, who has researched gender and weight. "Studies have repeatedly found that women diet much more than men do and that their body images are poorer," she says. "When men are overweight, they usually think they look fine, and when women's weights are normal, they tend to think they're fat."

One such survey was conducted in 1986 in London, England, and involved 348 boys and girls ranging in age from 12 to 18. The researchers found that hang-ups about body size and shape made even the youngest girls in the group go on sometimes extreme diets and feel tremendous guilt about eating, whether or not they were even overweight, while the boys tended to be blissfully unconcerned about such matters.

It's a pattern, regrettably, that often lingers long into adulthood for women and may, in the most extreme cases, lead to such eating disorders as anorexia nervosa and bulimia. Yet men's overly casual attitudes about their weight, coupled with the way their extra pounds tend to settle in their chest and stomach, can result in serious health problems of their own, including heart disease, stroke and adult-onset diabetes.

Nutrition and the Nanny

Fat parents, fat kid, right?

That's all too frequently the case. And that's not too surprising, considering that a child shares both his parents' genes and their lifestyle. The big shockeroo is that a man's size can be affected by the baby-sitter he had when he was a kid.

In a study conducted at Boston's New England Medical Centers, director of clinical nutrition William E. Dietz, M.D., found that a man with two thin parents had only a 14 percent likelihood of becoming obese at any point in his adult life. A man whose folks are overweight, on the other hand, had an 80 to 85 percent chance of following in their footsteps.

Dr. Dietz also found that if a boy had thin parents but an overweight baby-sitter who took care of him for any substantial length of time, his chances of becoming overweight jumped to 65 percent.

The moral of the story? Genetics play a part in determining a man's risk of developing a weight problem, but what he learns as a boy about food and eating are highly influential as well.

"The media constantly give women the message that they should not be overweight," notes Eck.

Being an overweight woman in the 1990s is a no-no, plain and simple. Roseanne Arnold and especially Elizabeth Taylor—who went on and humiliatingly off the diet wagon in full public view—remain the butt of perpetual jokes, though we're much kinder to less-than-svelte male stars such as John Goodman and Willard Scott.

As a result, the typical overweight man can usually get away with thinking of himself as "solid" or "husky" or "portly," none of which sounds nearly as bad as "fat."

Real Men Don't Cook

The one who ruled the kitchen in the '50s—the woman—still does decades later. Sure, you'll see a male weekend pancake flipper or a summertime king of the barbecue grill, but the vast majority of meal planners and meal makers are women. And unless a wife is whipping up healthy, low-fat dishes for the family, a married man may not be eating the way he should. If he's single, he's even more likely to have poor eating habits.

A man who feels the pressure of work, family and other obligations may

The Right Choices

Eating on the run? Grabbing a quick snack? Just because you're moving fast is no excuse to drop your nutritional guard. Here's a few smart alternatives to all those high-calorie waist stealers.

Instead of . . .	Have . . .
Half a pepperoni pizza	2 slices of regular pizza with a big green salad
A bran or corn muffin	A bagel or English muffin
A handful of cashews	2 handfuls of popcorn
Fast-food chicken nuggets	A fast-food broiled chicken sandwich
Fettuccine Alfredo	Pasta with veggies in a light olive oil or tomato sauce
16 oz. of red meat	6 oz. of red meat (or better yet, turkey or fish) plus a large baked potato and steamed veggies

find himself grabbing coffee and doughnuts on the fly and a couple of slices of pizza instead of a healthier sit-down lunch. Or maybe he does sit down at noontime—to big, calorie-laden business lunches at fancy eateries, making it hard for him to stay trim. What's more, many men's jobs take them on the road, where fast food is the rule of the day. Being in the air isn't any better; airline food can be mediocre to bad, from both a taste and a caloric standpoint.

Equally unfortunate is the severe shortage of time for exercise in the harried man's schedule. Little wonder the waistband is starting to feel snug.

When the busy working guy finally does get a few minutes to himself, he often spends it in front of the TV set with a couple of beers, or after work with the guys, along with a bowlful of cashews and a few happy hour drinks.

Alcohol is one of the overweight man's greatest foes. Not only is it high in calories—around 100 to 150 per drink—but it also impairs judgment and weakens the resolve to do the right thing. So even if a man is planning to have a green salad with a touch of Italian dressing and broiled fish at the restaurant, a glass or two of wine or beer can lead to an oh-what-the-hell attitude: He lowers his guard and switches to the prime rib and a green salad drenched in blue-cheese dressing.

Moreover, alcohol in the system slows down the body's fat-busting process, so that whatever you do eat will be harder to burn off.

Real Men Don't Diet

For most men, *diet* is definitely a four-letter word. Going on a diet, whether that means toting up calories or grams of fat, weighing a fillet of sole on a food scale, or baring your soul in a weight-loss support group, is simply not considered a "guy" kind of thing to do.

Furthermore, "diet" invariably translates to "deprivation" in the male mind, and men generally do not take kindly to being told that they can't eat their usual favorites or hefty portions. So most overweight men would prefer to hang on to their extra pounds rather than do anything that seems as "un-masculine" (or that smacks of deprivation) as go on a diet.

Fortunately, there's also plenty of good news for the overweight man who finally decides to take the plunge and do something about his spare tire. Compared with women, guys have it made. Why? An overweight male can eat more food and still lose weight more quickly and easily than his female counterpart because a man:

- Is usually physically bigger.

- Has a higher percentage of muscle versus fat, which enables his body to burn more calories per pound of body weight.

- Will more often than not reach his goal weight . . . and stay there.

"Your Perfect Weight 52-Week Plan," on page 177, is designed to help everyone, female and male, achieve their weight-loss and fitness goals. However, overweight men—because their lifestyles and attitudes are often quite different from women's—can benefit from these additional tips from Dr. Shaevitz's Lean and Mean Program for Men.

DO learn a bit about nutrition. Ignorance is not bliss when it comes to your weight and your health. Bone up on the basics, such as what makes carbohydrates, proteins and fats different from one another, and a few examples of foods found in each category. Skimming this book is an excellent place to start.

DO recruit your family's help. If your wife is already on a diet plan and up until now she's been preparing separate (i.e., bigger, more-caloric) meals for you, ask her to begin serving you the same low-fat/low-calorie dishes she eats. She'll probably be thrilled to see you taking an interest in slimming down. Not surprisingly, it's been proven that men who follow their wife's lead in eating healthier meals have an easier time with their own weight loss. And if you can help with the cooking, so much the better—for your marriage and for your own education about nutrition.

What about the kids and their high-fat snacks you're trying so desperately to avoid? That's tougher, but a gentle request from you to not chomp on the Chee-tos in your presence just might do the trick. After all, your children will benefit by learning how to eat better. They'll want to see you slim and healthy, too.

DON'T let yourself feel deprived. One of the surest ways to lose your diet motivation is to put yourself on a weight-loss plan that makes you feel as though you're starving yourself or making some supreme dietary sacrifice. The reality is that to be successful in your weight-loss efforts, you can't continue to eat whatever and whenever you ate before—that's what got you overweight in the first place. But if you build into your weekly menu some of your favorites including, for instance, a small steak and dessert, you'll be far more likely to see your weight-loss program to completion and keep the weight off for good.

In addition, don't be fooled into thinking that losing weight necessarily means itsy-bitsy portions. With a few simple switches in what you're eating—from high-fat and sugar-packed items to healthier complex carbs (like potatoes and pasta) and low-fat protein sources (like shellfish and poultry) proteins—you can still eat hearty serving sizes that will leave you feeling satisfied.

DO go easy on the alcohol. No one's saying you have to lock up the liquor cabinet and throw away the key, but for the reasons previously stated it's a good idea to cut back on the alcohol as much as you can. Try drinking only half as much and half as often as you usually do. Swap regular beers for the light varieties. Switch from high-calorie mixed drinks to wine. Just making these few changes will produce a substantial calorie deficit, and you'll see the pleasant results on the bathroom scale.

DON'T let job obligations be an excuse to blow your diet. It's easy to say, "How can I possibly stay on a diet and go to all these conferences (translation: cheese Danish, bagels and cream cheese), cocktail parties (alcohol and hors d'oeuvres), business dinners (wine, steaks and rich desserts) and plane trips (nuts and high-calorie meals)?" Yet with a little forethought and planning, you can take care of your business and your body at the same time.

At breakfast conferences, for example, skip the sweet rolls and choose a bagel instead. At cocktail parties, work the room with a noncaloric drink in your hand, such as club soda with lime, and nibble on the crudités. At business meals, avoid alcohol and heavy desserts and focus on light salads (without creamy dressings); broiled or grilled fish, chicken or lean meats; and steamed or lightly sautéed veggies. For dessert, have sorbet or fresh fruit.

As for those notorious airline meals, which neither your waistline nor your taste buds will appreciate, special order a meal ahead of time (which will include mostly fruit or veggies and some protein, such as cheese) or bring your own healthy snack.

DO exercise regularly. Exercise is discussed at much greater length in "Exercise: Your Secret Weapon," on page 58. For now, just remember that sustained weight loss—for women and men—is virtually impossible without an ongoing exercise program, and that if you don't continue some regular aerobic workout (ideally supplemented with some resistance training), any weight you've lost will almost certainly return.

But start slow. Dr. Shaevitz has repeatedly found that out-of-shape men—unlike out-of-shape women—tend to plunge headfirst into a fitness program, attempting too much too soon. So before you do anything else, get your doctor's okay. Then, begin a brisk-walking program, starting with 20 to 25 minutes a day, three to five days a week. If 20 minutes is too much for you, start with less. The important point is to start. Eventually, you should increase your time until you're up to 45 minutes a day, about five days a week. You may also want to try slow jogging or a stationary bicycle.

Insist that you don't have time for exercise? Try what Dr. Shaevitz himself does: Over his home stationary bike he has a reading light and a magazine rack, with a telephone and a remote channel changer nearby. Nearly every morning he does 45 minutes on the bike while reading a couple of newsletters, watching a few minutes of the news on TV and checking in once or twice with his office by phone.

Another nice idea: family exercise time. Bike riding with your wife, playing basketball in the backyard with the kids or even taking a sports vacation—where you can all swim, horseback ride or rock climb together—will not only boost your own fitness level but will also reinforce your commitment to a healthier lifestyle for your family.

FOR WOMEN ONLY

There are two key times in a woman's life when weight gain is all too typical and may not involve overeating: after she's had a baby and when she enters menopause. Even if a woman has never had weight problems before, these special times and the extra pounds that may come with them often throw her into a tizzy. This is especially true for women who have never put on extra pounds before.

But while experts say putting on weight is common both for new moms and for women entering menopause, there are ways to deal with the changes going on. And if you put on more pounds than you should, there are ways to maintain a slim, healthy body.

Battling Postpregnancy Weight Gain

That brand-new baby of yours is a cutie, all right. But why, oh, why do you still feel nearly as big as you did when you were pregnant? Baby fat may be fine on a baby, but not on you. However, now that you're a new mom with an infant needing constant attention, you've hardly got the energy to even think about dieting. Luckily, you don't have to—not right away, anyway.

But first things first. Let's take a look at the weight you put on over the past nine months. "Nowadays it's considered okay to gain anywhere from 24 to 36 pounds during pregnancy, based on a woman's prepregnancy weight," says registered dietitian Joann Heslin, co-author of *The Pregnancy Nutrition Counter*. "If you start out fairly thin, then your weight gain should come in at the high end, and if you weigh more, you should still gain about 22 to 24 pounds."

Let's assume you hit those numbers, more or less. You leave the hospital, go home, hand the baby to your husband and collapse. Perhaps two or three days later, you'll get up the nerve to step on the scale. Well . . . you knew the news wouldn't be good, but it's not too bad, either: You're 10 to 20 pounds

---

Breast-Feeding Bonus

One of the nice things about breast-feeding—besides the way it lets you get close to your newborn—is that it may actually promote weight loss.

In one study done in Philadelphia, 24 new moms—some who breast-fed exclusively, some who fed their babies formula exclusively and some who did a combination of the two—were studied for six months after giving birth. Those women who breast-fed, even only part of the time, were closer to their prepregnancy weight and had lost many more inches from their hips compared with the mothers who fed their babies formula.

---

heavier than you were before you became pregnant. That weight consists primarily of your heavier uterus, which may have expanded from about 2 ounces in weight to as much as 24; extra breast tissue; extra blood, which might have increased by about 4 pounds; and maternal stores—anywhere from 8 to 11 pounds of fat and fluid your body accumulated during your pregnancy.

And while you're not thrilled that you can't zip your prepregnancy jeans right at this very moment, here's the best news of all: If you don't substantially increase your eating and if your activity level stays constant (and with a new baby at home, it's bound to), these extra 20-or-so pounds should drop off on their own within three to six months.

Don't Sabotage Yourself

However, warns Heslin, you can't afford to become complacent. "Sometimes a woman will become so depressed about being heavy—if she's about 13 pounds more than usual, then she's up one dress size. That's when the 'diet saboteurs' come out," she says. "I teach nutrition classes to pregnant women, and I try to alert them during their last trimester to be aware of the tendency to sabotage their ability to lose weight. Sometimes all you need is awareness."

Once you've had a baby, you're fully aware that your life is no longer the same. Even if you were fairly active before, you're going to be a lot more tired than usual, and when you are, you're going to want to sit down, not jog around the park.

"You may think you're physically active because you're getting up six times a night and doing four loads of laundry. But," says Heslin, "that's just fatigue, and, unfortunately, it doesn't burn the same number of calories as running for the commuter train or taking an aerobics class does."

Chances are you're going to be eating more, too. "Not necessarily because you're depressed—although you may be experiencing postpartum de-pression—but mainly because your life is topsy-turvy," says Heslin. "You're at home, and if you worked before, you may feel isolated. Also, if it's your first baby, you may feel unsure about dealing with it. So to help you get through it all you may reward yourself orally. If you're nursing the baby at 3:00 A.M., you just may find yourself reaching for a doughnut."

That's where the need for awareness comes in. If you must nibble at those times, make a better choice—a piece of fruit, for example, or a glass of skim milk. These snack attacks need not be damaging to your waistline.

What about your diet if you're breast-feeding? Eat the way you would if you were still pregnant, advises Heslin. The old recommendation that breast-feeding moms should take in as many as 2,500 to 2,800 calories daily is out of date; these days doctors recommend 2,000 to 2,100 healthy calo-ries. If before your pregnancy you were consuming two servings of low-fat milk, increase it now to three, and aim for about six ounces of protein daily. Like everyone else, try to keep your fat intake to about 30 percent, which will ensure that the remaining 70 percent will be loaded with healthy veg-gies, fruits, starches, low-fat dairy products and protein choices. (Naturally, you'll want to first check with your doctor, in case she recommends a dif-ferent diet and/or vitamin supplement for you.)

For mothers who are not breast-feeding, 1,800 healthful calories should be adequate for most women—pretty much what you'll get if you shoot for the lower serving sizes from the Food Guide Pyramid (see page 54) devised by the U.S. Department of Agriculture (USDA) in 1993.

You've Got to Keep On Moving

And don't forget exercise! We're not talking about running a mara-thon—you shouldn't be doing anything too vigorous for at least six weeks following your delivery. But if your doctor okays it, there's no reason you can't start a program of brisk walking as soon as 48 hours after having your baby. When you feel up to it, take your baby for an hourlong walk every day.

"Put her in the carriage and push it uphill, or strap her into a baby bike seat and pedal around the neighborhood," urges Heslin. "Work up a moderate sweat. Not only will it help you lose weight but you'll also be serving as a healthy role model for your child." If the pounds aren't coming off at a steady two to four pounds a month, she recommends that you increase the time you spend exercising rather than cutting back too much on your calories.

Firming exercises are important now, too. According to Marion Mc-Cartney, a certified nurse-midwife at Maternity Center Associates in Bethesda, Maryland, and co-author, with Antonia van der Meer, of *The Midwife's Pregnancy and Childbirth Book*, you can begin doing some simple floor exercises as early as the day after a vaginal delivery. (Check with your doctor if you've had a cesarean; you'll need to be much more careful.)

Start with stomach crunches: Lie on the floor, with the small of your back flat on the floor. Slowly bring your chin to chest, then slowly return your head to the floor. No matter what your workout routine may have been before your pregnancy, *go slowly*. Do one stomach crunch the first day, two the next, and so on. Continually asking yourself, "How am I feeling?" will help you pace yourself properly.

Above all, remember that having a baby is a terrific but draining experience, so be good to yourself. "Even if you're determined to lose weight now, this doesn't have to be a period of total deprivation," insists Heslin. "The act of motherhood automatically means some losses—lost sleep, maybe a lost job, lost social contacts. . . . You may even lose contact with your husband because you're so overwhelmed. Of course, the baby is wonderful, but you may still want something to make you feel good."

Often, that means something sweet—but that doesn't have to mean completely sabotaging your diet. So one day, have some frozen low-fat yogurt sprinkled with raisins. Suck on a piece of hard candy or a lollipop, or eat a few jelly beans. A few handfuls of presweetened breakfast cereal gives you a quick sugar-fix and is a lot less harmful to your weight-loss program than an almond-studded chocolate bar would be.

"Sometimes, after being a new mom for a while, you want to be a baby yourself," says Heslin. "So . . . baby yourself."

Don't Let Menopause Put On the Pounds

If you're on the verge of menopause—or have already reached that plateau—you've certainly observed some changes going on in your body and mind. On the plus side: no more worries about becoming pregnant and, as many women report, there's that feeling of finally being comfortable with who you are. The flip side of menopause? It often means a few unpleasant symptoms including hot flashes, fatigue, bouts of the blues—and extra pounds.

Not every woman gains weight as she goes through menopause, of course. "There are some women who actually lose weight after menopause," according to Lila Wallis, M.D., founder and first president of the National Council on Women's Health. "But predominantly you see weight gain—about five to eight pounds if you're not overweight to begin with, and more if you are." And this seems to be the case regardless of whether or not a woman is undergoing estrogen replacement therapy (ERT).

Dr. Wallis explains the reason for this weight gain as "simple arithmetic."

"Women tell me, 'I don't eat any more than I did before, but I'm gaining weight.' And I say, 'Right! You didn't increase your intake, but your caloric requirements have dropped.' As people age, they tend to expend less energy," explains Dr. Wallis. "And unless they decrease the number of calories they take in accordingly, they'll gain weight."

So, sound eating habits are more important than ever at this stage of your life. A low-fat, nutrient-rich diet is in order—and "Your Perfect Weight 52-Week Plan," on page 177, is a good place to start. Aim for a slow, steady, pound-or-so-a-week weight loss. Don't attempt to cut back on your calorie intake any further than that, because it may cause your metabolism to slow down even more and weight loss will be far more difficult.

Battling the Blues

Dr. Wallis warns women who are going through menopause to be particularly careful of not letting their moods rule their diet. "A lot of obsessive eating is due to depression," she points out. "Women without many interests may fixate on food and it may now become one of their only pleasures." Although ERT isn't for every woman, one of its advantages, she adds, is to help elevate mood, which could make sticking to a sensible diet easier.

Experts agree that keeping active is at least as important for a woman after she's gone through menopause as what she eats. Happily, as women get older they often turn to physical activity of their choice. And a *Prevention* magazine survey reveals that that's exactly what many women are doing. Of the 16,500 who responded to the questionnaire, a whopping 80 percent of women over 65 say they exercise at least three times a week, and 40 percent of them work out almost every day.

And if they can . . . you can. To help your body become a more efficient fat burner, develop a regular exercise plan, if you haven't already. Stick to your favorite activities, whether that means swimming, biking, fast-walking or dancing, and do them as many days a week as possible. Not only will it help you shed pounds but it will also strengthen your bones and boost your adrenal glands' production of estrogen precursor. What's more, the lift you'll get from your workouts may ease some of your symptoms, such as the hot flashes and "the blues." "Exercise is a great antidepressant," says Dr. Wallis. "It makes you feel better immediately, as well as later on."

The best prescription of all for losing weight and staying slim forever? "Keep moving!" urges Dr. Wallis. "Don't just sit frozen in place, walk around! Not just when you're going somewhere, but also when you're watching TV, when you're planning something, when you're thinking. You think better when you walk anyway. And don't walk as if you're made of porcelain—use your arms, twist your torso, look around. You expend more energy by being alert and active."

And if you're alert, active, full of energy—and thin!—your age will be the last thing on your mind.

HIS/HER GUIDE TO WEIGHT LOSS

Launching a weight-loss program with your spouse sounds so promising at the outset. But a few weeks later, you find yourself wondering why it isn't working for either of you. It could be because you're both going against your gender's built-in grain.

Research is beginning to show that what switches off her appetite might be a turn-on for his. Or what sends her straight to the gym might leave him sitting on the couch. When it comes to food and fitness, each gender has its own preferences and behaviors. And the point is, if you wouldn't wear your spouse's Levi's, why try to fit into his or her weight-loss plan?

Once you know where your own gender's best fat-fighting potential is, you can use it to tailor a weight-loss program that works for you. So here's a rundown of some of the most important (and surprising) his/her differences and how you can turn them to your advantage.

He Likes It Flaming
She Likes It Reliable

When it comes to food, men like it hot. In one study, spicy foods—hot peppers in particular—rated high on the list of tastes men prefer. Researchers think this may be more about sensation-seeking than it is about biology.

For women, it's healthy foods that score high. Among the favorites: yogurt, vegetables and fruits. Experts can't say for sure whether women love these tastes or just tend to love what's good for them. Either way, fostering this food preference puts you a step ahead when it comes to losing weight.

His strategy: Say *sí* to salsa. This spicy convergence of tomatoes, hot peppers, cilantro, garlic, onion and other savory tastes adds zest to a meal without adding fat. Use it everywhere, especially where you used to load up on cheese, sour cream or other high-fat condiments, advises Morton H. Shaevitz, Ph.D., and author of *Lean and Mean: The No Hassle, Life-Extending Weight Loss Program for Men.*

Get creative about using salsa as an ingredient or topping. Put it on a baked potato or in omelets. Use it as a marinade for chicken or as a salad dressing. Just open a jar and pour it on—most packaged salsas contain little or no fat (although you'll want to check the label to be sure).

If salsa isn't your style, there are other hot and flavorful options, says Dr. Shaevitz. "Mushrooms, onions, green peppers, vinegar and mustards are good ways to give food excitement without calories."

Her strategy: Go wild with a good thing. While he's firing up his potato with hot peppers, rely on your more subtle favorites to spruce up yours. Try topping potatoes with nonfat or low-fat yogurt and vegetables. And take those veggies out of the ho-hum by cooking them in some chicken broth or by sautéing them with a little garlic and a bit of onion.

Capitalize on your taste for fruit by bringing it into the main course. Registered dietitian and American Dietetic Association spokesperson Evelyn Tribole, author of *Eating on the Run*, recommends a family favorite: fruit pizza. She creates hers on a homemade, low-fat, whole-wheat pastry crust, but any low-fat crust will do, she says. It's only three steps to the finish from there: Mix fat-free cream cheese with nonfat or low-fat ricotta, and spread that over the baked crust. Add kiwi or other fruits—peaches, berries or other seasonal favorites—as if they were pepperoni. Zap some marmalade in the microwave and brush it on top with a pastry brush and eat.

His Mirror Says Arnold Schwarzenegger
Hers Says Fat Lady at the Circus

He looks into the mirror and sees burly and strong. She looks in and sees her hips stretched out to the size of Nebraska.

What it's about is body image, and surveys show that high numbers of Americans are turning their reflections into fun-house mirror distortions. The problem is, basing a weight-loss program on what you think you should look like or weigh undoes the efforts of both genders.

Many overweight men think they look fine. In fact, 40 percent of overweight men "felt at about the right weight," according to one *Prevention Index*, a survey of the nation's health. Others may weigh in on target according to the height and weight charts, but they have potbellies and no buns. Either way, what looks healthy from the outside might not be so on the inside—their heft may be heightening their risk for heart disease.

On the female side of the chart, the desire to be superslim may lead her to aim for a body weight far below what she's genetically programmed to be. Look at the facts: According to *Prevention's* Healthy Women Survey, 73 percent of the women who responded felt they needed to lose pounds to achieve a healthy body weight. Yet only 44 percent of the surveyed women were actually overweight.

Both genders can avoid spinning the wheels of their diet plan by turning away from an *ideal* weight and setting their sights on a *healthy* one.

His/Her strategy: Change your thinking. Don't let your weight determine your behavior. Let healthy habits determine your weight. That is, take your focus off what you believe your body should weigh and learn what's healthy for it to weigh.

"We don't think that everybody should be the same height. There's no biological reason that everybody should line up in a row and be the same weight. It's just not the way biology works," says diet expert C. Wayne Callaway, M.D., associate clinical professor of medicine at George Washington University Medical Center in Washington, D.C., and a member of the Dietary Guidelines Advisory Committee to the USDA and the Department of Health and Human Services. Some men can be perfectly healthy at 210 pounds, while others will be metabolically obese at 180 because their cholesterol levels will be way out of balance, with triglycerides climbing and HDL levels plummeting (HDL is the good kind of cholesterol). It all depends on what your body's made to handle.

To determine what's healthy for you, set a new standard by looking inside. First, check your health statistics. According to the National Institutes of Health's National High Blood Pressure Education Program, you should make sure your cholesterol is under 200, your blood pressure is under 140/90 and your blood sugar levels are normal.

Next, look at fitness or performance. Can you do what you need to do and feel good? You don't have to be able to do everything your 22-year-old aerobics teacher does. But you should be able to walk briskly without being short of breath and be able to talk at the same time.

Finally, ask your doctor if your current weight will put you at risk for obesity-related diseases in the future.

If your inner health isn't where it should be, work with your doctor, registered dietitian or exercise physiologist to establish smart eating and exercise behaviors that will get you healthy and keep you there. When you do that, you might find yourself at a lower (or higher!) weight than you thought was ideal. If you feel good, you move well and your health is on target, why let the number on the scale determine what you do or how you feel about yourself?

His Gut Wants to Gain It
Her Hips Want to Hold It

Why is it that he can get a potbelly and lose it in no time, while her fat seems to settle on her hips and thighs for the duration, even though she's losing weight?

In a word, estrogen. Women have a greater number of fat cells on the hips and thighs than do men, and it's part of estrogen's job to take fat there and keep it there. In fact, the average female body wants 120,000 calories stored up as fat so it can deliver the next generation, even in a famine.

Guys, on the other hand, get fat in the belly first because, some experts believe, the fat cells there are more metabolically active. Bellies gain weight quickly, but give it up quickly, too. As short-term energy stores, they were especially handy in hunter/gatherer days when quick access to body fuel got you safely out of the reach of what might have been hunting you.

If you're thinking that belly fat is the kind to have, think again. Big bellies can swell your risks for numerous diseases. "So far, nearly everything that's been studied that's associated with obesity—heart disease, stroke, diabetes and high blood pressure—has to do more with belly fat than hip and thigh fat," says Dr. Callaway.

Doctors determine risk with what they call the waist-to-hip ratio (WHR). The higher the ratio, the greater the risk. That puts men with "spare tires" at higher risk than so-called pear-shaped women. Women who are naturally "apple-shaped," or women past the age of menopause whose fat has redistributed farther north, fall in between.

Both genders can burn this excess fat with aerobic exercise. While you can't spot reduce, you can choose exercises that tone your trouble spots, making them appear trimmer once the weight is gone.

His strategy: Smoothing your stomach is a threefold process. First, cut down on what's building it up. Research shows that the gut grabs fat when you drink alcohol, smoke or are under stress.

Second, reduce what's already there with aerobic exercise. You'll need at least 20 to 30 minutes of continuous aerobic exercise three times per week to get things moving. Remember that you not only have to exercise enough to release fat into the bloodstream but also have to keep going long enough to burn it.

Third, put the crunch on it. Abdominal crunches, or sit-ups, won't do much to burn off fat. But they will tone the area so it looks tighter and firmer when the fat is gone.

Her strategy: Aerobic exercise is your best bet for fighting fat, too. Make your workout time do double duty by choosing fat-burning exercises that also tone your trouble spots. Walking, jogging, stair climbers and cross-country ski machines are good ways to get the large muscles in the legs and hips in shape so they'll look tighter and slimmer when the fat is gone. To give those areas even more tone, ask the gym fitness instructor to show you how to use the leg machine that works both the inside and outside muscles in your legs.

Finally, stay tuned to subtle changes. While his gut seems to be just dropping off, keep in mind that you lose weight more uniformly, so your body gets smaller without changing shape dramatically.

He Loses 20 Pounds
She Loses 15

Over the same amount of time and with the same amount of physical activity, he can actually lose more pounds than she can, says George Blackburn, M.D., chief of the Nutrition/Metabolism Laboratory at New England Deaconess Hospital in Boston. As he puts it, "The man would be a V8 engine and the woman a V6."

Men burn calories faster for two reasons: First, they're usually heavier to begin with and are burning more calories all the time. (It takes more energy to carry 200 pounds one step than it does to carry 150 pounds the same distance.) Second, guys have a greater proportion of fat-burning muscle, or fat-free mass, than women do. Healthy young men have about 12 to 19 percent body fat; older men have about 15 to 22 percent. Women, on the other hand, have between 19 and 26 percent when they're younger, which rises to 22 to 30 percent in older women.

His strategy: Don't get smug. When you compare percentages, not pounds, you'll see that you're making the same relative weight reduction as she is. If you weigh 200 pounds and lose 20, you're losing 10 percent of your body weight. If she's 150 and loses 15, she's done the same thing. Don't let too much ride on the initial quick drop, says Dr. Callaway. Men tend to feel really great when the numbers are dropping, but when things level off, in comes boredom. Once the challenge is gone, you'll return to your old way of eating and put the pounds right back on. Here again, instead of focusing on the numbers, focus on how you feel.

Her strategy: Nowhere is patience more a virtue than in weight loss. Not only do you burn calories more slowly because you're smaller, you may also have slowed down because you've tried to lose weight before—28 percent of you started doing it seriously at age 17 or younger.

"There's some evidence that the more you diet, the better you get at starvation," says Dr. Callaway. When frequent dieters cut their intake, their bodies prepare for starvation. Cells may clutch hard to the energy already in them and gobble up more when they get it. That makes it tougher to lose weight and easier to gain it back. You can break the cycle, however, with realistic weight-loss expectations of a half pound to one pound per week.

To avoid feeling discouraged, don't compare the numbers on your scale with his. If you have to compare, use percent reductions.

He Craves Meat
She Craves Sweets

Wouldn't it be great if when a craving hit, it was for apples or carrots? No such luck. Two recent studies, one on obese men and women, another on normal-weight people, suggest that men favor or crave meats and cheeses, and women prefer sweets and desserts—all fats, fats, fats.

Researchers can't yet pinpoint whether cravings are about texture, taste or emotions, says cravings expert Marcia Pelchat, Ph.D., research scientist at Monell Chemical Senses Center, in Philadelphia. Past studies don't definitely show whether substituting low-fat or nonfat versions for your favorite high-fat foods will keep your weight down, but it's certainly worth a try. By knowing where your weaknesses are, you can plan substitutions that may put your fat intake at the right level. Letting it settle at about 25 percent of your total calorie intake will help you avoid eating fats your body can't use (and fats it sticks into storage). It can also put a hold on heart disease by reducing high serum cholesterol.

His strategy: First, switch to ground turkey or chicken breast instead of beef, and you'll find big fat savings. In a three-ounce serving, ground turkey has about 8 grams of fat. Ground beef has about 13.

Then, slice the portion size. "Most recipes tell you to use one pound of meat. There's nothing magic about one pound. You can usually cut that down without missing it," says nutritionist Tribole. In any case, trim off the fat—one study shows that men are less likely than women to trim the visible fat from their meat, but it only takes a second to do.

Her strategy: Studies show that when premenstrual syndrome hits, so does a craving for chocolate. Your best defense is to decide ahead of time what to do about it, advises Thomas A. Wadden, Ph.D., director of the weight and eating disorders program at the University of Pennsylvania in Philadelphia.

You can decide to allow yourself a certain amount on the two or three days you're particularly craving it. Or if portions are difficult, remove chocolate from your house and just go out for a treat when you want it, he says.

By the way, the second biggest fat trap in the female diet is salad dressing. Although women haven't been shown to crave it, they definitely eat it. Studies show that women with the highest fat intakes ate regular salad dressing in larger portions and more frequently than did women with lowest fat intakes.

Try nonfat bottled dressings or make your own low-fat ones. Puree favorite ingredients such as mustard, garlic, Worcestershire sauce and minced, sun-dried tomatoes into nonfat cottage cheese or plain, nonfat yogurt. Tracy Ritter, chef-owner of Stamina Cuisine, in San Diego, recommends a vegetable-based dressing made of steamed carrots. Simply puree them with defatted chicken stock and rice-wine vinegar. Some fresh ginger, lemon juice and a sprinkle of hot-pepper sauce finishes it off with zest.

He Gains Weight with Friends
She Gains It Alone

For both sexes, who's at the table may be just as important as what's on it. Dr. Shaevitz has observed that men do most of their overeating in social situations; women do it in private. Whether they're around other men or just Mom, men get encouraged to eat a lot—a "lumberjack appetite" can be a desirable male trait.

Women, in contrast, may eat less in public to appear more feminine, says Dr. Shaevitz. That works to their favor when they're out, but what they do at home is another story.

"Women are so busy taking care of other people that the one thing they do to 'care for themselves' is eat something that tastes good," says Dr. Wadden. In fact, women are nearly twice as likely as men to eat a special dessert to indulge themselves. When women are around food all day or are too busy to sit down and eat, it's easy to pick up too many calories.

"The psychology there is that if you're not sitting down, it doesn't count," says Dr. Wadden. "Unfortunately, it does."

His strategy: Keep talking. "View the evening as a social event with food present, rather than an eating event with people present," says Dr. Shaevitz. Make your focus the people, not the food, and you'll find that you can keep both your weight-loss plan and your social life intact. Chances are, people will remember how charming you were, not how much you ate.

If, however, you're in a situation where there's extreme pressure to eat a lot, fill your plate high. Just substitute less-calorie-dense foods for the standard fare. Beef up a meal, so to speak, with two baked potatoes, lots of vegetables or extra bread.

If lunches out lead healthy eating astray, find a standard meal that's 500 to 700 calories. Men have to avoid having a dinner meal at lunch and then again in the evening, says Dr. Wadden. Good lunch options include a good-size salad with turkey or chicken in it, or a turkey sandwich that's easy on the mayo.

Her strategy: Give priority to yourself. Then make yourself dinner.

When your schedule is tight, don't try to find time for yourself. Make it. Getting out of the kitchen will pick you up better than a hot fudge sundae will. "If you can get 15 minutes to do something for yourself, whether that's going for a walk in the evening, reading a book for a few minutes or watching a show on television, that's more helpful than just eating," says Dr. Wadden. Plus, you won't feel bad about it later.

When you do need to be around food—if you're preparing it for the family—remember that a bite here and there can soon hit heavy below the belt. Stock the kitchen in your favor by keeping good foods in clear containers and fat-filled snacks in opaque, hard-to-reach ones.

Decrease your temptation to snack when the kids do by feeding them ready-made snacks or ones in single-serving packages. Contribute what's left to Mother Nature. You can't feel guilty about tossing leftovers when they help out the compost heap.

He Exercises to Get Bigger
She Exercises to Get Smaller

Both of you know that exercise is essential in any weight-loss program. To get it, it's natural for him to head to the weight room and her to take up aerobics, says Dr. Shaevitz. That's a good start, but you're both missing weight-loss opportunities unless you reach to the other's side of the gym.

His strategy: Add aerobics. This not only melts fat but also helps stave off cardiovascular disease in the process. According to the American Heart Association, being sedentary has as negative an effect on your heart's health as high blood cholesterol, high blood pressure or smoking.

Aerobics doesn't mean wearing a cute little outfit and going to class three times a week. It means getting out and moving. In a study of more than 18,000 people trying to lose weight, walking was the number-one favorite way to get physical activity. Walkers over the age of 40 also weighed less than the people trying to lose weight who reported no activity. For exercise, start with one-half mile and try to increase the distance by a half mile each week.

Make walking a way of life, says Loretta DiPietro, Ph.D., epidemiologist and assistant fellow at the John B. Pierce Laboratory at Yale University School of Medicine. "If you're going to drive, park your car a little farther away and walk to your destination. If you take mass transportation, get off a little sooner and walk two or three stops. Take the stairs rather than the elevator. If you have to start by taking them down, then take them down and the elevator up. People ask, 'What difference is that going to make?' But think about the cumulative effect. If I deposit $5 a week in my checking account, over time, it adds up."

Her strategy: Borrow his barbells. When those 18,000 dieters were questioned about their exercise programs, weight training wasn't mentioned as a strategy for weight loss. If weights aren't part of your workout, you're missing an important way to boost your fat-burning ability. The more muscle you have, potentially the more fat you burn—even when you're not at the gym.

Three days a week is all it takes to bump up your metabolic rate, your strength and your percentage of muscle (called lean-body mass). An added bonus is that weight-bearing exercise may help ward off osteoporosis, too.

"A woman can make phenomenal gains in strength with very little change in the overall size of her muscle," explains Sydney Lou Bonnick, M.D., research professor at the Center for Research on Women's Health at Texas Women's University in Denton, Texas. Dr. Bonnick has designed exercise programs especially for women at the clinic. "So if she's worrying about her appearance as a result of strength training, she should know that what you tend to see is a decrease in the size of her hips and thighs. The amount of fat goes down and cancels out the increase in the size of the muscle. So she really doesn't get bigger, but she does look better."

Women who have moved into the weight-training arena tend to stick with it, says Dr. Bonnick. "When they realize how good they feel and how much better they look, you can't get them out of the gym."

He Likes a Solo Win
She Prefers Teamwork

"Men approach weight loss almost like a competitive sport," says Dr. Wadden. "When you say that group A of dieters is going to compete against group B, you'll always find that the men in group A take on group B as fiercely as they can."

Women, on the other hand, help pull each other toward the finish line. One woman can be another's personal cheerleader, support system and healthy-recipe file all in one. "Women enjoy discussing their feelings about food, about difficulties they're having controlling their eating, and they're more likely to share helpful comments," he says.

His strategy: Make a bet. Capitalize on your competitive nature by setting a weight-loss goal with a friend. Then check in with each other every week.

Your best bet is one that encourages healthy eating habits. See who can stick to a challenge of the week, such as cutting down on fat intake or pruning the number of sugared sodas consumed in a day. That way, you're banking on healthy new habits, and you won't fall prey to "lose-it-fast" behaviors that can get you to your goal but can't keep you there.

"In order to lose a half pound a week, it's best if you can do it by changing your behaviors over time," adds Dr. Callaway. There's some evidence that if you lose weight slowly, your metabolic rate doesn't decline in order to conserve energy. As a result, you don't set up the biological signals for bingeing that occur when you starve and refeed.

Her strategy: Find a buddy. Set aside time to trade strategies, recipes and food-preparation tips. Better yet, share what works while you're out for a walk. Capitalize on your cooperative nature by cooking together. Or use teamwork to find the lowest-fat food selections at the grocery store. Or trade shopping lists if impulse buys are your downfall.

KEEPING YOUR KIDS SLIM

You're concerned about your weight, and you're pretty careful about what you eat, avoiding high-fat fare as much as you can. You even try to work in an hour or so of walking every other day. But you may be forgetting something.

Your kids.

You know, those small creatures with insatiable appetites for sugar, salt and Nintendo. Right now they're just tater tots, but they might slowly be turning into couch potatoes, not only getting chubby but also piling up all the heart disease risk factors associated with the sedentary lifestyle you're trying so hard to avoid. Of course, it's not all their fault—or yours. Plenty of factors are contributing to the fattening of America's youth.

- Physical education has all but disappeared in high schools.

- Kids are less inclined to walk or ride bikes to school, even if they live just blocks away.

- Television has become the electronic opiate of the teenage masses, with kids infusing 15 to 25 hours of TV and video games into their heads each week.

- The family dinner table has been replaced by the drive-through window, with "You want fries with that?" becoming the toughest culinary decision.

So it's no surprise that kids are fatter than ever. In fact, a study found that children weighed an average of 11.4 pounds more in 1988 than in 1973, even though they were eating the same number of calories and less fat. Ten-year-olds jumped from 75 pounds to 86 pounds, without getting any taller! And, sadly, it doesn't look as though the situation's likely to improve any time soon.

"We're churning out unhealthy kids, who may tragically become unhealthy adults," agrees fitness guru Kenneth Cooper, M.D., president of the Cooper Aerobics Center in Dallas and author of *Kid Fitness*. "We're already finding higher blood pressures and evidence of premature coronary heart disease among the young right now."

That news may sound alarming, especially if your kids are already overweight and underactive. But you can fight the trend. You can help get your kids—whether they're tots, teens or somewhere in between—on the road to a slim body and a healthy lifestyle they can follow for life.

Eating Slim, Kid-Style

While you can't control what your kids eat when they're at the mall, away on trips or at a movie with their friends, you can—and should—take command at home. You can turn your house into a healthy sanctuary from all the greasy fast-food and sugar-packed snacks that assault your child away from home. Here's how to offer kids maximum nutrition to help them grow up but not out while they're under your roof.

Shop smart. Improving your child's eating patterns means getting the upper hand at the supermarket. Studies show that more and more children are responsible for making food purchases and preparations, with less parental supervision. And that presents problems. The key: selecting, and helping them select, the right foods to fill the fridge and the cupboards.

Give kids choices . . . within reason. "Parents should be in charge of what children are offered, and then children should be in charge of what they choose to eat from what's being offered," says William E. Dietz, M.D., Ph.D., pediatrician at the New England Medical Center in Boston. Then you don't have to infringe on your children's sense of independence, which will only cause them to rebel when they're away from you.

Secure the snacks. Make sure there are plenty of healthy no- and low-fat snacks on hand. Sliced fruits, vegetables, unsalted air-popped popcorn and nonfat fruited yogurt can be given easy access. The sports bars athletes use as low-fat, high-carbohydrate boosters can be cut up into smaller portions and used as snacks as well. They come in chocolate and other tasty flavors.

Be a role model. If you want children to eat healthy and slim down, you'd better be prepared to toe the line yourself. "A parent who sits on the couch and asks her child to get her a bowl of cheese dip and then expects him to eat fruit had better think twice," says Ronald Kleinman, M.D.,

The Pudgy Problem

There's nothing worse for an overweight child than hearing the coach or gym teacher yell, "Scrimmage! Shirts on one side, skins on the other!" If it's tough to get kids involved in exercise, it's even tougher for those with a weight problem. "Overweight children are often not accepted by their peers and become wallflowers, participating in even less activity," says Kenneth Cooper, M.D., president of the Cooper Aerobics Center in Dallas and author of *Kid Fitness*. "Some just get embarrassed to death."

Luckily, there are many neighborhood fitness programs geared specifically for overweight boys and girls. Some, like those found at local YMCAs, are free, and others may cost you, but even so, insists Dr. Cooper, "It's worth it." For instance, Shapedown helps overweight young people ages 6 to 20. It promotes safe short- and long-term weight loss, improving self-esteem and increasing knowledge of nutrition, exercise physiology and weight-management principles. It's offered by hundreds of hospitals, HMOs, medical centers, private practitioners, clinics and health departments across the country.

Another program, the Body Shop, is distributed by the American Institute for Preventive Medicine and is available at approximately 100 hospitals throughout the United States. A ten-week program for kids that focuses on diet, exercise, weight loss and self-esteem, the Body Shop also offers a support group for their parents.

chairman of the American Academy of Pediatrics Committee on Nutrition and chief of pediatric gastroenterology and nutrition at Massachusetts General Hospital. "But if you stock your house with healthy foods and your child sees you eating them, there's a good chance he'll eat them, too."

Learn from the enemy. "Look at commercials to see what kids are being told to eat or what's fun to eat, and interlace those items with foods they should be eating for better health," suggests Liz Applegate, Ph.D., a nutritionist from the University of California, Davis, author of *Power Foods* and mother of two growing kids. If you completely cut your kids off from the popular stuff, they'll go wild on junk food the minute they're old enough and have a little change in their pockets.

But be careful: Don't confuse your children by using sugar and fatty items as treats and then turn around and tell them how bad those foods are. "Integrating these foods into a healthy diet shows kids that they can have a little of them, but in a controlled, responsible manner," says Dr. Applegate.

Pay attention to breakfast. One way to keep a kid from snacking too much on the wrong things is by serving him a good breakfast. Filling him up with wholesome cereals and breads that have little fat and are no sweat to prepare can make your child less likely to pig out the rest of the day. What's more, getting him into the breakfast-eating habit early in life means he won't have to learn it when he's 40—after the cardiologist orders him to.

And you needn't serve your children the usual bowl of boring old bran flakes. Says Dr. Applegate, "I let my kids have both kinds of cereals—the sugary kind and the high-fiber kind. We pull out five boxes and mix them up." That interesting blend may keep 'em coming to the breakfast table instead of gobbling down a candy bar on the bus.

Dress up a waffle. "I put light whipped cream on low-fat frozen waffles, and my children think it's a sundae," says Dr. Applegate. "I'll toss strawberries on it so it fools them into eating their fruit. If you separate the foods out, they're less likely to eat them. I make a face on the waffle, using whipped cream as hair and strawberries as eyeballs. It's an exciting way to provide variety using things they will eat."

Slim by skimming. Start reducing the fat in your child's diet by weaning her off whole milk after age two. You can start by dropping down a notch—to 2 percent, then 1 percent, then onto skim.

"By substituting skim milk for whole, you're cutting out eight grams of fat per glass," says Dr. Cooper. "And you're actually giving your kids more calcium, too—302 milligrams per eight-ounce glass, compared with 291 milligrams from whole milk." And don't worry if your child craves chocolate milk, it doesn't add to her fat intake, though it does add sugar. "If your child isn't eating a high-sugar diet, chocolate milk is fine," says Dr. Applegate. "It may get a child who hates milk to drink it."

Freeze to please. Sure, fruits are cool and colorful, but to most children they're borrr-ing. So turn them into kid-pleasing desserts by chucking them into the freezer. Grapes, when frozen, are transformed into fun-to-eat mini ice pops, loaded with juice. Frozen bananas, strawberries, watermelon and cantaloupe are other great choices. Just cut the fruit into pieces, spread them on a flat pan and put them in the freezer for an hour. When frozen, pop the pieces into plastic bags, where they'll be ready when the snackers ambush the fridge.

How to Make a Brown Bag Appealing

Pity the typical brown-bag lunch. Most kids empty the contents, trade what they don't want and toss the rest. You can help prevent this pattern by making healthy, low-cal lunches with plenty of kid appeal. Here's how.

Pick fruit first. Pack apples, bananas, peaches, melon chunks—whatever your children like best. Fruits that have excessive juice can be packed in a plastic container. Even kids who don't generally like fruit will probably eat boxed raisins and dried fruits.

Skip the sandwiches. Baked or broiled chicken pieces, low-fat soup in a Thermos bottle, turkey slices or cubes of low-fat cheese are other appetizing alternatives.

Counter that snack attack. Include a container of low- or nonfat yogurt or fat-free pudding, a homemade low-fat muffin or some fat-free potato chips to help kids steer clear of fattening, commercial snack items.

Block that punch. Avoid packing punch or fruit beverages, which are little more than colored water and sugar. Instead, serve natural, 100 percent fruit juices.

"I'm not a firm believer in the typical lunch consisting of a sandwich, a piece of fruit and a drink," says Dr. Applegate. "Kids like to nibble. They eat one thing, put it down, blab to a friend and pick up something else." The more items the better, she says, but with much smaller serving sizes. "I give my daughter fresh-cut vegetables, caramel-flavored rice cakes, dried fruit, a sports drink (milk in a Thermos is usually not touched—it's boring), maybe a quarter of a sandwich and a slice of nonfat process cheese. She eats everything instead of trading away the big three lunch items and scarfing dessert."

Dancing the Fast-Food Shuffle

You don't have to blow the diet—yours or the kids'—just because you're at a fast-food restaurant. "They may be tugging at you, telling you what they want, but *they* aren't ordering. You still have control," says Dr. Applegate. Here are a few things you can do to keep down the fat and calories when the kids insist on a fast-food meal.

Try a little take-in. "We go with a bag of crunchy vegetables like cucumber slices," says Dr. Applegate. "While we wait in line for our burgers we munch on the veggies. I also bring sports bars—they're lifesavers. Kids treat them like candy bars, and they're a great way to avoid the fatty stuff that's out there."

Look for lower-fat items. If the kids are craving a cool, sweet dessert, fear not: The low-fat frozen yogurt cones are often the lowest-fat items on the fast-food menu. Low-fat milk is also available. And order the basic burger—"The cheapest one almost always ends up being lower in fat," says Dr. Applegate.

Share and share alike. "It's very difficult to go into a place with all the smells and see everyone else eat and say, 'We're here but we can't have that.' It doesn't make sense to kids," says Dr. Applegate. "So we'll divvy up our food, such as french fries, to reduce the amount of fat we're all getting. And we'll pass around the low-fat shake, taking turns sipping."

Overcoming the Yuck Factor

You know eating more veggies is a key to losing weight and keeping it off. But try telling that to a kid who thinks the four food groups are burgers, fries, soda and desserts.

Leave it to a pro football athletic trainer to figure out how to do it. Dean Kleinschmidt, president of the Professional Athletic Trainers Society and head athletic trainer for the New Orleans Saints professional football team, has found the trick to getting his kids to not just eat their vegetables but actually *love* them. He brings on the veggies as soon as possible, while the children are still open to new tastes. He also sets a good example.

"For the past ten years, the focus at home has been on having more vegetables," he says. "I have a ten-year-old son, and from the time he was three his favorite meal has been fettuccine and broccoli. Our two-year-old daughter is also into vegetables."

Is Kleinschmidt trying to raise a generation of vegetarians? No way, he insists. "We serve grilled chicken and veal and even pork sometimes," he says. "But these kids eat vegetables and grains and *like* them, and it's because we started them early."

Don't Forget the Physical Fix

The scientific evidence is in: Kids don't need strenuous exercise to be thin and gain important health benefits. They do need to exercise, however.

The basic prescription is simple. To maintain fitness, children and teens should set aside three 30-minute periods per week for some kind of sustained aerobic activity—walking, jogging, dancing, cycling or any continuous activity they find fun. "If they're already involved in a vigorous school sport like basketball, gymnastics or soccer, you can drop that down to 20-minute periods," says Dr. Cooper. The key is to have your children identify an activity they enjoy and encourage them to do it as often as they can.

Whether your kid is now fairly active or whether he's already showing signs of turning into a BarcaLounger-and-beer aficionado, you can help him get fit and stay slim at every stage of his development. Here, according to Dr. Cooper, is what kind of exercise your child may need at each age.

Birth to 2 years: This isn't a critical time for maintaining or improving fitness. Kids are highly active on their own (just ask any new mom!) and don't need any extra exercise. For now, stacking toys or blocks, rolling and retrieving objects, playing games and crowd-pleasing attempts at walking are all these energetic tots normally need to do.

2 to 5 years: Here's a time when you can join in and help develop certain skills involving hand-and-eye coordination. Teach your child to kick, throw, catch or bat a ball. These skills do more than provide the groundwork for other abilities they'll develop later—they're also fun.

5 to 8 years: Start encouraging your child to exercise aerobically with walking, playing soccer and basketball with friends, or other playground sports. Group play and even some milder team sports are possible options. "Getting your children involved with other kids helps keep exercise fun and can prevent them from losing interest later in life," says Dr. Cooper.

8 to 10 years: Now kids can get more actively involved in more vigorous activities. Let them investigate all sorts of sports and games to find out which one suits them. Tennis, bowling, volleyball and soccer are all popular, fun, low-risk activities available at most neighborhood youth centers. "At this time some children may find team sports attractive, while others may not," says Dr. Cooper. "All kids are different. But if they do get involved, allow them to choose what they want to do and play down the competitiveness, which can turn them off."

10 to 14 years: Here's where the adolescent slump can rear its lazy head, with the tendency to turn slothful reaching its peak. It's especially important now to provide the support and enthusiasm needed to help your child stay interested in exercise.

14 to 17 years: "If you haven't gotten your kids used to a regular pattern of exercise by this time, it'll be a real uphill struggle," warns Dr. Cooper. Since most older teens have already reached their growth potential, you can help encourage a strength-training program—for both boys and girls—by purchasing a basic weight set. Weight training may appeal to older teens by creating tangible physical rewards (muscles get bigger) that offer psychological benefits. Weight training also helps avoid the competitive pressures of team sports that alienate those who aren't as skilled as others. If your child does take a shine to strength training, make sure there's always strict supervision by a knowledgeable adult.

Keeping Motivation Going

Tell a kid, "Get plenty of exercise," and chances are the response you'll hear will fall somewhere between a groan and mocking laughter. Forget lip service—the key is motivation. Here are a few strategies to keep exercise fun and continually interesting for your child—and you.

Let the kid take charge. Exercise imposed from above will be deep-sixed in no time. Let your child freely choose her activities. Encourage her

Building a Better Body Image

Can a teenager feel better about her body and maybe even avoid developing an eating disorder via regular exercise? Medical research suggests the answer is a definite yes.

In a report presented at the American College of Sports Medicine, researchers looked at girls ages 13 to 17 who participated in a school athletic program. They were found to be more satisfied with their bodies, their overall appearance and their level of fitness when compared with a similar group of girls who didn't participate at all. More important, these active girls were less preoccupied with their weight compared with the other girls.

Although the researchers didn't look specifically at the incidence of eating disorders such as anorexia or bulimia among the study subjects, the results strongly suggest that regular exercise may be one active, powerful way to offset negative feelings, the kinds of feelings that may lead girls to dangerous eating habits.

to select the kind she likes, not necessarily the activity you excelled in when you were her age.

Make it an event. Have at least one fun fitness outing—a hike or bike ride, for example—scheduled for the weekend. That way exercise becomes less of a chore and instead becomes something fun the kids can look forward to.

Get peers involved. Organize weekend or after-school events that get your child's friends and classmates into the act with ice-skating outings, touch football or Frisbee.

Set a good example. Research has established that a parent's actual involvement in his own sport or exercise has a positive effect on the kids. (Call it the trickle-down theory of fitness.) Think about it: How can you ask your kids to keep in shape and cut down on TV watching while you're notching a permanent imprint on the den couch? If you don't want to actually play, you can get involved as a sponsor or coach for your child if he's on a team or just show up and become an interested spectator.

Select a substitute. If your child is involved in an organized activity and you can't be there to offer support, find someone else who can go to the games. A relative, older sibling or close neighbor can substitute and cheer your kid on.

Lend support. If she's beginning an organized activity, monitor her physical and emotional well-being. Be alert to physical complaints or any

Boning Up

For young girls, the looming threat of osteoporosis later in life makes it imperative that they get regular doses of weight-bearing exercise, such as walking, running, dancing and most competitive sports, to supplement their dietary intake of calcium. Resistance exercises, such as light weight lifting and calisthenics, are also good. The "fracture threshold" is the level below which a bone might be likely to break spontaneously, and the goal is to get as far above that threshold as possible. That way, when bone declines later in life, as it inevitably will, there's a sizable deposit of bone to draw from.

"Most young girls have less than optimum bone strength, and by the time they're 25 to 35 years old they have reached their maximum bone density," warns Kenneth Cooper, M.D., president of the Cooper Aerobics Center in Dallas. But by getting enough exercise and calcium during the early years, young women can rise way above the threshold that makes bone vulnerable. "Exercise doesn't have to be intense—just fun, all-around weight-bearing activity may do the trick," says Dr. Cooper. "That way women may not have to start worrying about that threshold until they're 90 years old."

major emotional change. Is she sullen or depressed since tennis or basketball started? Is she feeling sick right around practice and suddenly feels better when she knows she doesn't have to go?

Have your child teach other children. As your child forges ahead in an activity, whether it's golf, bowling or softball, encourage him to teach others how to play. "You'd be surprised how that child takes pride helping other kids," says Dr. Cooper. In a way, you may help create a chain of healthy instruction in your neighborhood, where each child teaches a friend, who teaches another and so on.

DINING-OUT GUIDE

Does the sight of a restaurant menu fill you with delight . . . or dread? Is dining out your chance to enjoy a fine, relaxing meal (that you don't have to cook yourself) in the company of friends? Or does it become the occasion for hours, or days, of remorse because you blew your diet?

If the thought of restaurant dining scares you, you're not alone. Put the average dieter in her own kitchen, surrounded by food she's purchased herself and plenty of scales, books and measuring cups to help keep her mind on her waistline, and she usually manages just fine. But put her in a restaurant—be it anything from French to fast food—and more often than not she panics. Is this, she worries, when she'll wipe out in one sitting the results from all those weeks of grim discipline and hard work?

It needn't be.

Forget the idea that you can manage your diet only when you're doing the cooking. After all, you have to live in the real world, and restaurant dining is a wonderful part of it! Indeed, eating out is more popular than ever: The National Restaurant Association reports that in 1991 every American eight years old and older ate on average 198 meals per year away from home. You may not be visiting restaurants quite that often, but if you want to there's no reason to let your diet be a deterrent.

Furthermore, restaurateurs have become increasingly sensitive and responsive to the public's growing demand for low-fat, low-calorie meals and many have adjusted their menus accordingly. This is why you see more and more restaurants—especially those that cater to businesspeople who dine out much more than most of us—offering special "heart-smart" and weight-conscious dishes prepared with fewer saturated fats, less sugar and more fresh fruits and vegetables.

But even our favorite fast-food chains have gotten into the low-fat act. McDonald's, for instance, removed most of the fat from its McLean Deluxe, with just 9 percent fat in its beef patty (compared with 20 percent in other McDonald's beef patties and up to 30 percent in the ground beef you'd find in the supermarket). Their breakfast selections now include fat-free muffins, whole-grain cereals and 1 percent milk. And, adds a McDonald's nutritionist, "because we want customers to have all the facts on our food so they can fit it into their overall meal plan, we post nutrition information in the lobby of all our restaurants, and we distribute brochures with calorie counts, fat counts and complete ingredient information."

The Skinny on Savvy Restaurant Dining

Eateries of nearly every kind are trying their best to prove that you can enjoy their dishes without sending your diet down the tubes. Still, some places are better than others for people trying to shed some pounds. "In general," says Aliza Green, a Philadelphia restaurant consultant and former chef, "dieters should steer clear of old-fashioned American or 'home-style' restaurants, as well as classic French, which will have pretty rich dishes, and 'continental' restaurants, which usually feature heavy sauces and big portions of starches and meats."

Her recommendation? Ethnic eateries, including Thai, Chinese, Italian, Mediterranean, Greek, Turkish, northern African and the like. "In most ethnic places you can get a lot more vegetables, grains and lighter sauces, and the more authentic the restaurant, the better." Of course, she warns, "you still have to be careful. For example, fettuccine Alfredo, which is loaded with cream and butter, is the most popular dish in some Italian restaurants! But if you look you can find a nice piece of fish or a roasted-pepper antipasto, and bread that tastes good enough that it doesn't need butter."

There are certain key words and phrases on a restaurant menu that generally spell trouble for dieters, according to Myron Winick, M.D., former director of the Institute of Human Nutrition at Columbia University in New York City. These include:

- Buttery, buttered or butter sauce

- Sautéed, fried, pan-fried, breaded, glazed or crispy

- Creamy, creamed, in cream sauce or in its own gravy

- Au gratin, Parmesan, in cheese sauce or escalloped

- Au lait, à la mode or *au fromage*

- Marinated, stewed, basted or casserole

- Prime, hash, pot pie or Hollandaise

Brain Food

You're at the office, you look up at the clock: 11:30 A.M. It's an hour before your lunch date, and you haven't had a morsel to eat since breakfast at 6:45. You're so famished you could eat the eraser right off the pencil, not to mention every doughnut on the coffee wagon.

You've just found out why you should never, ever go too long between healthy meals or snacks. "Glucose, your brain's energy source, runs out after about five hours, compromising your brain power," explains registered dietitian and nutritionist Evelyn Tribole, author of *Eating on the Run*. You'll begin to feel a hunger so intense that you'll be willing to eat anything and everything.

It helps to plan a healthy lunch at work, advises Tribole. Pack your own if you tend to get so caught up in work that you forget to go out, she says. And as extra insurance, take some nutritious "grazing" food along to tide you through the day. Carry along tiny boxes of raisins, rice cakes or small containers of tomato juice to keep in your lunchbox or desk drawer when you need a quick work-time pick-me-up.

However, there are plenty of other safe eating options at your favorite restaurant. Just look for these words or phrases in the description.

- Pickled

- Tomato sauce or cocktail sauce

- Steamed

- Poached

- In broth or in its own juice

- Garden fresh

- Roasted

- Stir-fried

Here are a few other tips for savvier restaurant dining.

Speak up. Don't be afraid to make special requests—in this day of health- and waist-conscious eating, it's quite common. In fact, nine out of ten restaurant owners surveyed by the National Restaurant Association said

Selecting the Best of the Best

If you're smart in your meal selection, there's virtually no type of restaurant that's off-limits for those trying to lose (or maintain) weight. The chart below will give you a good idea how leaning toward certain items and away from others can mean big fat and calorie savings in your daily food budget. Yes, it's definitely possible to eat more at your favorite restaurant *and* weigh less.

Instead of . . .   **Have . . .**

AMERICAN

Bacon, lettuce and tomato sandwich (335 cal./16 g. fat)	Lobster salad sandwich (270 cal./11 g. fat)
Chef's salad, no dressing, 1½ cups (260 cal./15 g. fat)	Garden salad, no dressing, 1½ cups (50 cal./2 g. fat)
Sirloin steak, 8 oz. (523 cal./27 g. fat)	New York steak, lean, 8 oz. (478 cal./22 g. fat)

CHINESE*

Kung pao chicken (490 cal./25 g. fat)	Stir-fried chicken with vegetables (245 cal./14 g. fat)
Moo shu pork (630 cal./38 g. fat)	Beef and green pepper stir-fry (290 cal./11 g. fat)
Pan-fried soft noodles (680 cal./36 g. fat)	Shrimp chow mein (240 cal./5 g. fat)

FAST FOOD*

Burger King Bacon Double Cheeseburger (510 cal./38 g. fat)	Burger King Hamburger (260 cal./10 g. fat)
Domino's Deluxe Pizza, 2 slices (500 cal./20 g. fat)	Domino's Cheese Pizza, 2 slices (375 cal./10 g. fat)
Hardee's Chocolate Shake (390 cal./10 g. fat)	Hardee's Cool Twist Chocolate Cone (180 cal./4 g. fat)
McDonald's Chicken McNuggets, 6 (270 cal./15 g. fat)	McDonald's Chunky Chicken Salad (150 cal./4 g. fat)
Pizza Hut Super Supreme Pizza, 1 slice (276 cal./10 g. fat)	Pizza Hut Veggie Lover's Pizza, 1 slice (192 cal./8 g. fat)

they would, if customers requested it, happily serve dishes with sauce or dressing on the side and cook with vegetable oil or margarine instead of highly saturated butter, lard or shortening. And eight out of ten of these eager-to-please restaurateurs add that they would gladly bake or broil your

Instead of . . .	Have . . .
Taco Bell Taco Salad, without shell (481 cal./31 g. fat)	Taco Bell Tostada (170 cal./7 g. fat)

FRENCH

Crème brûlée, 4 oz. (325 cal./25 g. fat)	Orange soufflé, 4 oz. (155 cal./8 g. fat)
Duck à l'orange, ¼ duck (835 cal./69 g. fat)	Orange-glazed cornish hen with wild rice stuffing, 1 hen (560 cal./ 26 g. fat)
Veal cordon bleu, 4 oz. (440 cal./27 g. fat)	Chicken divan, 6 oz. (385 cal./18 g. fat)

ITALIAN

Cannoli (530 cal./35 g. fat)	Zabaglione, 4 oz. (120 cal./4 g. fat)
Pasta with cream sauce and prosciutto, 12 oz. (906 cal./18 g. fat)	Pasta with fresh tomato, basil and garlic, 12 oz. (520 cal./11 g. fat)

MEXICAN

Beef burrito with sour cream (431 cal./21 g. fat)	Chicken burrito, 6" tortilla (334 cal./12 g. fat)
Chicken chimichanga (605 cal./35 g. fat)	Chicken fajita (190 cal./8 g. fat)
Red beans with pork, 3 oz. (320 cal./19 g. fat)	Refried beans, ½ cup (130 cal./2 g. fat)

SEAFOOD

Breaded and fried clams, 6 oz. (342 cal./19 g. fat)	Steamed clams, 20 small (155 cal./1 g. fat)
Breaded and fried shrimp, 6 oz. (412 cal./20 g. fat)	Seasoned shrimp, 6 oz. (154 cal./2 g. fat)
Broiled swordfish steak, in olive oil, 8 oz. (600 cal./45 g. fat)	Poached salmon, 8 oz. (368 cal./14 g. fat)

*All sizes are typical entrée servings.

chicken or fish rather than fry it. Just say the word.

Play the trade-off game. "When you know you'll be going out to a nice restaurant for dinner, 'bank' your calories by eating a bit less than usual at breakfast and lunch," urges Carole Livingston, author of *I'll Never Be Fat*

Again. Carole lost 40 pounds 20 years ago and never saw them again, despite her membership in the Wine and Food Society and her hundreds of visits to fine restaurants around the world. When you've "banked" a few calories, you can go out, have the foods you enjoy and not feel guilty about it.

Don't be penny wise and pound foolish. Never go to a one-price, all-you-can-eat restaurant. Ever. (Need we say more?)

Say yes to soup. Soups—including vegetable, bean and clear soups—are often good choices. In an Italian restaurant, for instance, try *tortellini in brodo* (meat-filled pasta in broth). But avoid soups beginning with the words "cream of."

Bury Caesar. Don't let the word "salad" on a menu lull you into thinking that it's automatically a wise choice, says Green. Caesar salad, for instance, is the most popular salad in American restaurants—just about every one of them features it, some with variations such as grilled chicken or shrimp on top. "But it's one of the worst things you can order," she says. "These days, chefs don't use raw eggs when they make the Caesar salad dressing, they use mayonnaise and cheese in the dressing, and plenty of it. And the croutons are fried in oil. It's a very rich dish."

Beware of salad bars. Similarly, salad bars may look like safe havens for dieters, but watch out! Ladling on those creamy, high-fat dressings, sprinkling on handfuls of croutons or bacon bits, and gobbling down those mayonnaise-packed potato and macaroni salads can turn your "light" lunch into a caloric nightmare.

Be wise about size. Don't think that just because you paid for the food it means you have to finish every morsel. "Restaurant portions are 'unisex,' so they're usually too big for most women," reminds Green. So ask for a doggy bag and take the extra food home for another meal.

Ban the butter. If there's bread and butter on the table, ask your dining companions if it's okay to move it to their side of the table. Better yet, have the waiter remove them altogether.

Lose the race. Have an (unspoken) competition with your dining partners to be the last person to finish eating. Men and women with weight problems tend to eat fast and are usually the first ones in any given group to be done. For once, experiment to see how slowly you can eat. Bonus: You'll enjoy the conversation and the food so much more.

Take two for one. For a change of pace, try ordering two low-fat appetizers instead of a main course. The practice is not as uncommon as you may think. Don't feel pressured into ordering in "order." Make your own menu. It's okay to graze.

Ask questions about the menu. Some people are better off not looking at the menu to avoid confusion. If you've been watching what you eat for any length of time, you already have a pretty good idea of what you can have and what you can't. Ask for specifics about the specials; even if they don't have exactly what you want at the vast majority of restaurants you can still get baked or broiled poultry or fish, a simple pasta dish, steamed vegetables and fruit for dessert. Remember the menu is there to tempt you; you're there to make choices.

Order first. Be the first one at the table to order. You'll be less tempted to have some of the other, more fattening dishes your companions may choose.

Forget the umbrella. You don't have to skip alcohol altogether—a glass of wine during dinner or some champagne as a cocktail is fine. However, stay away from any alcoholic beverage with a straw or a little paper umbrella in it or one that's a primary color. Fruity mixed drinks and heavy after-dinner cordials are packed with sugar and calories.

Satisfy your thirst. Drink plenty of water throughout the meal and you'll eat less. Order a bottle of mineral water for the table, or ask the waiter to bring a pitcher of tap water.

Go native. In a Chinese or Thai restaurant, use the chopsticks (especially if you don't use them well!). Why? It slows you down.

Be a skeptic. In diners or family-style restaurants, be careful about ordering the so-called dieter's specials, which, ironically, may have excessive amounts of protein and calories. Just because a hamburger comes with a side scoop of cottage cheese does not make this a smart choice for waist watchers. If anything, you'd be far better off ordering the burger or the cottage cheese à la carte, with a green salad or some steamed veggies on the side.

Specify moo. Ask the waiter to bring you milk (better yet, low-fat milk) for your coffee. Unless you ask, you can expect to be served cream or half-and-half.

Get your just desserts. Here's the $64,000 restaurant question: "What's for dessert?" Sure, there's always fresh fruit or sorbet. But if you want something a bit more daring, try a hot fruit soufflé, which is made primarily of fresh fruit and egg whites. Or if you must have Death by Chocolate, it needn't spell death for your diet: Simply order one serving for the entire table and take just a forkful or two. You'll find it surprisingly satisfying.

Cut loose occasionally. As a general rule, dining out doesn't mean leaving your diet at home. However—and this is not a contradictory statement—everyone, including someone who's trying to lose weight, is entitled to have exactly what she wants in a restaurant from time to time. If you're going out to celebrate your 25th anniversary or your son's college graduation, have that piece of chocolate cake or that extra glass of champagne. As long as you're mindful of your weight-loss program and return to it immediately, you can have a "sinful" restaurant meal occasionally.

SPECIAL SITUATIONS

Thanksgiving. Vacations. Birthdays. Fiftieth anniversary parties. Easter.

If you're the type of person who prays for fudge, not flowers, on Valentine's Day and who associates Halloween with colorful candies instead of colorful costumes, then you know that these joyous times are usually accompanied by an overabundance of high-fat, high-calorie food. Sometimes you successfully resist temptation.

And sometimes you (ahem) don't.

So if you should happen to get on the scale on January 1 or the day after you return from a week in the Caribbean, don't be surprised if you notice that you've suddenly acquired a few extra pounds. You may not be happy about the result of your holiday pig-out, but rest assured you've got lots of company. According to a survey by *USA Today*, some 43 percent of adults gain about six pounds during the five-week Thanksgiving-to-New-Year's period.

Why is weight gain so often a part of holiday time and vacation time? If we've been following a weight-loss program and exercising faithfully, we tend to regard these periods as dietary escapes, as times to let ourselves go.

Many people seem to approach weight loss almost as a form of punishment. And with that kind of attitude, it isn't surprising that so many view vacations and holidays as the perfect excuse to throw caution to the wind and indulge in mindless and high-calorie eating.

Another explanation: When you've saved and shelled out a lot of money for your holiday, you're determined to get your money's worth. For many that includes eating their fill, and then some. Unfortunately, cruise ships and vacation spots boasting all-you-can-eat menus tend to bring out the glutton in us. "I've paid for this food and I'm going to have it!" is the typical thinking. So is, "Everybody gains weight during vacations—why should I be any different?"

The Pleasure-Time Survival Guide

Well, perhaps now you should begin to think about being different, particularly if you have a frustrating history of yo-yo dieting. We're not talking about depriving yourself. The key is simply to begin to think of holidays, special occasions and vacations as fun days when more and better-than-usual food is available. You can have some treats, and enjoy yourself as much as everyone else, if you decide ahead of time to sample them in reasonable quantities.

Keep your usual healthy way of eating as a guide, then add those things you really want, in moderation: a half slice of key lime pie for dessert, or one complete-with-an-umbrella cocktail (not three) before dinner, or two small barbecued ribs, balanced with a green salad, at the poolside cookout. Often a taste of "forbidden" foods is enough to give you what the diet experts call "mouth satisfaction" without blowing your weight-loss program. You can then return home feeling as though you did indeed have a special night or week, and your waistline won't have suffered a bit.

Remember, too, that vacations and family get-togethers provide the perfect opportunities to increase your usual exercise regimen. Who wouldn't want to go swimming in a crystal-clear lake or play volleyball on a beautiful beach or do some golfing on a championship course?

Instead of sleeping in every morning, try a brisk prebreakfast walk in the mountains or on the beach or wherever you happen to be—you'll enjoy the workout and the lovely change of scenery. If you've developed a fondness for resistance training, you'll want to take advantage of your hotel's fitness facility, be it state of the art or a spare room equipped with some free weights and a stationary bike. These days it's hard to find hotels that don't feature some sort of modest gym.

And even if your vacation plans consist of little more than a weekend of visiting friends or family, there is still fun and calorie burning to be had. Try getting everyone together for a morning run with the dog, a jog along the beach or a brisk after-dinner walk.

That, of course, is the ideal holiday scenario: reasonable eating and solid exercise. But what happens if, during that cruise or that reunion, you go completely AWOL from your diet. (You know you'll have to face the bathroom scale eventually, but you opt to forget about it until the moment of truth.) The trick to emerging from this food fest without permanently losing your weight-loss motivation is to accept that you've slipped a bit, and then get on with your wholesome new way of low-fat living.

Immediately resume your usual food-and-fitness program, no matter how many days you've been away from it. Overindulged during the Christmas and New Year's holidays? One clever remedy is to use January to get a jump on your spring cleaning—wash the windows, scrub the floors, overhaul those closets. Not only will you be getting the year off to a fresh, clean start but you'll also burn off those extra holiday calories like mad.

Most important: If you've overindulged, be kind to yourself. Mentally beating yourself up over how much you ate and how little you exercised is pointless. "Guilt is not a motivator," says Atlanta-based registered dietitian Kathleen Zelman, a spokesperson for the American Dietetic Association.

TIPS FROM TOP SPAS

People from every corner of the world, from dukes to dentists, fly thousands of miles and spend thousands of dollars to drop a few pounds and get pampered for a week at a luxury spa. While these pages can't offer you the sensuous pleasure of an herbal wrap or a soothing massage, they can provide you with the best diet tips culled from the spiffiest spas in the country.

The New Age Spa, Neversink, New York

Focus on losing inches rather than pounds. As you reduce the fat in your diet and step up your level of exercise, you may find that your weight may actually remain the same, although you look better and feel better and your clothes are looser on you. What's going on? Explains Werner Mendel, New Age's owner, "As you convert your body fat to muscle, you may not lose pounds because muscle weighs more than fat. But you will look and measure differently."

Eat a good breakfast. On-the-go people think they're being calorie wise by skimping on breakfast or skipping it completely. But that's a surefire way to sabotage your diet, says New Age's fitness director, Sandra Brown. "Breakfast here at the spa is self-serve—we have everything from hot and cold cereals to baked apples to yogurt and cottage cheese to whole-grain breads—and we encourage guests to have a good breakfast. They may be hiking or taking aerobics classes, and they need that fuel." You need it, too.

Love yourself first—the rest will follow. "If you can, through meditation or yoga, learn to love yourself, then proper eating and exercise will kick in thanks to your higher self-esteem," insists Mendel. "That's really the most important ingredient for health and well being: self-love."

147

Norwich Inn and Spa, Norwich, Connecticut

Make changes in your diet gradually. If you're trying to limit the amount of meat or poultry you eat, for instance, don't cut it out altogether; start by going from a whole chicken breast to half a breast, urges spa chef Bernice Veckerelli. "Also," she adds, "once a week have a meatless meal, featuring pasta or grains and vegetables, or maybe a lentil-and-brown-rice pilaf. Little by little, increase the number of these dishes." Slow but steady adjustments in your mealtime strategies will bring you greater success than attempting overnight changes, she insists.

Don't let yourself get bored. "Eat a variety of foods," says Veckerelli, even if you're having weight-loss success with certain tried-and-true items. "A lot of time people think that dieting means nothing but grapefruit, or fruit and cottage cheese, and eventually they get bored and hungry." But if you make a point of experimenting at mealtime and especially try to increase your intake of whole grains, fruits and vegetables, which are very filling and satisfying, you'll perk up your palate and be more apt to stick to your weight-loss program, too.

Canyon Ranch in the Berkshires, Lenox, Massachusetts

Enjoy what you eat. "According to a lot of studies, there's a great deal of guilt and fear associated with eating," says registered dietitian Kathie Swift, nutrition director of Canyon Ranch in the Berkshires. "But food should not just be good for us but also good-tasting. After all, taste is the first determinant of our food choices." So your diet should include many of those things you naturally enjoy eating, prepared in healthful ways and served in reasonable-size portions. "Build the pleasure principle into your eating," she urges, and you'll find weight loss much easier.

Focus on mindful eating. "Explore the 'whys' of what and how much you're eating, so you can determine whether you're eating in response to a real physiological need or to an emotional one," says Swift. Greater food awareness, she adds, usually means greater diet success.

Safety Harbor Spa and Fitness Center, Safety Harbor, Florida

Buy smaller until you've learned to eat less. "If you found that you only had inch of shampoo left in the bottle, you might add some water to it to get few more days out of it," says Joe Kiley, former executive chef at Safety Harbor Spa. "So it stands to reason that if you had smaller amounts of food, you'd probably learn to stretch them, too. If you buy olive oil by the gallon, you don't care how much of it hits the frying pan. But if the bottle has only a few ounces in it, chances are you'd use the oil with a lighter hand." It may not be the most economical way to shop, Kiley admits, but your waistline will thank you for it.

Watch out for anything that breathes. Animal fats and animal proteins are the major sources of cholesterol and saturated fats, notes Kiley, so "make sure you don't have a lot of them. If you're buying chicken, for example, divide it into four-ounce portions for each dinner serving and freeze the rest. Then if somebody wants seconds, just say, 'You can't have any more—it's frozen! Wait till tomorrow.'"

Learn to make healthy substitutions in your favorite recipes. Kiley reports that one of his spa clients recently asked him how she could make a low-fat Caesar-salad dressing at home. "I had her identify the unhealthiest ingredients in a typical Caesar-salad dressing—egg yolks and oil. Then I pointed out to her that those two ingredients are the major components of mayonnaise, and so she could substitute a low-fat mayonnaise for them in her recipe." Similarly, she could swap some part-skim cheese for the Parmesan and Romano usually found atop Caesar salad.

Some substitutions may not be instantly identifiable, notes Kiley. But the more you learn to analyze the nutritive value of your favorite foods by reading food labels and checking a food-nutrient guidebook, the easier it'll become.

The Palms, Palm Springs, California; The Oaks, Ojai, California

Do yoga. "One reason people overeat is that they're stressed," states registered dietitian Eleanor Brown, for 15 years a food consultant and yoga instructor at both the Palms in Palm Springs and the Oaks in Ojai. "Many people are nervous eaters—they don't even know they're doing it. Everyone is looking for peace, but you'll find it's there all the time if you can just relax your body and mind. Getting rid of tension in a positive way will keep you from eating out of tension."

As Brown notes, just about every city offers at least one yoga class (try your local Y for starters), although you can also learn yoga through reading a book or watching a video on the subject.

Write down your fitness goals. "It's been proven that if people write down their goals and read them over frequently, they'll achieve them," says Brown, who started following her own advice seven years ago at age 50. "I used to think that journal keeping had to be done in some big book, but it can be done in just a tiny, spiral-bound notebook. It's easy. It's just a matter of writing your monthly goals, then making a notation of what you will do that day to reach those goals. Then the next day, review how you did."

Not losing weight or following your exercise regimen as well as you'd like? Says Brown, "If you're not achieving your goals, it doesn't mean you're a bad person. Maybe your goals were too high. So rewrite them."

Le Pli Health Spa and Salon
at the Charles Hotel, Cambridge, Massachusetts

Eat many small meals instead of three big meals each day. "If you put a little coal into the furnace several times a day, rather than a lot of coal all at once, it will burn more efficiently," explains Liz Carlson, fitness director at Le Pli. "It's the same with your body. It'll have a hard time trying to digest large amounts of food at once, but if you eat small meals several times a day, your metabolism stays active all day and becomes a more efficient calorie burner."

A typical menu Carlson recommends goes something like this.

Early morning: oatmeal and fruit

Midmorning snack: a slice of toast and fat-free yogurt

Late-morning snack: pretzels and a small banana

Lunch: a turkey sandwich on whole-wheat bread with lettuce, tomatoes; carrot sticks

Midafternoon snack: pretzels

Late-afternoon snack: tomato juice and nonfat crackers

Dinner: fish and rice or pasta; small green salad; two servings vegetables

You should also drink plenty of water throughout the day.

It's best, Carlson adds, if you don't eat much, if anything, past 6:00 or 7:00 P.M., "when your metabolism is starting to shut down in preparation for sleep. You usually don't have much reason after that hour to expend too many calories through exercise, and if you have too many calories in your body then, they're more apt to be stored as fat."

La Costa Hotel and Spa, Carlsbad, California

Customize your weight-loss plan. At the world-famous La Costa Spa, head dietitian Karen Ladman works individually with guests to create a personalized eating plan. "We do a computer analysis," she explains. "They come in to me and say, 'This is what I've been eating,' and we feed that information into a computer. Then I go over the printout with them, indicating what I'd have them change, instead of giving everyone a set program."

You can do something similar at home. Take inventory of what you tend to eat in a typical day, and see where you can make healthy changes by reducing fat, by adding more complex carbs (switching your white rice for brown, for instance) and by making certain you're getting three to four servings of veggies and three to four fruits. "It's important," adds Ladman, "to look at your own likes and how can you can individualize your diet. There's no one thing that works for everybody."

The Greenhouse, Arlington, Texas

Limit alcohol. Alcohol can harm your diet in a number of tricky ways, warns registered dietitian Cindy Wachtler, a former nutritionist at the renowned Cooper Clinic in Dallas and currently a nutritionist at the Greenhouse spa. "People think that because it contains no fat grams, they can have as much as they want, and yet the body utilizes it much the same way it utilizes fat," says Wachtler. What's more, she adds, it impairs your good sense.

"Drink a glass of wine before dinner and suddenly the food looks better and tastes better, and your judgment of quantities will diminish," she says. "You have to approach it with respect, because it does things to your body that you're not aware of."

Green Valley Spa and Tennis Resort, St. George, Utah

Get out of the deprivation mentality. "In order to experience a lifetime of good health and ideal body weight, you must be able to enjoy the process, not just the results," says Green Valley Spa owner Alan Coombs. "If you look upon exercise as work and reducing fat consumption as deprivation, then your efforts at losing weight will always be a battle and either you'll fail or your success will have been won at a terrible price."

The Phoenix Spa, Houston, Texas

Go ahead—play with your food! In fact, it's a terrific idea if you're trying to limit your intake, says Angie Day, the Phoenix's executive director, until its closing in late 1993. "When you go out to a restaurant, order food with lots of 'play' potential, things that keep your hands busy and take longer to eat—hot soup, for example, or lobster in the shell," she advises. "They'll satisfy you and you may not eat as much as you would of some other dishes."

Eat before you eat. "Have a light salad—maybe with some cucumbers and tomatoes and a little nonfat dressing—before you go to a party or a restaurant," urges Day. "That way, during cocktail hour you'll have a full stomach and you won't be tempted as much to pick on the more fattening hors d'oeuvres."

Wear something tight fitting when you go out to eat. "Being a little uncomfortable is a nice little reminder that you're trying to lose weight, and it will keep you from overeating," insists Day. "It's a trick that works for me—absolutely."

Satisfy your need for the taste you're really craving. Have a hankering for something crunchy, like potato chips? Then eating a banana or drinking a glass of tomato juice just won't do it for you; afterward you'll still long for that crunch. So, advises Day, make sure you have a crunchy something that won't blow your diet—a small bowl of bite-size shredded wheat, for example. "When choosing a snack," she says, "identify the taste and texture you truly crave and look to satisfy that need."

20 Unexpected Reasons Why Weight Loss Fails

You're determined to drop that weight, and this time you're doing everything right. You're cutting fat-packed foods from your diet as much as you can. You're stoking up on fresh fruits and veggies, whole-grain breads and cereals. Plus, you're exercising more consistently than you have in recent memory. So then, why aren't you shedding those pounds? It's maddening when you honestly believe you're putting forth your best effort and it's still not being rewarded as you feel it should be.

Your diet dilemma could have of a number of explanations; it's just a matter of understanding what's going on and making a few simple switches. Check the list below and see which, if any, apply to you. Make the necessary adjustments, and before you know it, your weight loss will soon be back on track.

1. Being too rigid. "Many people believe that being perfect in their diet will guarantee success, but it's actually more important to be flexible than to be rigid," says registered dietitian Judy E. Marshel, director of Health Resources of Great Neck, New York. Say that your favorite restaurant, where you could always count on having a delicious, low-fat meal, suddenly goes out of business, and now you have to explore other, unfamiliar ones, and you're afraid to adjust your menu. Your attitude may then be, "Well, if I can't have what I was planning to have, I'll have whatever I want." And that, explains Marshel, may set up a new cycle of overeating and dieting.

Because life is bound to throw you a curveball every now and then, you might as well get used to the notion that you and your diet will have to adapt. An unexpected change in plan need not mean the beginning of the end of your weight-loss program.

2. Not eating enough! Your metabolism is a tricky devil. Eat too much, and it won't be able to burn all those calories, so, natch, you gain weight. Eat too little, and your metabolism—perceiving that you're starving yourself and desperate to help your body hang on to the calories you are consuming—slows to a crawl. Result? Little or no weight loss.

Studies have repeatedly shown that drastic calorie-cutting diets don't work, not in the long run and sometimes not even in the short run. All the pros today agree that it's just as vital to eat sufficient quantities of the right foods (fruits, vegetables, grains) as it is to cut back on the wrong ones (fats, sugar, alcohol). Warns Marshel, "If you don't consume enough calories, even if you're on a weight-loss plan, you may see a slowing down or even a total cessation of your weight loss."

3. Not satisfying those cravings. "In order to lose weight succesfully," says Ronna Kabatznick, Ph.D., psychological consultant to Weight Watchers International and a specialist in weight control, "you have to have a certain level of inner satisfaction, which you get by eating things that make you feel good. If you don't eat those things, you'll walk around feeling deprived on a psychological level and deprived on a physical level, and eventually you'll binge or start eating more of the things you don't particularly want."

So if you're a chocoholic, for instance, appease your need for the sweet stuff with a fat-free frozen chocolate pop or a low-fat chocolate shake whipped up in the blender. Even half of an honest-to-goodness chocolate bar every once in a blue moon won't hurt. Giving yourself a little of what you crave now and then will actually help you choose the rest of your meals more wisely.

4. Falling off the wagon. Diets may not work as well the second, third or fourth time around. When you embark on a weight-loss diet for the very first time, your body typically sheds some water, some fat and some muscle mass. But anytime you put weight back on, your body only regains fat, which is harder to lose than muscle.

So if you're a diet veteran, don't be surprised if it's taking longer and requiring a greater effort to make those extra pounds go away. New tactics might be in order. If, say, your diet is now about 30 percent calories from fat, try cutting back to the 25 percent range. Additional time on the stationary bike or the jogging path each week may also be needed to coax off that unwanted weight. Be patient—your persistence will pay off.

5. Disregarding seasonal and activity changes. "People who go on diets think that they have to follow the same food plan in every situation—summer or winter, during vacations—but it's not true," says Kabatznick. "Some days you're more active than others, some days you may eat out more. Also, you should have extra food in winter because it's cold and you need more calories to keep your body warm." So take your activity level and the seasons into account and vary your diet accordingly for the best possible weight-loss results.

6. *Taking certain medications.* Unfortunately, if you have health problems that require certain prescription drugs, they may slow down your weight loss. For instance, corticosteroids, used to treat rheumatoid arthritis, tend to cause water retention and stimulate the appetite. Check with your doctor to see how you can make the appropriate adjustments in your diet while continuing your medication. In all likelihood, a stepped-up exercise program will do the trick.

7. *Changing body needs.* As you age, your body just naturally requires less energy (that means fewer calories) to maintain its current weight. So whatever may have worked before in helping you shed pounds may not quite do the trick with each succeeding birthday. Be prepared, therefore, to either reduce your caloric intake a little or increase your level of exercise.

8. *Losing your perspective.* "Many people invest so much in the idealization of having a thinner body that when that thinner body is nearly theirs and their fantasies don't come true, they get disappointed," explains Kabatznick. What happens then? Usually some unconscious overeating here and there, or a slow, subtle loss of interest in exercise. No wonder the extra pounds are still hanging around.

"If you're realistic," says Kabatznick, "you'll know that losing weight means you'll have a thinner body and a healthier lifestyle, but it won't change who you are."

9. *"Invisible" eating.* "They're the little things you're not even aware you're eating—that piece of candy in your purse, that extra pretzel, those foods that come with sauces that you just accept," notes Carole Livingston, author of *I'll Never Be Fat Again.* "You think it's okay to have them, but it's not okay unless, of course, you want to keep your weight stuck where it is."

10. *Those old devil moods.* "When I'm unhappy, my eating habits can be poor, and I may eat more of something that I shouldn't, like ice cream," admits Marie Simmons, author of *The Light Touch.* Sooner or later, your emotional state is going to do a number on your appetite, if you let it. Should you suddenly find yourself doing more and more unconscious snacking by the light of the refrigerator door, check your mood. Then figure out how to improve matters without using food as a crutch.

11. *Underestimating portion sizes.* "When I ask people in my classes, 'What's a half cup of spaghetti?' most people don't know. On a plate, it looks pretty paltry," notes registered dietitian Joann Heslin, co-author of *The Pregnancy Nutrition Counter.* "I try to help them distinguish between the classic portion—a half cup to one cup of spaghetti, for example—and the traditional portion, which is a plateful. The traditional portion is often really two portions. The same goes for meat. The classic portion is four ounces of bone-less meat, fish or poultry—a piece about the size of your palm. If you think about how much meat you ate last night, you probably ate more."

The moral of the story: Without becoming fanatic about portion sizes, start developing your awareness of how much you're eating.

12. *Taking baby steps instead of big ones.* "It's actually easier for many people to make dramatic changes in their eating than small ones," insists Dean Ornish, M.D., who heads the Preventive Medicine Research Institute in Sausalito, California. For example, he says, "If you continue to eat red meat and merely reduce your portion sizes, you'll feel deprived and you'll never really lose your taste for it." As a result, you'll still crave it, keep eating it, and probably have a hard time dropping those pounds. "But if you give meat up completely, not only will you be eliminating a lot of fat from your diet but after a while you won't even miss the taste."

13. *Getting fooled by fats.* "Dietary fats are the biggest deterrent to weight loss," reminds Bernice Veckerelli, a chef at the Norwich Inn & Spa in Norwich, Connecticut. "People are so programmed to think about re-ducing their cholesterol, so they may have margarine instead of butter, but they forget that one tablespoon of fat is one tablespoon of fat." Conse-quently, she says, many people believe that as long as they're sticking to heart-healthy fats such as olive and canola oil, they can have lots of it. But if you do, those pounds just won't come off as you'd like them to. "If you need to lose weight, you automatically will, once you start to watch your fat intake," Bernice promises.

14. *Swimming!* Swimming seems to fit the description of a great total-body exercise, yet it doesn't measure up to other exercises when it comes to fat burning. Researchers aren't quite sure why. Many studies suggest that your appetite increases as your body temperature decreases, so swimming in cold water may cause you to eat more. And there is a chance that in re-sponse to the colder temperatures of the water, your body will hoard fat for insulation instead of burning it for fuel.

But it may be possible to turn swimming into a fine fat burner by ap-plying the interval training concept: Instead of swimming for 30 minutes straight at a low-to-moderate pace, after about a 10-minute warm-up, pick up your pace for four laps. Then drop back to a recovery pace for another four laps. Keep alternating until you have about 5 minutes left. Then finish your workout at your recovery pace. And if that doesn't work, switch to an-other aerobic activity that's been proven to heat up the body and burn fat, such as walking, cycling or cross-country skiing.

15. *Getting bottled up.* Check that label on the bottle of light beer—zero in the fat column. There's none there, right? That doesn't make it okay. One study found that alcohol may impair the body's ability to burn fat. Maybe that's why people who down more than two drinks a day tend to pad up around their middles. Other studies suggest that drinking a brew with a meal tends to make you overeat.

"I find that when I get a dieting man to stop drinking, it makes it easier for him to deal with food, plus he can eat a lot more," says Morton H. Shaevitz, Ph.D., director of the Institute for Family and Work Relationships in La Jolla, California, and author of *Lean and Mean: The No Hassle, Life-Extending Weight Loss Program for Men.*

16. Being a member of the Clean Plate Club. Some habits die hard, and many of us simply can't get used to the notion of deliberately leaving food behind, especially when we've paid good money for it in a restaurant. But as you're downing every last morsel on your plate, keep in mind that you're probably eating more than your weight-loss diet calls for.

17. Combining fat and sugar. You're in the mood for a treat. That's fine every so often and in reasonable quantities. Just make sure it's not cheesecake or any other combination of fat and sugar. The decadent duo works to increase your waistline like this: When sugar hits your bloodstream, your body releases a flood of insulin in response. That insulin triggers your fat cells to open. So the fat in the cheesecake that follows goes right into storage. If you must eat fat, at least try not to combine it with sugar.

18. Letting down your guard. Something's different in your environment or everyday routine. Changes in your daily life, both subtle and obvious, may be responsible for your weight-loss slow-down. Did a new pastry shop—conveniently located on your way to and from work every day—just open? Did you move to a new city and, in the process, lose your support circle? Has an injury or temporary disability sidelined you from your normal exercise regimen?

You may now be taking in extra calories (or not burning off those you typically burn) without even realizing it. Build awareness into your daily activities, even the ones you may not automatically associate with food. Once you do, you may find you're losing weight at a better rate.

19. Eating to please another person. "Go on—have some! It's good!"

For every time you successfully sidestep that offer, there may be one or two you simply can't resist. Your determination to eat only when you want to may be solid, but it takes a steely will to refuse to try one of your daughter's homemade brownies, or to keep from disappointing your husband when he says he wants you to share some pizza and beer with him after the movie. Diet saboteurs lurk everywhere, and although they may insist they want to see you thin, they may also want you to eat when you'd just rather not. For your weight's sake, learn how to say no, graciously and firmly.

20. Calling it a "diet." Yes, you want to lose weight. But as Jim Fobel, author of *Jim Fobel's Diet Feasts*, points out, "'Diet' sounds like deprivation, and you will set yourself up for failure. Think of what you're doing as making a healthy lifestyle change.

MAKEOVERS
TO LAST A LIFETIME

Sometimes the best way to learn how to lose weight and keep it off is by following the sensible examples of others who've done it successfully. Here are five inspiring real-life stories of women and men who changed their eating and exercise habits and collectively lost hundreds of pounds. In the process they shed both a host of health problems and a debilitating negative self-image.

A Walk on the Slim Side

At 42, Leslie Arnim is a diet expert. She knows all the weight-loss plans that don't work for her, but happily, she discovered one that works like a charm.

When she weighed 360 pounds, she was still trying diet programs like Weight Watchers. (She needed to lose 15 pounds before her weight would even register on their scale.) Even though the organization helped Leslie lose her fat, her frustration grew.

"I was craving foods and feeling deprived," she recalls. "I hated the idea of living the rest of my life with a food scale in my purse and a weekly food diary to fill out!" That's when Leslie decided to join the *Prevention* Walking Club, launching a walking habit that has helped her shed 170 pounds and has taken her from a size 56 to a size 14. Best of all, she's stayed there.

"When I first started my walking program, my knees and hips hurt terribly. I consulted my doctor, and he said it was probably because of my weight. He said that the pain was actually not as dangerous for me as the fat. I just needed to keep at it, slowly."

Leslie's pain came and went. "It seemed as though every time I lost another 30 or 40 pounds, the aches would start again." But as she soon came to realize, "My body was simply adapting to the changes brought about by my weight loss.

"The walking club logbook really helped me during those painful days. I would write down how far I walked and how I felt. Just keeping a record really improved my mood and kept me in touch with my accomplishments," she says. Today her knees are fine, her hips no longer ache, and she has no sign of osteoarthritis.

As far as her eating habits are concerned, "I eat when I'm hungry," she says. "Some days I eat a little more than I need, sometimes a little less. It all seems to balance out. I did a lot of reading about eating and emotions, and I got some counseling on how I had always used food to soothe myself. These days I watch my emotions more than I watch my calories. It works!"

And because Leslie dropped her weight slowly over a two-year period, her face stayed relatively wrinkle-free. "But I had lots of sagging skin on my belly and thighs. I used to look like one of those Chinese dogs, all wrinkly," she says. "But I haven't had any cosmetic surgery, and my skin actually seems to be shrinking as I continue to walk and work out."

She likes to reserve her evenings for walking, "but sometimes I get caught up in everything, and I slack off and the weight comes back a little," she admits. "Then I fall back on the walking club. Reading the newsletters helps inspire me and get me motivated again. I use lots of walking tapes to keep from being bored.

"These days my routine is varied," Leslie adds. "Some days I walk, some days I do aerobics and some mornings I just lie in bed and smile at my muscles!"

Join the *Prevention* Walking Club. For just $3.95 you'll receive our Walkpower booklet with helpful hints for beginning your walking program, a yearlong log and an awards coupon with colorful stickers to chart your progress. And look to *Prevention* magazine every month for tips and inspiration from "Walker's World." For information about the *Prevention* Walking Club, write to: *Prevention* Magazine, 33 East Minor Street, Emmaus, PA 18098.

He's Having the Last Laugh

As an overweight child, John Passadino, of Bellerose, New York, discovered that fat was funny. In school he'd clown around about his hefty shape to get his share of laughs—and the spotlight. But at 29, the computer analyst-turned-part-time-actor-and-comedian finally realized his weight was no laughing matter.

At 5'7" he had reached 212 pounds. His cholesterol had climbed to 375, his legs frequently cramped up and his breathing was labored. That was when he decided to get serious about weight loss. With a little self-education, he was able to write himself a new routine for living, with a sensible diet and exercise at center stage. And the results would make anyone smile.

"When I was growing up, people always said, 'He's eating, God bless him! He's healthy!' Or else, 'Eat the fat. It'll keep you warm in the winter!' So I did eat the fat, and lots of it. I ate hamburgers, hot dogs, cakes and candy. No wonder I was the fat kid in class. None of the girls were ever interested in me. That was why I became the class clown—to get attention."

By the time John was in eighth grade, he hit 163 pounds and went on the first of many crash diets. "I lost a lot of weight, but by high school I'd put it all back on. After that I tried a lot of other crash diets—like a grapefruit or a one-meal-a-day diet—to lose weight for special occasions, such as weddings. I'd lose about 20 pounds, but afterward my weight would go right back up."

As the computer analyst began to moonlight as a comedian, he found that he could use his jowly appearance to get laughs. But all the while he was afraid the audience was laughing at his body, not his jokes. "I was afraid to lose weight for fear of losing laughs," he admits.

By June of 1988, his 212 pounds were causing major physical problems for John. "I was experiencing muscle cramps in my legs. My breathing was so labored people could hear it when I talked to them on the phone. And when I had my cholesterol tested, it was 375."

John's doctor told him that his weight was putting him at risk for developing diabetes and that his elevated cholesterol was making him a candidate for heart disease, warnings that didn't surprise him. "My father had suffered his first angina attack in his late forties," John recalls. "I kept looking at all his medications and thinking, Am I going to have to do this when I'm in my forties? This is crazy! It's time to make a permanent change. And that's just what I did."

The comic had to learn a whole new act. He'd never learned how to eat right, so he had to completely educate himself about nutrition. "My first step was to get some books on health and nutrition from the library," he recalls. "I learned how much I should be eating to maintain my weight as well as how much less I'd have to eat to lose some." The biggest revelation to John? "I realized I would have to drastically cut my fat intake."

He set out to lose a modest five to ten pounds, and began by cutting out fatty red meats in favor of skinless chicken. He swapped ice cream for fruit, and swore off the egg yolks that were helping to keep his cholesterol count high.

"I also knew from my reading that I had to exercise if I wanted to lose weight and keep it off," he says. "But I had never been active in my life—my weight had turned me off to exercise.

"So I started out slowly. I began riding a stationary bike for just five minutes a day. It was so easy that each time I finished, I felt as if I hadn't done anything! But I knew I would burn myself out if I did too much too soon. So I stuck with just a five-minute ride every day for two weeks."

By the third week, John was up to 10 minutes a day. The following week, he rode for 15 minutes. Not only did he begin losing weight very easily but he also suffered no hunger pangs at all. Within a month of starting his exercise program and fat cutback, he'd lost 10 pounds. And after three months, he was riding the stationary bike for about 40 minutes a day and was thrilled to see his cholesterol reading drop down to 213.

"Once I saw results," says John, "I really got into losing weight and cut back my diet a little further. I started drinking low-fat milk instead of whole milk and eating low-fat yogurt and cheeses instead of the higher-fat versions. But I allowed myself pizza once a week as an incentive to keep going."

By January 1989, he had stepped up his exercise program, too. "I began weight lifting to tone my muscles, and I even started jogging. I started out slowly, jogging for just 15 minutes. Then I worked up to a half hour. Within six months, I was jogging for 40 minutes at a time.

"I was rediscovering my body," he adds, "and it felt great to be able to do all the things I'd never been able to do in the past, such as play paddleball and ride my bike. I didn't turn into an athlete, but I did feel more coordinated. And I never would have thought of jogging before I started my program! But then my joints started hurting. I had read that walking was as effective as running, so I scrapped the jogging and took up walking instead."

In addition to his regular walking regimen, he started taking the train to his comedy and acting jobs, getting off at an earlier stop and walking the rest of the way. The walk was about 30 to 40 minutes each way, and John would do it two or three times a week. By that spring he was down to 150 pounds, and his cholesterol had dipped to 196.

The following year John became a total vegetarian, excluding even dairy products. "I became very fanatical about my diet, and I was trying to squeeze too much exercise into my already tight schedule. As a result, I was under a lot of stress. So I decided to relax a little, in both my diet and exercising."

By then he could easily afford to let up. In June 1990, when he stopped trying to lose weight and started trying to maintain, he weighed only 138 pounds. "I really looked too thin then, and not just to my mother, who insisted I was sick! So I put myself on a maintenance plan that I continue to follow today. I drink skim milk and eat nonfat yogurt. I eat egg whites, but still no yolks. I have fish twice a week—mainly tuna and salmon and sometimes scallops or shrimp—rather than meat, and occasionally beans and rice." He also tries to avoid sugar and alcohol.

John has relaxed his exercise program, with no adverse effects. Now he walks at a brisk pace four times a week for 30 to 60 minutes. If the weather is bad, he opts for 45 minutes on his exercise bike, and he does calisthenics three or four times a week.

The results have been great. The cramping in his legs is gone, and he can breathe easily now. He boasts a 32-inch waist, and his weight is a steady 145. What's more, his cholesterol stays within a healthy 190-to-210 range.

As for his career, "I'm happy to say my weight loss has actually helped, rather than hurt, my comedy," John says. "Once I lost weight, I realized I would have to rely on my talent to be funny—there was no fat to do it for me anymore. As a result, I think I'm funnier now than I ever was!"

Pumped Up, Slimmed Down

Mark Cuatt is half the man he used to be—less than half, in fact! At the age of 19, Mark weighed 465 pounds. Today, at age 22, he's a solid 225.

How do you lose 240 pounds? you may be wondering. "The same way you lose 5 or 10 pounds," says Mark. "You learn to eat smart and you start to get some exercise. If it worked for me, it'll work for anyone."

Mark woke up one day and felt a sense of determination to change his life that he likened to a religious experience. "I'd been on diets before, but somehow I knew it would work this time. It was a strange feeling how certain I was that I wouldn't cheat anymore.

"I'm not sure what triggered it," he continues. "All I knew was that all my friends were either getting married or going off to school, and I was being left alone. Good friends are hard to come by when you weigh 465 pounds; I didn't make new ones easily. I definitely felt discriminated against because of my size, both socially and at work. But through it all, I was determined to change."

After seeing a doctor to rule out thyroid or other physical problems, the first thing Mark did was to cut out snacks. "As a kid, our refrigerator worked on the open-door policy: I could eat whenever and whatever I wanted. So I decided to change that and eat three balanced meals a day—no snacks.

"Then I started to read everything I could get my hands on about nutrition. I concentrated on cutting fats rather than calories." Today he eats six small meals a day with a total of about 30 grams of fat, which enables him to maintain his weight easily.

The second part of Mark's program was exercise. Walking was the most convenient, and literally the only, exercise he felt comfortable doing. "I walked the first day until I felt tired—about a half mile. Gradually I worked up to a mile, then two, then three. Six miles a day was my maximum. By that time I'd lost a lot of weight and I felt comfortable riding my exercise bike.

"Finally, I joined a gym and began to lift weights—I'd gotten so thin, I felt I needed to build up my body a little. Today I'm a competitive bodybuilder. I work in a gym, and I'm looking forward to getting my master's degree in nutrition. What a change!"

Mark admits that he encountered lots of emotional ups and downs on his road to a healthy lifestyle. "And I still do. When I weighed 465 pounds, people used to stare and laugh at me when I went to the mall. Now I get stares because I look good and because I'm a bodybuilder, but at times I still feel like people are staring at a fat guy. That's when I feel all the old emotions. I have my weight under control, but sometimes my self-image is scrambling to catch up."

But that's a process he's willing to deal with because the rewards of fitness have been so great. Meanwhile, he warns those attempting to imitate him that the first two weeks will be the hardest. "That's when I craved everything. I was going through withdrawal. How did I cope? Whenever I got a craving, I went for a walk or hopped on my exercise bike."

Now, says Mark, staying trim is a snap. "I don't have any food cravings or feel any frustration or deprivation. The old junk foods just don't appeal to me anymore. And exercise is a permanent part of my life."

A Crossing Guard at the Crossroads

Nancy Myers of Parkersburg, West Virginia, was at a crossroads in her life. On the verge of turning 40, the 5'2" crossing guard had reached a milestone with her weight: 240 pounds. And her back was feeling the brunt of it. With her cholesterol creeping upward, too, she believed that if she didn't slim down soon, she'd never do it. So she stepped into action. Nancy moved from life on the sidelines to life in the fast lane, and bypassed her usual fare for leaner cuisine. The result? She dropped 105 pounds, and seven years later she hasn't turned back.

"I had always heard it was impossible to lose weight after 40," says Nancy. "And there I was at 39 weighing 240 pounds."

She had been heavy all her life, and as a young woman she had tried to lose weight "all the wrong ways. I took diet pills. I took laxatives. I made myself throw up. When you're a teenager without any dates and you think it's because you're too fat—I weighed as much as 170—you'll try anything to lose weight."

Sometimes she succeeded, only to regain the lost weight and then some. But as she got older, she gained more steadily. When she got married and had her first daughter, Nancy gained 50 pounds; with her second daughter, she gained even more.

"I wasn't active at all," Nancy admits, "and my eating habits were pretty poor. I could sit down at night and eat four or five peanut butter and jelly or bologna sandwiches. And I loved all kinds of fattening sweets like cakes and pies. I thought, I'll drink diet soda to balance out the calories. But the truth was, I didn't care how much I gained."

However, once her daughters got a little older, she started working as a crossing guard at a grade school, and then it was a different story. "People I did not even know started making fun of me," Nancy recalls sadly.

"Strangers would holler things like, 'Don't walk on the sidewalk! You're gonna crack it!'

"I acted as if it didn't affect me, but it did. And my weight was starting to affect my health, too." Nancy had such severe muscle spasms in her lower back (worsened by her weight) that she had to be taken to a hospital several times. Though her blood pressure was a safe 120/80, her cholesterol, at 233, was definitely high.

But the turning point for Nancy came the day before Valentine's Day 1985, when she walked up the stairs at her home and found she could hardly breathe. "I decided that was it. It was time to try to lose weight for good. The following day, I gave all of my Valentine's candy away!"

Next, Nancy started cutting out all the fattening sweets she used to eat—the candies, cakes and pies—as well as eliminating salt. "I used to pour salt on every bite of food I took," she says. "But I knew from reading about health that salt makes you retain water and can raise blood pressure in people who have a tendency toward hypertension."

She also began eating three balanced meals a day: cereal with fruit for breakfast, a salad for lunch and a chicken or fish dish for dinner. "I cut red meat and lots of other fats out of my diet. I'd never used a lot of butter, but I started using low-fat salad dressings rather than rich ones. And I began cooking differently. I used to fry everything, so I switched to broiling or microwaving, adding no fat whatsoever."

Nancy still loved sandwiches, but she went from those made with fatty meats to tuna sandwiches without mayonnaise, topped instead with lettuce and tomato, all on reduced-calorie bread. "In fact," she says, "I found I loved to eat plain tomato sandwiches!"

For snacks she turned to celery, bananas or apples and, every once in a while, artificially sweetened candies to satisfy her sweet tooth. She also drank plenty of low-fat milk, which satisfied her between meals. "But," she adds, "I knew dieting alone wouldn't help me keep off weight. So I started to exercise, too."

She understood the value of exercise because she had seen the good it had done for her husband. He had had a weight problem himself until the year before Nancy started her diet, and jogging had helped him shed 65 pounds. Nancy had never gone jogging with him because she was afraid of hurting her bad back "and I thought I was too fat. But when I started my diet, he suggested that I try walking. That I knew I could handle."

She started out walking two to three miles twice a day, between her crossing-guard shifts. Then she'd walk again in the evenings with one of her daughters, who's very active and encouraged her mom in her new fitness regimen. "I started out slowly, figuring it would be difficult for me to breathe," says Nancy. "But I found I could do it, no problem!"

Soon she started speeding up and increasing her distance. After several weeks, she was walking five miles three times a day, every day except

Sunday. "The more I walked, the more I enjoyed it! And after a few months of walking and eating right, the pounds just melted off. Instead of making fun of me, people were stopping to compliment me!" By June Nancy had lost 80 pounds.

But that same month her weight loss reached a standstill. "And since I was still determined to lose more weight, I decided to join my husband and try jogging. I still felt fat, and I didn't want anyone to see me, so I went to a nearby cemetery that's two miles around. At first, I could only jog down the hills and walk the rest—my breathing was very uncomfortable. But slowly I built up my endurance and I got used to breathing correctly. Soon I could jog the whole two miles!"

It took about three weeks for Nancy to get off her weight-loss plateau, and she started dropping weight again. Over the next three months, she lost 25 more pounds. "I also ran a two-mile race with some hills that, to me, seemed like mountains. I didn't place, but I did finish, and that was my goal."

Nancy discovered that she loved jogging so much that she joined a runners' club. "I started running races and even won a few trophies in my age division. I'm up to running a nine-minute mile!"

By the time Nancy reached her 40th birthday that August, she was down to about 120 pounds. She had a big celebration "but without a cake!" she says, with no hint of disappointment.

That fall, her weight dipped to below 120 pounds and she started feeling underweight. "So I started eating a little more of the right foods, like skinless chicken, salads and fruits. I even allotted myself some sweets, like low-calorie cake. By doing that, I built my weight back up to 135. I looked much better."

All her hard work paid off. At 40, Nancy was a totally different woman. "When school started in the fall and I returned to my post as the crossing guard, people didn't even recognize me. The mailman who'd passed me for four years didn't know who I was!" she laughs.

Now, seven years later, her weight is holding at 135. Her back problems are gone, her blood pressure has dropped to 108/72 and her cholesterol is down to 200. She works evenings now, so she's switched to afternoon jogs—four to eight miles a day. And instead of hearing nasty comments from strangers, Nancy hears wolf whistles!

"I find that I can eat a lot more now and stay slim as long as I continue to eat a low-fat diet," says Nancy. "I feel great about myself now. I'm never turning back!"

Getting Over "Heartbreak Hill"

When the Reverend St. George Crosse weighed 419 pounds, a parishioner told him, "Some people are Chihuahuas, Reverend Crosse, and some are St. Bernards. You happen to be a St. Bernard."

"My parishioners didn't seem put off by my girth," says Crosse. "I thought people liked you to be big—they associate size with authority. And so many church functions involve food. Everyone is always trying to feed the minister!"

But preaching in the enthusiastic style his parishioners loved left Crosse exhausted and fearing a heart attack. "I had to sit down immediately after my sermons," says Crosse. "I would get so tired and out of breath.

"One day, at a reception following a funeral, I overheard a woman saying, 'How can he teach us to control our spirits when he can't control his appetite?' I figured a lot of other people might be saying the same thing. Then, when two of my close friends had heart attacks and strokes, I decided it was time to do something about my weight."

The first thing Crosse needed was to find determination and self-control. For that, he turned to God. "I had been abusing my body. I prayed for forgiveness and for self-control, as an addict might." His search for an appropriate weight-loss program led him to his dog, Bronco. "He eats when he's hungry, stops when he's full and never stops exercising," says Crosse. "I decided the same thing should work for me."

He soon learned that this was a good place to start, but it wasn't enough. So Crosse began cutting out fried foods, salt and sugar. "I learned to eat lots of fruit and salads during the day. I would eat my main meal, which was also low in fat and well balanced, with my wife in the evening," he says. Then, to attain a 200-pound weight-loss goal, he began a protein-sparing, modified-fasting program under the supervision of his physician. And Crosse began to walk.

"At first, I'd just walk around my multilevel house—a few steps here and there kept me huffing and puffing. I could walk for only ten minutes or so.

"Then my wife and I started walking together outside. The biggest challenge was a hill by our house we nicknamed 'Heartbreak Hill.' On the way back up the hill to our house, I'd have to stop halfway because my back ached so terribly."

Gradually, Crosse worked up to 4 miles every weekday, with a 12-mile walk on Saturday. And Heartbreak Hill stopped hurting.

"My weekday walks are often on a treadmill because my job in Washington doesn't allow me the time to walk in my neighborhood. But on Saturday mornings, I walk six miles out and six miles back. I like to walk alone because it gives me the chance to practice my sermons. Sometimes my wife joins me for a while, but my pace has gotten a little too brisk for her."

The rewards for his pilgrimage? Today, at 53, Crosse is a healthy 234 pounds. "At 6'2", I'll always be a big man," says Crosse. "But now I'm healthy. I have energy. My blood pressure and cholesterol levels are healthy. And my daughters are willing to dance with me!"

In fact, his two daughters help keep him on track. "They care enough about me to let me know if I'm putting on a little weight," says Crosse, "and I appreciate that. I've reconciled myself to the fact that keeping my weight down is a lifetime journey for me. As part of my modified-fasting program, if I regain more than 10 percent of my goal weight I return to my meal-replacement program and, with the help of my physician, eat healthy foods and increase my daily walking.

"That's the great thing about walking," he adds. "On Saturdays, I always pass a tiny, old woman who must be in her nineties. She's going slow, but she's going. Walking is something I'm sure I'll be able to do for a very, very long time."

KEEPING IT OFF FOREVER

Beverly's lost 29 pounds, and now she's smiling like the cat who just swallowed the (low-fat) canary. She has boundless reserves of energy, she looks terrific in shorter skirts and though she's been slowly losing for seven months, the compliments are still trickling in. She even gets an appreciative wolf whistle from her husband every now and then.

Beverly's a happy woman, no question, but she's also a little scared. After all, she's reached this stage before, and she wasn't able to maintain her weight loss then. In fact, when she regained her weight she put back even more than she had taken off. (Sound familiar?) Her determination is high at the moment, but will it last?

Meeting the Biggest Challenge

The truth is, Beverly's right to be concerned. Any diet veteran will tell you the same thing: Weight loss is simple. Weight maintenance is much tougher. For one thing, after the initial euphoria dies down, real life inevitably intrudes.

"In the beginning, there are a lot of factors helping to keep you motivated, such as getting compliments as you lose weight," says Susan Zelitch Yanovski, M.D., an obesity expert at the National Institute of Diabetes and Digestive and Kidney Diseases in Bethesda, Maryland. "But as time goes on, people stop commenting on how good you look, and there might be stress at work, or family problems—things that happen day to day. It's very difficult to keep up that level of motivation over a lifetime without some reinforcements."

"What works today doesn't necessarily work tomorrow," adds Joyce D. Nash, Ph.D., a clinical psychologist in the San Francisco Bay area and the author of several books on weight maintenance, including *Now That You've*

Lost It: How to Maintain Your Best Weight. "Our health changes, our metabolism changes. And we always have to adjust to transitions in life: going off to college, which is often a source of weight gain, especially for females, or having a first child, or divorce, or menopause. Life changes can impact our weight level, so we must constantly adapt to our environment."

Saying No to the Yo-yo

If in the past "handling" life changes has usually meant pigging out, that's out. Forget falling back on your "Oh, well, I can always lose it next time" excuses. The diet yo-yo is a no-no. Why?

Researchers have discovered that there may be negative health consequences of having fluctuating weight. That was the conclusion reached by Kelly D. Brownell, Ph.D., a Yale University psychologist and obesity expert who reported the results of a 32-year study on weight fluctuations and their consequences.

What's more, if it seems as though it gets harder and harder to drop the weight each time you try, you're right. That's because whenever you lose weight, you lose fat and some lean muscle mass; whenever you regain weight, you add only fat. As a result, with each subsequent diet effort, you're struggling with even more tough-to-shed fat than you had the last time around.

It may also be psychologically stressful to be on and off (and on and off) diets. Which is why Dr. Brownell insists, "People should not undertake a diet unless they are really ready not just to lose the weight but to keep it off indefinitely."

Strategies for Success

So assuming you're in the process of accomplishing mission number one—weight loss—and are about ready for mission number two—weight maintenance—there's something you should know. That is: While it'll be a challenge, it will not be a mission impossible. Look around. People do manage to shed pounds and keep them off, and you can join that select and slender club!

The key to successful weight maintenance: commitment to a new, slimmer way of life. We all say we want to be thin, and most of us are committed enough to do what's needed to lose that extra weight. But unless we're ready to permanently change those habits and attitudes that got us overweight in the first place, we're likely to see those pounds creep back on.

A tall order, but you can do it! Just follow these steps for a forever-slim body.

Get real about your weight goal. If you're aiming for a weight that's too low for your height and build, or if you come from a family of big people, or if you are over 50 and have been heavy for some time, getting to and remaining at your goal weight may be a constant struggle. Keep all these factors in mind as you fine-tune your goal.

"Once you establish a weight that's both healthy and one you can live with, you have your target," says Dr. Nash. "It's actually a range; for example, my healthy range is 128 to 140 pounds. If you maintain your weight within an appropriate range, you'll avoid a major relapse, and I don't consider movement within the range a major relapse."

Sound the three-pound alarm. Indeed, you'll never have a major relapse if you sound what Dr. Nash calls the three-pound alarm and take immediate action once you see you're that much outside your range. Similarly, if your eating behavior should temporarily go out of kilter—say, if you overdo things at the restaurant tonight—compensate right away by cutting back a bit on your food and exercising more.

"That way," says Dr. Nash, "self-regulation goes on all the time. What we want to do is to avoid waking up one morning to find we're 40 pounds away from a healthy weight."

Make a commitment to yourself. Tell yourself (and mean it!) that this time you're losing the weight for good. You might find it helpful to actually write out a brief statement, a contract with yourself, spelling out what your health and weight goals are during this period of maintenance and how you intend to achieve them. Your contract might include such terms as, "If I overeat at the company banquet tonight, I'll ride my bike for an extra 60 minutes this week." The terms don't have to have a negative edge to them, they can also include positive rewards, such as, "If I stick to my strength-training program for four straight weeks, I'll reward myself with a new CD."

Refer to this contract whenever you feel your motivation slipping.

Keep low-fat in the forefront. Continue to focus on the variety of low- and nonfat foods that helped you reach your goal weight, and plan on maintaining this healthy program with some adjustments here and there. Add some extra food to your menu during the first week, a bit more during the second week, and so forth. Fine-tune your fat and calorie intake until you see your weight stabilize.

Continue to check nutrition labels at the supermarket, and aim for no more than 25 percent of your calories from fat. And make sure you include some of your favorite foods each day to avoid feelings of deprivation.

Keep up that workout! By now you've probably become a lot more active than you were at the start of your diet, and if you've chosen activities you enjoy, you'll find it no problem to continue your regular aerobic workouts.

Aim for a minimum of three 30-minute sessions weekly, increasing that schedule if you start to notice a few pounds creeping back on. And as soon as you start getting a bit bored with your jogging, stair-climbing or whatever, switch to something new. Don't forget your twice-a-week resistance training either.

"Exercise can also be used more specifically for relapse prevention," note Dr. Brownell and Carlos M. Grilo, Ph.D., in a report on the importance of exercise in weight loss. "First, planning exercise during vulnerable times—

Weight-Loss Winners: What's Their Secret?

Some people shed pounds and keep them off, seemingly with ease, while others struggle for a lifetime to maintain their ideal weight. How do you separate the winners from the, er, gainers diet-wise?

"In my research, I've looked at the differences between successful maintainers and those who relapse at one time or another, and I have found two significant differences in the way the maintainers think," explains Joyce D. Nash, Ph.D., a clinical psychologist in the San Francisco Bay area and the author of *Now That You've Lost It: How to Maintain Your Best Weight.* "First, they stay aware of what they're doing. They don't go 'unconscious' or on 'automatic pilot.' " Which means they know just when they're about to have more pasta than is good for them, or that they need to get back to their walking program.

"Those who don't maintain their weight use denial—'It won't hurt me to have it this one time'—or a variety of excuses," says Dr. Nash. "This gives them permission to engage in behaviors that undo their weight-loss success."

Successful maintainers have a set of guiding principles they refer to on a regular basis, says Dr. Nash. "People need guiding principles to hold the decision power for them. Things like, 'I don't eat that' or 'I want to stay away from too many fat calories.' The diet or program you're following usually defines the rules for you. This is a strategy that shifts your attention away from the immediate situation to a superior set of values."

Having an established set of values that you refer to regularly will remind you of the goals you're trying to achieve, and help keep you on target.

lonely weekends or periods of high stress—represents an excellent preventive coping strategy. Second, using exercise during a tempting situation is likely to be effective. If you are home alone, feeling bored and wish to eat the junk food in the cabinet, going for a walk instead can prevent the overeating, weaken the temptation, burn calories and lead to increased confidence. Third, the use of exercise after a high-risk situation, regardless of whether overeating occurred, can also enhance maintenance."

Not bad for a simple walk around the park!

Write it down. "After people lose their weight, they often start relaxing in terms of their eating and exercise pattern—first a little, then a little more. And eventually they may relax completely," notes registered di-

Talking to Yourself

Those little voices that you hear in your head may be driving you . . . off your diet.

The things that you tell yourself both during and after a concerted weight-loss effort can have a powerful impact on your long-term success, says Joyce D. Nash, Ph.D., a clinical psychologist in the San Francisco Bay area and the author of *Now That You've Lost It: How to Maintain Your Best Weight.*

The trick to keeping your self-talk from undermining your accomplishments is to talk back. Any time you catch yourself putting down your own efforts, you need to be ready with a quick comeback.

Here's how it works.

"I'm gaining weight—I might as well quit."

"No, I need to reevaluate my strategy and make the right changes. If I keep making healthy choices, the weight will come off."

"I was meant to be fat."

"Genes are not destiny. Even if I have a fat family, I can minimize a tendency to fatness by adopting a healthy lifestyle."

"If it weren't for my (job, kid, etc.) I could lose weight."

"My job (or my kid) may be demanding, but I just need to be more creative in finding a way to deal with this."

"She (or he) insists that I eat."

"I won't let myself be pushed around. I need to stand up for my well-being and say no."

"I deserve a little treat now and then."

"Yes, I do deserve a treat now and then, but it doesn't have to be food. How about a bubble bath or a long walk in the woods?"

"It's not fair that others can eat what they want and I can't."

"I have to work with my metabolism and my needs, no matter what others do. It's not fair to my body to make unhealthy choices."

"I'll start tomorrow."

"Today is the only time I've got—there are no guarantees about tomorrow. If I don't start now, it may be too late tomorrow."

etitian Judy E. Marshel, director of Health Resources of Great Neck, New York, and a member of the American Dietetics Association. "They've grown used to their slimmer body, which was once so new and exciting, and now keeping it slim through exercise and a sensible diet seems like too much trouble."

The cure for sagging motivation? Write it down! "Your Perfect Weight Success Diary," on page 275 is a great place to start, but a simple spiral-bound notebook is equally fine. Jotting down that frozen yogurt bar you nearly forgot you ate while watching TV, or the Jazzercise class you skipped because you had the flu last week, will help you stay focused on your fitness program and keep you going.

Be your own cheerleader. As we mentioned before, once the praise drops off, the pounds often pile back on. Says Marshel: "A person who gets accustomed to hearing compliments during her journey to her goal weight will stop hearing them once she gets there. And if you're not an inner-directed person—someone who can motivate herself and doesn't wait for outside pressures or influences—you'll have a harder time keeping your weight off without that outer support."

The trick, then, is to be your own best diet buddy. Constantly remind yourself of your weight-loss achievements by reviewing the positive steps you took to get you to where you are now. Periodically dig out some "before" pictures of yourself for a quick ego boost. Treat yourself to a small gift every month that you're within two or three pounds of your desired weight. You deserve it!

Develop stress-management techniques. You may be feeling on top of the world now that you're finally at (or very close to) the weight you want to be. But face it: You're not always going to feel this great. The day will soon come when you and your spouse get into an argument, or your teenage son dents the car, or your boss criticizes your work. You're going to be awfully tempted to take out your aggression on a family-size bag of chips, but not if you plan your bad-mood strategy.

How will you foodlessly handle your anger/stress/sadness/boredom when it inevitably strikes? Make a mental or written list of pleasurable activities, such as going for a walk, calling a friend, working on a hobby or soaking in a warm, scented bath. Take your pick, and steer clear of food.

Prepare for special occasions. You won't always be in situations that you can easily control, such as your kitchen. Life is, after all, full of restaurant dining, vacations and other good times. In fact, Dr. Nash's research reveals that nearly twice as many people found positive situations more challenging to their diet than negative emotions. "Any kind of socializing occasion presents a challenge to weight management," she says. "There's often the inclination to say, 'What the heck! This time it won't matter.'"

Again, planning will head trouble off at the pass. If you know that special events with bigger-than-usual meals are coming up, prepare for them by cutting back a little before and afterward, and plan on dining sensibly at the party or restaurant. If drinking alcohol tends to make you careless about your eating habits, stick to club soda with lime, or some fruit juice.

Memorize a diet mantra. Says Dr. Nash, "People have told me about a phrase they repeat to themselves: 'Nothing tastes as good as being thin feels.' This is great—it's a little aphorism that keeps reminding them of their long-term goal."

Take a refresher course. Periodically, urges Dr. Yanovski, "look and see what you're doing or, more likely, what you've stopped doing. Exercising? Keeping food records? Watching the fat in your diet? If you've dropped out of a weight-loss program, check in again. Or call a nutritionist for a booster session or two. You need to realize what kind of help you need, and when you need it."

Forgive yourself if you slip up. Face it: You're a food lover, and only human. You're not always going to be able to control your eating and your weight perfectly, so don't beat yourself up if you have a minor (or even a major!) relapse. If you've put back a couple of pounds—something everybody, no matter how vigilant, does sooner or later—don't get disgusted and throw in the towel. Instead, remind yourself how far you've come with an I-did-it-before-and-I-can-do-it-again attitude. Learn to focus on the bigger picture, get back to your good habits, and the extra few pounds will soon be gone.

Remind yourself why you dieted in the first place. Once you've reached your desired weight, you no longer have a weight-loss goal, but rather a *lifestyle* goal. There's no immediate reward to look forward to; what you're now embarking on—weight maintenance—is a lifetime endeavor.

As Marshel says: "During maintenance, there isn't that psychological reward of getting on the scale and seeing a smaller number each week. Now your goal is to see the same number all the time, and for some people it's not nearly as satisfying." When all is said and done, your focus has to shift so it seems worth the constant effort. For example, there's the psychological reward of waking up each morning knowing your clothing will fit.

But remember, you've just devoted the last weeks or months of your life to a program designed to enhance nothing less than your looks, your health, your self-esteem and your happiness. Aren't these things important enough to hold on to forever?

Part Three

ONE YEAR
TO YOUR
PERFECT WEIGHT

YOUR PERFECT WEIGHT 52-WEEK PLAN

You've undoubtedly heard the expression, "Today is the first day of the rest of your life." Well, think of today just that way, for you're about to launch not another diet but a whole new way of living that will ensure you a slim body, radiant good health and feelings of eating satisfaction. Sound too good to be true? Not at all. It's possible, and it's something more and more people are getting into because they've finally come to a stark realization: Dieting doesn't work, but a combination of low-fat food and regular exercise does.

A little less ice cream here, a little more walking there—that's really all it takes to shed that excess weight for good. In these pages we'll be showing you the way to go, through a combination of savvy food swaps and easy low-fat meal preparation, stepped-up activity, including a weekly walking goal, and quick tricks to help you stay psyched for success.

If you aim for a 500-calorie-a-day deficit—the number of calories you need to burn (or avoid) to achieve slow but steady weight loss—you should expect to drop about a pound a week. Six months from now you can be 20 or 25 pounds lighter, not from a diet, but from your brand new lifestyle.

Your Perfect Weight 52-Week Plan is designed for everyone, whether you have been totally inactive and have a substantial amount of weight to lose or fairly active and have just a few pounds you'd like to shed. As you'll see, while the exercise portion of the 52-week plan gets progressively more challenging week by week, you will not have to exert yourself beyond your capabilities. It's meant to be a program you can comfortably follow for life.

Each week you'll be given new food and fitness activities to try. Aim to build as many of them into your daily routine as you can. The symbols beside them—a fork, sneakers and a head—will tell you at a glance whether the activity deals with eating, exercising or boosting your motivation.

Oh, one more thing. With Your Perfect Weight 52-Week Plan, you won't need any fancy workout equipment, food-measuring gizmos, shiny spandex leotards or computer-generated menus. You will, however, need one indispensable item without which the plan cannot possibly succeed. It's called *commitment*—the determination to change your eating and exercise behavior for the better. But with such a wonderful, important goal ahead of you, how can you not feel a powerful sense of commitment? After all, you're not simply going to lose 20 or 30 pounds, you're going to be changing your life for the better, forever.

Let's get started!

7/24/95

WEEK 1

Day 1: Set some goals
Exercise goal: Take a ten-minute walk

Question: How can you know if you've succeeded at something if you don't know what your goal is? Answer: You can't. Which is why Your Perfect Weight 52-Week Plan gives you weekly goals (and during Week 1, daily goals) to help you focus on and take the reins of your weight-loss success.

What's so great about goals? They're specific and they're measurable, so that by the end of the allotted time you've given yourself, you've either achieved your goals . . . or you haven't, and you can aim to do better next time. No one's expecting perfection here, by the way, but setting goals actually makes it easier to accomplish what you set out to do.

Day 1 is the ideal opportunity to establish your overall goals for fitness and slimming down. We'll also be offering minigoals in the coming weeks on food, exercise and motivational themes to help you keep going to the weight-loss finish line.

Changing Your Ways

Remember, you should set behavior goals rather than weight-loss goals, because you can control your own actions far more easily than you can control what happens to the arrow on the bathroom scale. With this in mind, your goals might include such items as:

- To reduce my fat intake to 25 percent of my daily calories within three months

- To do some kind of exercise for at least 15 minutes each day

- To write down everything I eat and drink every day

- To avoid eating after 8:00 P.M.

- To do 15 minutes of additional exercise any time I've eaten more than I planned to

- To replace my usual morning coffee-and-Danish with a low-fat snack

You get the idea. Think about which of your particular habits have caused your potbelly or love handles and what needs changing the most, then write them down. We'll show you in the days and weeks to come how to make those crucial changes, and you're bound to be pleased at your future weigh-ins.

Weigh to Go

And speaking of weigh-ins . . . weigh in today! Don't be afraid, even if it's been a long while since you and that square metal guy sitting on your bathroom floor have made physical contact. Remember, it's not where you start, it's where you're headed that's important. And on this journey, you'll be sleeker and slimmer next week, next month, next year than you are today.

For now, jot down your weight on the line on page 180 or on the first page of "Your Perfect Weight Success Diary," on page 275. You should plan on weighing yourself and recording that number just once a week—no more, no less.

By the way, if you're unsure as to what weight you should be aiming for, this is a good time to reread "Setting Your Goal Weight," on page 12.

Whatever number you choose for yourself, realize that over the next few months this number may very well change as the pounds come off and your weight starts to stabilize. That's fine—you're aiming for a weight range you can live with forever, and you may not know what that range is at this moment.

Even more important, start to think of all these numbers as guidelines for measuring your progress, not as things to make you feel good or bad about yourself. If Your Perfect Weight 52-Week Plan does nothing else but get you to stop obsessing about the scale and start focusing on your ever-improving eating and exercise activities, it will have helped you accomplish a great deal.

Take a Walk

Once you've got your goals on paper, go for a walk.

In the days and weeks to come, you'll enjoy a growing awareness of the joy of daily activity and how crucial it is to your weight-loss program. Tomorrow you'll find out just why walking is the perfect exercise—regardless of the shape you're in today or hope to be next year—and how you can use it as the basis of your workout program.

For today, though, simply put on your most comfortable shoes and take a pleasant, ten-minute stroll. If it's your first such walk in a while, really enjoy it. Pay attention to how it makes you and your body feel. You're going to be doing a lot of this from here on, and you're going to love the almost magical way it will help you peel off pounds and keep them from returning.

Date: _**7/24/95**_

Weight: _**186.7 Doctor's scale / 178 home**_

Day 2: Pick an exercise program
Exercise goal: Take a 15-minute walk

Today we're going to focus on one of the three key components of Your Perfect Weight 52-Week Plan. The three keys are low-fat eating, exercise and motivation.

Today the spotlight shines on—you guessed it—exercise, the simple yet profound ingredient for lifetime slimness.

In order to make exercise a part of your life it simply has to be something you enjoy doing. You need to ferret out all the ways you enjoy being active, and make those things the foundation of your weekly workout regimen.

Now is the perfect time to decide to get back into a once favorite sport (swimming? bike riding? ice skating?) or try something brand new (jazz dancing? in-line skating? water aerobics?). The key is for you to feel like it's really fun.

If, for openers, you'd rather try something more basic, there's always walking. There's no need to apologize for selecting walking as your exercise of choice. Walking is a great exercise for everyone in terms of ease and comfort. It's also something you can do regardless of your current fitness level.

Because walking is such an ideal form of exercise, that's the activity we'll focus on in this program. In these pages you'll be given a weekly walking goal as part of a 52-week plan created by Casey Meyers, a St. Joseph, Missouri–based walking coach who lectures and conducts walking clinics for the Cooper Wellness Program at the Cooper Aerobics Center in Dallas. Meyers is the author of *Walking: A Complete Guide to the Complete Exercise.*

Move That Body

Meyers discovered the joys of walking in his fifties, and today, at age 66, he's one of its biggest boosters. "Walking is the number-one exercise," he says. "It has the highest adherence rate and the lowest drop-out rate, and it's not injurious. One of the beauties of walking is that it literally massages your muscles while you do it, so you can pick up pace gradually and not experience any discomfort.

"And," he says, "if you're talking about walking for weight loss, then you're talking about a lifestyle change, moving away permanently from being sedentary to being active. In order to do something for rest of your life, it must be enjoyable, something you look forward to doing every day."

Incorporating a walking program into your daily life can actually improve your eating habits, thus putting a double whammy on body fat. "As you become a serious exercise walker," says Meyers, "you start to develop the mental discipline that will also help with the way you eat."

He should know: Not only has daily walking helped him shed 52 pounds but it also has helped keep them off. "In nine years my weight hasn't fluctuated by more than two pounds, even through the holidays," says Meyers with pride. Exercise, then, is critical to weight loss and beyond. "You must stay with it even after you hit your goal weight," Meyers insists. "Now's when you want to nail down the exercise habit for a lifetime."

Today, pick a favorite path or area you've always wanted to explore on foot. Increase your time from yesterday's brief stroll and walk for 15 minutes or so. Make sure you enjoy the walk. At no time in this 52-week plan should you push yourself to the point of discomfort. Go easy on yourself. You'll be gradually working up to longer, daily walks during which you'll increase not only your distance but also your intensity level to help give you a terrific fat-busting workout.

If at any point in this 52-week plan the designated goal feels like it's a bit much for you, simply alter it to suit your individual needs. It's okay for you to move at a slower pace, as long as you keep on moving.

Plan Your Next Moves

Start planning how much exercise you can reasonably expect from yourself as days go by. This week, Meyers suggests, you should walk a minimum of four days. And remember that the closer you come to daily exercise, the steadier your weight loss will be, the more easily you'll be able to maintain your goal weight and the more low-fat food you'll be able to eat without packing the pounds back on. (Pretty good incentives, no?)

Also, begin to think about when you'll be most apt to want to work out. Early morning, before your day gets crazy? As a lunchtime break? After dinner, strolling with a friend or family member? Will you plan extra exercise time on weekends to catch up, or are Saturdays and Sundays days you'd prefer to leave your walking shoes in the closet? It's up to you. Just be honest with yourself about what you can and can't expect from yourself. "Consistency is the most important aspect of your walking program," says Meyers.

As with your food, write down your exercise today—what you did and for how long. This is the basis upon which you'll be building your lifetime fitness program.

Day 3: Customize your food plan
Exercise goal: Walk 20 minutes (or take a break)

If you want to be thin forever, high-fat foods have got to go! Chances are they've been the single biggest contributors to your weight problem. Fat calories are harder to burn off than carbohydrates and protein, and are more readily converted to body fat.

You don't even get much bang for your caloric buck when you eat fats, because they weigh in at a big nine calories per gram versus just four for carbs and protein. So the sooner you start moving high-fat foods out of your diet and replacing them with fruit and vegetables, beans and breads, fish and low-fat dairy products, the quicker you'll see a slimmer, trimmer body.

Today, start by rereading "A Beginner's Guide to Cutting Fat," on page 19, and reviewing the "Fat Budget" table, on page 23. It will show you exactly how to trim your fat intake to a skinny 25 percent of total calories, without having to use a calculator or keep a running tally of calories.

And to help you start becoming more aware of your food preferences and patterns—say, if you're a chocoholic, or if you have trouble preparing a meal without nibbling your way through it—be sure to jot down everything you've eaten today, and review it sometime before bedtime. There's one more thing you can do to help you get off to a good start.

Clean Out the Fridge

This is a scary prospect for some people: the idea of throwing away food instead of sending it down the usual hatch. But you've got to make a clean sweep, literally and figuratively, if you hope to win the weight-loss game.

So, be brave today and go through your fridge, cabinets and pantry with a fine-tooth comb. What has to go? We'll give you some hints.

- Anything you sneak-eat after the family goes to sleep

- Anything you tend to eat in unnaturally large quantities

- Anything you've been known to keep hidden in the hamper

- Anything that leaves crumbs on the rug and grease on your fingers

- Anything your kids fight over

Admittedly, this procedure will be tough if you have a family that likes to eat a lot of the sugary, high-fat foods you're trying to avoid. But while you may not be able to simply dump all their favorites, your efforts to transform your kitchen from fattening to low-fat only means you'll be gradually improving their diets as well.

Go through each bowl and bottle, carton and container, even those bits of aluminum foil hiding in the back of your refrigerator since Arbor Day, and see what's in them. If you're not sure, read the food label on the package.

Anything overly high in fat and/or sugar? Get rid of it or, at the very least, keep it until your next trip to the supermarket where you can buy a low-fat, sugar-free equivalent. Then throw it out.

From here on in, you'll be grocery-shopping smarter than ever before, and, as a result, your cupboards and pantry will be stocked with foods your family likes and that will also do your diet good. After all, if it's not in your house, you won't eat it.

Do It Your Way

Designing a low-fat diet around your personal likes, dislikes and daily routine is the surest way to success on the scale—far more effective than your trying to conform to a cookie-cutter weight-loss regimen. "It's more important that your diet and exercise plan fit into your lifestyle than your lifestyle fit into your diet and exercise plan," says Ronna Kabatznick, Ph.D., psychologist with Weight Watchers International.

Losing weight your way means you don't have to resign yourself to celery-stick-and-parsley-sprig suppers. Happily, it means being able to have your favorites, in moderation.

"Completely eliminating your problem foods may set you up for failure," says registered dietitian Judith Stern, Sc.D., professor of nutrition and internal medicine at the University of California, Davis. However, she adds, "You have to determine what those foods are and find replacements for them if you can't control your appetite for them."

Now's the time to get even specific about how and when you'll be eating in the days and weeks ahead. Read the list of statements below. Wherever they apply to you, check and use the accompanying tips to help you begin to create your own perfect, custom-made diet plan.

I rarely plan when or what I'm going to eat.

_____Always keep the kitchen stocked with the makings of one or two of your favorite dishes, before they run out.

_____Keep a couple of low-fat frozen meals in the freezer.

_____Once every few weekends, make a hearty grain-and-veggie casserole, a pot of soup or a big bowl of ratatouille and freeze it so it'll be ready to microwave for a quick lunch or supper.

I eat too much at mealtime.

_____Fill your plate in the kitchen, then immediately wrap and freeze the remainder.

_____Use portion-controlled, low-fat frozen meals.

_____Serve your meals on salad plates instead of dinner plates—you may feel as though you're eating more.

I'm a snacker.

_____Stick to low-cal, low-fat snacks like fruit, raw veggies, tomato juice, rice cakes and frozen-fruit bars.

_____Eat more complex carbohydrates (pasta, bread, rice, potatoes) at mealtime for a greater feeling of fullness.

_____Drink water. Your "hunger pang" may really be thirst.

I eat on the run.

_____Depend on grocery store salad bars (skip the mayo-soaked macaroni and the cheese chunks), frozen low-fat meals, microwavable potatoes topped with low-fat cheese or yogurt.

_____Stick to the lowest-fat choices at fast-fooderies, such as grilled chicken sandwiches (hold the mayo) and salads with low-fat dressings.

_____Carry low-fat mini-meals in your purse or briefcase: an apple, bread sticks or low-fat cheese, for example, or a pear, a small bottle of mineral water, a whole-wheat pita stuffed with cut-up veggies.

I sample while I cook.

_____Sip ice water while you stir and chop.

____Chomp on raw veggies or air-popped popcorn.

____Stick to low-fat, low-calorie meals and your nibbling won't do much harm.

I'm always the first one finished.

____Put your fork down between bites.

____Choose slow-to-eat foods—lobster, shrimp in the shell, artichokes, watermelon.

____Make a game out of being the last to finish.

Remember that however you adjust your eating habits, one thing remains constant: Low-fat is where it's at!

Enjoy Your Walk

If you choose to walk today (you'll notice that you have the option to skip a day), step it up to 20 minutes. Don't worry about breaking any speed records, just go at a pace that's comfortable for you. The main thing is to move.

Day 4: Buy new walking shoes
Exercise goal: Walk for 20 minutes

Today start by quickly reviewing yesterday's food-habit checklist so you can plan your eating accordingly. Will you be cooking dinner for the family tonight? Then make sure you choose one of your low-fat nibbling options. Expecting a stressful, nonstop day? Then pack a healthy snack or two to take with you so you don't find yourself staring ravenously into the face of some vending machine at 3:00 P.M.

Get the Right Shoes

It's also high time to do a footwear inspection. If you're going to get serious about exercise, then that old, worn-out pair of sneakers just won't cut it. The $50 or so that you invest in a good pair of walking shoes will make your feet feel so comfortable they'll be itching to hit the road every day. So today, replace those shoes if you need to.

What exactly makes a walking shoe a walking shoe? Every pair has the same key characteristics: a firm heel counter to keep your heel from wobbling, a beveled heel to keep you steadier and make it more comfortable as you come down on your heel, resiliency in the sole to cushion your foot, good arch support and a sturdy lacing structure to help prevent your foot from leaning in or out.

These things are only the basics. Any special features, such as different types of leather and mesh composition, waterproofing, varying sole thickness, a variety of styles and colors, will be determined by the kind of walker you are (or expect to become). What surfaces will you be doing most of your walking on? Will you be walking in all types of weather? Be sure to inform the salesperson of your particular needs before plunking down your credit card.

Here are for more tips to ensure you of the best possible fit.

Always get your foot measured. You won't be a size nine in every shoe, in every brand.

Never plan on "breaking in" your shoes. If they don't feel great in the store, don't take them home.

Buy shoes that are roomy enough. Your walking shoe must have adequate space for your foot to flex as you walk. What's more, your foot can swell to a whole size larger when you walk.

Make sure the heel doesn't fit too snugly. You should be able to slide a pencil between your foot and the back of your shoe for proper fit.

Take along your socks. When you're out shopping for shoes, don't forget to bring a pair of thick socks like the ones you'll be wearing on your walks. Need some new socks? Opt for synthetics over cotton or wool. The man-made fibers are best for absorbing perspiration and keeping feet drier and odor-free. These socks also retain their shape longer.

And what better way to christen your new walking shoes and socks than by going for a walk! As you can see from today's walking goal, you're going to walk for 20 minutes.

A fit walker can cover a mile in 20 minutes of brisk walking. You might want to lay out a mile-long course for yourself as another means of measuring your progress.

How can you tell when a mile is up? If you're an urban dweller, it's around 20 short city blocks. Otherwise, measure out a mile using your car odometer. (Because you're going to eventually work up to three miles a day, you might want to make a note of the two-mile and three-mile marks as well.)

And on cold or rainy days, plan on doing your fitness walking at an indoor high school or college track (one-quarter mile in circumference) or at a mall (ask someone in the know the distance around the mall).

Today just walk for 20 minutes and see how close you come to walking a full mile. Don't be concerned with speed. If it's nice outside, enjoy the day and the sights along with way, as well as how fit and energized your new walking program is making you feel.

Don't feel you have to push for the mile. Simply note your accomplishment and realize that you'll soon be walking that mile and then some . . . and enjoying it.

Day 5: Have a body-trimming breakfast
Exercise goal: Get fit around the house

Attention all you breakfast-skippers: What you don't know can hurt you and your chances of losing that excess weight.

Those of you who can't stomach early morning food might logically dub breakfast a dispensable meal. You might even conclude that avoiding those A.M. calories is the perfect way to jump-start your diet for the day. But your logic would be cockeyed, say the experts. Worse, you might actually be sabotaging your diet because skipping breakfast may make your metabolism sluggish, increasing snacking later in the day and ultimately leading to weight gain.

Here's the scoop: Some dietitians theorize that while you're asleep your whole body slows down and you burn calories at a reduced rate. It's not until you get up in the morning, start moving around and eat something that your metabolism perks up. Going without a morning meal keeps your body's "furnace" cold longer, so you ultimately burn fewer calories.

Learning to Love Breakfast

Because exercise is a great way to use up extra calories, a healthy breakfast and a light morning workout make an unbeatable weight-loss combo. Whether you eat before or after morning exercise is up to you, says registered dietitian Marilyn Majchrzak, food development manager of the Canyon Ranch Spa in Tucson. "Some of our guests eat a little something before their morning hike; others wait until afterward," she says. "But if people don't eat anything at all in the morning, they tend to fizzle by 10:00 A.M."

"Beginning the day with a healthy breakfast actually gives you the energy to perform at your peak all day long," says James M. Rippe, M.D., director of the Exercise, Physiology and Nutrition Laboratory at the University of Massachusetts Medical Center in Worcester.

And just what constitutes a "healthy" breakfast? One high in complex carbohydrates, says Majchrzak. Complex carbohydrates are found in breads, cereals and vegetables. "We often serve sweet potato waffles, for example," says Majchrzak. "They contain whole-wheat flour and filling sweet potatoes."

Foods high in complex carbohydrates tend to have another plus: fiber. Traditional breakfast foods like whole-grain pancakes, muffins and cereals are loaded with fiber. "Fiber creates an appetite-suppressing effect," says registered dietitian Diane Grabowski, a nutritionist with the Pritikin Longevity Center in Santa Monica, California. "It keeps you satisfied longer."

One more thing about eating breakfast: It's the easiest meal to put together. It's also the one meal of the day in which you are in control over your food intake. Once your day gets going, you don't know what you'll encounter—business lunches, dinners with friends and on-the-run snacks can be a nutritional grab bag. But if you get yourself off on the right foot in the morning, it helps set the tone for the whole day. So today, plan on having a good breakfast and making it the start of every day, from here on in.

Burn Those Calories

And, if you like, you can take another 20-minute walk today. If you're not in the mood, get your workout at home instead. Remember that house-work—vacuuming, washing windows, hauling laundry up and down the basement stairs several times—is exercise, too. So do get some calorie-burning in today—and maybe a cleaner house to boot!

Day 6: Take note!
Exercise goal: Walk one mile (or take a break)

If you haven't already done so, today is the day to really get to know "Your Perfect Weight Success Diary," on page 275. It will, over the next weeks and months, become an invaluable ally in your weight-loss campaign.

All this week you should have been jotting down the foods you've been eating, the type and duration of your exercise and, on Day 1, your starting weight. You will also notice that there are spaces in the diary for recording your body measurements. We as-sume you're not too happy with your numbers right now, but that's okay—you'll see them improving dramatically in weeks to come. Perhaps even more important, you'll see your clothes fit better, your energy level rise and, in all likelihood, better cholesterol and blood pressure readings at your next visit to the doctor.

And, speaking of the doc, if you're taking any kind of medication (there's a space to record that as well), remember that certain medications can cause weight gain or water retention. Tell your physician about your weight-loss program. She can explain precisely how your medicine may affect it. You'll still lose weight, of course, but it might be at a slightly slower pace.

Pay Attention to Feelings

Besides the numbers and meals you'll be recording, the diary also indi-cates spaces for you to write down your moods at the times you ate, the diffi-culties you may have had and the mealtime challenges you face. Whew! If it seems like a lot of work when all you want to do is to eat that turkey sand-wich in peace, you'll find that it gets easier and less time-consuming the more you do it. You'll find that it's worth the effort. Reviewing your notes each day will help you stay on track by making minor adjustments in your eating and exercise routine before they need to become major.

Did you have a substantial, low-fat breakfast this morning? Great!

Walk if You Want To

As for your exercise today, you see you have the option to skip a day of walking. That's because walking expert Meyers feels that it's fine to start your regular exercise program by walking four days the first week. But if you're eager to see quick weight-loss results, you can also keep the mo-

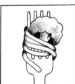

mentum going—and walk!

In the weeks to come you'll hear about other exercise options designed to give your weight-loss program a big boost, including strength training. But whether you decide that walking's the way to go for you or whether you want a more all-around workout, remember that consistency is the key.

Day 7: Focus on five magic foods
Exercise goal: Walk one mile

All week long you've been concentrating on low-fat eating and nearly daily exercise. Great start! But if you've been finding that every now and then you're feeling a bit ravenous, maybe it's because you haven't been filling up on the right kinds of foods. And *that,* warns George Blackburn, M.D., Ph.D., chief of the Nutrition/Metabolism Laboratory at New England Deaconess Hospital in Boston, "can stimulate your appetite and may cause you to binge."

If you start feeling desperate for energy and deprived, you're likely to backslide, to return to your old eating habits and your old, higher weight.

The solution is simple. Today and every day throughout Your Perfect Weight 52-Week Plan, focus on eating more of the five "high-octane" foods that are naturally low in fat, high in complex carbohydrates and high in fiber. These foods are:

- Potatoes and sweet potatoes

- Legumes, such as pinto beans, kidney beans and lentils

- Whole grains, such as whole-grain cereals, pastas, breads and brown rice

- Fruits, such as apples, bananas, berries and melons

- Skim milk and skim-milk products, such as low-fat cottage cheese and yogurt

These foods not only give you the energy you need to power through an active life but can also help you lose weight the "no-hunger" way. Here's how.

They help keep blood sugar levels stable. Dramatic swings in blood sugar from feasting and strenuous dieting can stimulate your appetite and cause you to overeat. These are hearty foods that keep you feeling fuller, longer.

They're low-cal. Because they have half the calories per bite as fatty foods, it means you can eat twice as much and still take in fewer calories than you would if you were eating fatty foods. (But, because high-octane foods are so filling, you'd probably be overstuffed if you tried!)

They naturally drive down your fat intake. All you have to do is make sure they're not prepared with too much fat or doused with rich sauces that offset their weight-loss benefits.

"Magic" Foods Melt Pounds

Here an example of how to go about using these five "magic" foods to create that important 500-calorie-a-day deficit. (This deficit, remember, translates into that one-pound-or-so-per-week weight loss you're striving for.)

- Drink one glass of skim milk instead of whole milk.

- Eat one bowl of oatmeal (whole-grain) instead of a croissant.

- Snack on an apple instead of a granola bar.

- Have oven-fried potatoes, baked with a bit of no-stick vegetable oil spray instead of french fries.

- Enjoy a bowl of bean-based vegetarian chili instead of chili with ground beef.

That's your 500 calories right there! These few changes don't even take into account your exercise routine, which can burn off another 200 to 300 calories a day.

Most of the calories you cut when you fill up on these high-octane foods are from fat. Don't worry so much about weighing and measuring how much you're eating. Simply choose these heartier foods first when you're hungry and stop when you're full. You know when you need to eat and when you've had enough.

And, be a little creative with your meals and snacks. Try low-sugar, whole-grain cereal in the evenings or for a snack, for example. That's also a good way to sneak more skim milk (something that's crucial for women, who need calcium to prevent bone loss as they age) into your diet. If you're fighting the switch from whole milk to skim, first go to 2 percent, then from 2 percent to 1 percent, then to skim.

Hit the Road

Of course, you'll need to walk off these five fabulous foods, so slip on those walking shoes and get moving!

And, as usual, be sure you write down everything you eat and drink—even water—in your success diary, or in a simple notebook.

Have any problems with your food this week? Check your diary to see how you were feeling at the time and plan how you can avoid a similar situation in the future.

One week down!

Congratulations!

WEEK 2: SIGN AN EXERCISE CONTRACT
Exercise goal: Walk five days, 1½ miles per day

Now that you've completed a full week of your 52-week plan, it's time to weigh in! If you've started trimming fat from your diet and you exercised four or more days last week, then you're probably down by a couple of pounds. Good for you! Record that number at the end of this section, as you will once a week from now on.

Chances are you're feeling pretty great about yourself and the way you're looking and feeling, and rightfully so—you're forming wonderful new habits that will last for life. Keep in mind that the first week of any new weight-loss program usually produces top-notch results, especially if you start out with a good deal of weight to lose.

In future weeks, your weight loss will likely taper off to a pound or so a week. And some weeks, you won't lose anything and might even gain half a pound or so. If that happens, don't be alarmed—it's all perfectly normal.

What you want is a nice, slow and steady, permanent weight loss. Keep eating that healthy breakfast and stick to low-fat, fiber-packed foods and you'll do fine.

Walking for Calorie Burn and Fitness

On Day 2, you'll recall, we talked about the weight-loss value of exercise in general and walking in particular. And for the past seven days you've been given a walking goal to aim for, which started off very slowly and easily. In fact, you may even feel as though you haven't been getting much exercise at all. Over the next year, you'll be building on your weekly walking success and working your way up to a substantial level of fitness that will do your ever-slimming body a world of good.

"Walking is a great exercise," says Art Mollen, D.O., medical director of the Southwest Health Institute in Phoenix, Arizona. "It works for most people and burns as many calories as jogging. If you walk at a moderate pace, seven days a week, you'll lose weight."

Yes, *daily* activity is what the experts agree is ideal for weight loss and maintenance. You want to get to the point where exercise is as much a part of your life as brushing your teeth or reading the morning paper. However, as you'll notice, this week's recommendation from walking guru Casey Meyers is to do five days, 1½ miles per day.

He wants you to start out slow and easy, gradually building you up to the ultimate goal of three miles a day, six or seven days a week, taking only 15 minutes to walk each mile, which is where you could well be by Week 41 of this program.

How was this program devised? "Most busy people can manage some exercise four days a week," says Meyers. "Gradually we increase the number of days of exercise by an additional day a week, till we get to six or seven. Then we fold in the *distance*, an extra half mile per week, until we're up to three miles each day. I like to use a base of at least a three-mile walk. Generally, you burn about 100 calories per mile, so to get a 300-calorie burn, that's a good distance to anchor the program on.

"Then you want to work on *intensity*," Meyers adds. "If you start off, say, doing a 20-minute mile—three miles in an hour, which is very conservative—you should slowly start to knock a minute per week off your walking time until you get down to a 15-minute mile, or three miles in 45 minutes. That's what the President's Council on Physical Fitness has determined will give you a good, moderate level of fitness and increase calorie burn."

It can't be emphasized enough that if at any point this walking program feels like it's too intense for you, simply adapt it to your own level of fitness. Add on time, distance and intensity as it feels right for your own body. If it takes longer for you to reach the goals laid out in this program, that's okay. The idea is to move your body regularly, day after day, and enjoy the changes that are taking place in your body.

Commit Yourself to Action

One way to ensure your commitment to your new exercise program is to sign an exercise contract with yourself. "We've used contracts in many different programs, from weight loss to cardiac rehabilitation," says Susan B.

Johnson, Ed.D., director of continuing education at the Cooper Institute for Aerobics Research in Dallas. "And we find they really help people focus on what they want and help them stick with it."

Your contract should state that you'll attempt to reach the weekly walking goals given at the beginning of each week in your 52-week plan. (Or, if you prefer, substitute another type of exercise. But be sure to pace yourself similarly.)

You should also indicate in your contract the consequences of meeting, or not meeting, your goals. If you succeed, you might promise yourself a trip to the movies, or some new, brightly colored sweats. If you don't meet your goals, you might decide to forgo a treat you enjoy. Be creative. Your contract should be signed and dated. Make photocopies and give them to another family member or a friend—ideally, someone who's trying to lose weight, too, who can relate to your goals and help cheer you on.

"There is something about writing down goals and sharing them with others that seems to really help people stick to them," says Dr. Johnson. "You may be surprised at how well this works."

Date: _____

Weight: _____

WEEK 3: BE A SUPER-SHOPPER
Exercise goal: Walk five days, 1½ miles per day

Grocery day! Yup, the time has come to replenish those refrigerator shelves and cabinets with the low-fat, high-fiber foods that will carry you (and your family) in good stead for the rest of your eating days. If you've had your healthy breakfast today, you can head off to market feeling satisfied and good about yourself, and therefore unlikely to do any impulse buying.

You may think your local supermarket holds few mysteries for you by now; after all, you've logged enough hours there to be a pro. You know exactly where the produce aisles are, exactly where the meat case is, and exactly when they put out the free samples in the deli department. But you'll be surprised to find what goodies you uncover, because now you're going to become a supermarket sophisticate, reading labels and comparison shopping and exploring new possibilities as you've never done before.

First, it's a good idea to go back and reread "Shop Talk: Developing Your Supermarket Savvy," on page 41, to pick up a few helpful hints. Here are a few more things to start paying attention to as you shop.

Make a list and check it twice. Make sure you get all the healthy, low-fat foods you'll need for the week down on paper. That way you'll be prepared for all the challenges that face you (plus, you won't have any excuses for not eating right). If you've come across a new low-fat recipe you want to try, be sure you have all the ingredients either in your kitchen or on your list.

Buy something new. Make a point of selecting one healthy, never-before-tried food—rhubarb, raisin-studded English muffins, raspberry tea—to give your taste buds a jolt. The more interesting you make your meals and snacks, the less you'll long for the fatty, sugary foods you used to eat.

Study nutrition labels. It may sound like a boring school assignment, but you'll be pleasantly surprised at how much simpler the government has made food-packaging information. The new Nutrition Facts boxes found on supermarket cans, cartons and bottles look and are much more user-friendly than their predecessors. Remember, you can keep fat out of your diet if you monitor the foods you buy and bring into your home—it's that easy.

Say yes to beef. Red meat need not be a no-no as long as you shop for the leanest cuts. If you keep in mind that meat marked "select" is the leanest (with "choice" your next best choice and "prime" the fattiest of the three), you can occasionally include steak and burgers on the menu with little harm to your diet.

Carry out the carbs. Remember the five "magic" foods we talked about last week, foods such as legumes, pasta and breads that keep you satisfied and slim? Review that list and make sure you fill your basket to the brim with them.

Scope out new sections. If you haven't visited the gourmet/imported food department lately, drop by! You're bound to find something intriguing to tantalize your palate. As always, read the labels carefully, and if you even suspect a lot of fat in that odd-looking container, keep on walking.

Check your calendar for the best buys. To everything, there is a season, and that includes fresh produce. Spring? Ask for asparagus and arti-chokes. In the summer, select juicy peaches, melons, berries and red, ripe tomatoes. Fall? Stock up on apples, pears and pumpkins. Come winter, gather parsnips and turnips to toss in a vegetable stew, not to mention sweet potatoes and butternut squash. If you choose produce when it's in peak season, you'll enjoy wonderful dishes bursting with flavor.

Don't forget that grocery shopping is exercise, particularly if you haul your groceries home by hand, and it's a nice supplement to your walking program. Perhaps you'll want to wait till this evening and walk off your dinner with a buddy, either a two-legged or four-legged kind.

Date: _____

Weight: _____

WEEK 4: DO SOME DE-STRESSING EXERCISES
Exercise goal: Walk five days, 1½ miles per day

The month's winding to a close, and you've been doing great! But you've got to admit that there have been some stressful moments, moments when had you not been quite as strong and on top of things as you are right now, a diet cave-in might have occurred.

Well, the sooner you realize it, the better: Stress is going to rear its head every now and then. What you don't want to do is to let your moods get the best of you. With a few smart stress-busting strategies at the ready, you can cope foodlessly with any situation.

Below are a handful of tension-reducing, energy-releasing exercises. Try a couple of them out this week and see if they don't make you feel calmer instantly.

Feel the stress. "Stress produces real physiological symptoms, and your first step is to figure out what yours typically are," says James S. Gordon, M.D., director of the Center for Mind/Body Medicine in Washington, D.C. Is it a tightening of the gut? Sweatiness? Restlessness? Hunger pangs? This awareness will help you begin to recognize the early signals of your food cravings so you can deal with them sensibly.

Work on your tension spots. Most of us barely have an inkling of where our tension lies. If you've been sitting at the computer for three straight hours, you may feel anxious and unconsciously grab for something sugary or greasy, when what you're really feeling is a case of tense muscles in the neck and shoulders. Dr. Gordon suggests that you deliberately increase the tension in your muscles (for example, scrunch your shoulders or tighten your fists), breathe in and out a few times, then relax.

Ask yourself: How am I feeling? What's upsetting you? Review your notes in "Your Perfect Weight Success Diary," on page 275—your most recent feelings, the events and/or people that are bothering you. Get a handle on exactly what's making you tense. How do your feelings relate to your urges to eat?

Move that body! Exercise is a terrific stress buster. The quickest remedy for frustration or a vile mood is to tie on your sneaks, grab that basketball or tennis racket, and go!

Try yoga or meditation. According to Dean Ornish, M.D., director of the Preventive Medicine Research Institute in Sausalito, California, these techniques "bring you into the present moment rather than let you dwell on the past or worry about the future. You begin to live life fully, as though each moment matters, which, of course, it does. The present moment frees us to change and to explore new patterns, pleasures and possibilities."

If you're new to meditation and yoga, get the basics via a video (some should be available from your neighborhood library), or sign up for a course at your local Y or adult education center.

As always, record your stressful periods and how you handled them in "Your Perfect Weight Success Diary," on page 275. Reviewing these pages each day will keep you and your diet on track. Chances are you're getting better and better with dealing with those tough times without immediately turning to food.

Date: _____

Weight: _____

WEEK 5: GET ACQUAINTED WITH RESISTANCE TRAINING
Exercise goal: Walk five days, two miles per day

How are you doing? Have you been keeping an eagle-eye on your serving sizes to make sure you don't overdo it? Sticking to sensible snacks? Eating breakfast each morning, even if it's just a bowl of cold cereal and skim milk minutes before you you race out the door, half-peeled banana in hand? Good!

And now that you've gotten into the walking groove and are clocking around seven miles a week, how are you feeling? Healthier? More energized? And are you heading to the mall or some such place for your foul-weather workouts? Wonderful! Keep it up. We want you to continue the walking, but this is the week you'll officially start resistance training, too.

Remember, walking and other aerobic exercise are crucial for calorie burning, and while resistance training doesn't burn calories, it's got all kinds of other fabulous benefits for dieters. Such as? Turning body fat into muscle, firming your body as you shed pounds and boosting your metabolism whether you're up and about or taking a snooze. Resistance training on a regular basis, along with your low-fat diet and your walking workout, is going to send your body fat scurrying!

Here's your chance, then, to finally get the flab out and the muscle in! No matter how successfully you've been slimming over the past month, adding resistance training to your weight-loss repertoire will give you an extra boost, both psychologically and physically.

Time to Get Acquainted

How much resistance training is enough to reap these benefits? Aim for two to three 20-minute strength-training sessions per week, in addition to your walking or other aerobics, suggests Wayne L. Westcott, Ph.D., strength-training consultant to the National YMCA and to the National Academy of Sports Medicine. If you're not already a member of a health club or Y, today would be a good day to go over to your local center, check out the machines and ask a few questions. Wear your workout duds under your street clothes—some clubs might be willing to give you a free mini-session on the spot. In future weeks we'll describe some of the best strength-training exercises using machines.

For today, though, you can do your first workout at home, and for that you'll need just one simple piece of equipment: a resistance band, which will be the key component of the following five simple routines. Before you begin, though, keep in mind a couple of points.

Take it easy. Don't hurry or jerk your body: Go slowly and concentrate on your form. And keep your back straight. Repeat the movements 8 to 12 times to make up one set. Do two to three sets per exercise.

S-t-r-e-t-c-h. To warm up, do about five minutes of slow, easy stretches. Don't neglect a five-minute cooldown period at the end, either.

Don't try to be Wonder Woman. Reread "Resistance Training: Pump Up Your Weight-Loss Power," on page 71, so you get a sense of what to expect in terms of results. Your workout should be progressively more challenging but should not cause you to exert yourself beyond reasonable limits.

Building a Beautiful Body

Now, on with the workout! Here are a few simple resistance-training exercises to help you get started.

Chest pull. Grab the band with your two hands and stand with your feet shoulder-width apart. Extend your arms straight out in front of you. Slowly pull your arms apart, stretching the band until your hands are on either side of you and parallel to the floor. Bring your arms back slowly. Repeat.

Outer thigh lift. Lie on your side with the band around your ankles. Lift your top leg slowly, with your heel turned up toward the ceiling as much as possible. (This will keep your foot from pointing, which will in turn keep your thigh lined up correctly for getting the full benefit from this exercise.) Now, lower your leg slowly. Repeat the sets on the other side.

Outer thigh press. Lie on your back with the band around your ankles and your hands under your buttocks. Spread your legs apart, stretching the band. Then bring them slowly back together. Repeat.

Leg extensions. Sit in a sturdy chair with the band around your ankles.

Hold one leg still and raise the other leg until it is parallel to the floor. Return to starting position and repeat. Alternate legs.

Standing arm row. Step on the center of the band with one foot. Grab the other end of the band in both fists. Now pull both fists up toward your underarms. Lower. Repeat.

Don't forget to start keeping track of your resistance-training sessions, right along with your daily walking and your eating. All these activities are working together to give you the slimmest, strongest body you've ever had.

Date: _____

Weight: _____

WEEK 6: ORDER UP WATER

Exercise goal: Walk five days, two miles per day

It's so simple, and yet so effective in helping you control your appetite.

We're talking about drinking water. "Drinking generous amounts of water is overwhelmingly the number-one way to reduce appetite," says George Blackburn, M.D., Ph.D., head of the Nutrition/Metabolism Laboratory at the New England Deaconess Hospital in Boston. 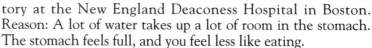 Reason: A lot of water takes up a lot of room in the stomach. The stomach feels full, and you feel less like eating.

Drinking water is also a good way to head off an urge to overeat. According to Dr. Blackburn, sometimes you misinterpret your body's need for water as a food craving. You grab that chicken leg or that slice of cold pizza, and not until it's down the hatch do you realize: "Hey, that's not what I wanted at all!" More often than you think, your "hunger pangs" are really your body's request for water. So the next time you get an urge to eat and it's not your normal mealtime, try a cup of water instead. You may find that your craving has subsided.

By the way, your body's constant need for liquid replenishment is understandable once you know how all that water is being used.

"Each day we take in about 3½ cups of water from the foods we eat—vegetables and fruit, for example, are about 90 percent water. The body also makes about ½ cup of water as a by-product of metabolism," explains registered dietitian Judy E. Marshel, director of Health Resources of Great Neck, New York. "However, each day we also lose 10 to 12 cups of water through climate, body processes, including perspiration and urination, and other factors."

Don't Forget to Wet Your Whistle

You don't have to be a genius to figure out that there's a critical gap here of about eight cups of water, which is why you're always being told to drink that much water every day—more if you're very active. By drinking a full eight glasses every day you not only keep your body healthy but you also feel more satisfied all day long. Another plus for dieters: Drinking water helps keep your skin smooth and supple as you drop excess weight.

How do you make sure you cover the waterfront?

Sip it slow. Don't gulp down an entire glass at a time as if it were medicine, or you'll never continue, advises Dr. Blackburn. Instead, sip three to four ounces at a time, throughout the day.

Get off to a wet start. "Make sure to drink at least some water just before each meal," urges Marshel. "It's a good way to take the edge off your hunger and keep you from overindulging."

Spike it! To give ordinary tap water some zing, add a couple of ice cubes and a squeeze of fresh lemon or lime.

Don't count caffeine. When you're figuring out how much water you're taking in, resist the temptation to include such caffeinated beverages as coffee, tea or colas in your daily total. "They have a diuretic effect," says Marshel. "Because they make you urinate more frequently, they're actually contributing to your body's water loss."

Turn on the tap. If you think you're staying healthy by sticking to bottled water, remember that not all bottled water is alike, or even that beneficial. "Mineral water, for example, comes from a natural spring, which is good. It means that the mineral content remains constant," says Marshel. "But seltzer water is just filtered tap water with some added carbonation, and club soda is filtered tap water with added carbonation, salt and minerals. So if you're spending a dollar or more for a bottle of club soda, what's the sense? It may be no more pure than your own tap water."

If your tap water isn't that good—say, you have an old house with old pipes putting contaminants like lead into the water—try spring water, well water or mineral water.

Make sure you're recording how much water you drink, today and every day, in addition to the meals and snacks you're consuming.

Has any stress been creeping into your life lately? If so, be sure to review some of the de-stressing activities described in Week 4.

And how's the walking going? Meyers, our walking pro, reminds you to make sure you keep a comfortable, sustainable pace. Never overdo it.

Date: _____

Weight: _____

WEEK 7: WATCH YOUR SERVING SIZES!
Exercise goal: Walk five days, two miles per day

Most eating plans ask you to weigh or measure your food, which is about as much fun as balancing a checkbook. That's what's so nice about Your Perfect Weight 52-Week Plan. You don't have to worry about measuring cups and food scales as long as you pay attention to the fat content of the foods you eat, and as long as you have a reasonable sense of what constitutes normal portions. This week you're going to start paying special attention to the portions you eat.

What is a normal portion? If you have a dieting history that ranges from skipping entire meals to eating entire boxes of Chips Ahoy! cookies, then you may not be able to judge serving sizes like folks without a weight problem can. They can eyeball a piece of flounder or a baked potato and know if they're looking at a serving for one or for a small family. If it's too much food, they don't eat it all. A simple concept, yes, but highly effective where it comes to weight control.

Generally, when you cut fat from your diet, you can eat more food. But it is possible to negate your diet efforts if you go haywire on the amounts of low-fat food you consume. If you're accustomed to eating pretzels by the bagful, frozen yogurt by the pint and pasta by the platter, the lists below will help you learn to eat reasonable-sized portions of all your favorites.

And don't forget that you can use the foods we measured here to help you figure out portions of similar foods. For example, the serving size for raisins can be applied to all dried fruits; orange juice is like all fruit juices; and an apple is equal to a pear, tangerine or any other similar-size fruit.

Legumes/Grains/Starch Vegetables

One serving equals:

• A slice of bread

• Two nonfat cookies

• Two rice cakes

• A small pita bread

• A fist-size baked potato

Two servings equal:

• A generous side dish of rice or couscous

• A generous cereal bowl of bran flakes (filled to the brim)

- A cereal bowl of oatmeal

- A whole bagel

- An English muffin

- A generous handful of pretzels

Three servings equal:
- A cereal bowl of low-fat granola (filled to the brim)

- A bowl of bean-based vegetarian chili

Four servings equal:
- A full plate of pasta

- One bag low-fat microwave popcorn

Fruits/Vegetables
One serving equals:
- Four carrot sticks

- A fist-size apple

- A small glass of vegetable juice

- A small glass of orange juice

Two servings equal:
- A side serving of broccoli

- One large banana

- A dessert dish of raspberries

- A generous handful of raisins

Four servings equal:
- An entrée-size salad

Low-fat Dairy/Fish/Poultry/Meat
One serving equals:
- Three egg whites

- A glass of skim milk

- A container of nonfat yogurt

- Two sandwich-size slices of low-fat or nonfat cheese

- A scoop of tuna salad with nonfat mayonnaise

- An extralean ground-meat patty (about ½" thick)

- 12 steamed mussels

- Fish fillet about the size of a deck of cards

Two servings equal:

- A dessert dish of nonfat frozen yogurt

- A whole chicken breast (skinless)

Properly portioning your meals at home shouldn't be much of a problem, but eating out, where portions are often bigger than the average woman (and sometimes the average man) usually eats, gets a bit trickier. Still, just because food is placed in front of you doesn't mean you have to eat it all. You're in charge, remember.

Of course, you're keeping up your walking, and writing everything down, too. Tempted to hop on the scale midweek to see how your weight is doing? Resist the urge! You may see weight fluctuations that don't accurately reflect your eating and exercise program. Wait until your officially designated weigh-in day.

Because you've stuck to your program for a full seven weeks, it's time for a nice, little reward for yourself, just as we suggested during Week 2. It can be as simple as a new tape to listen to on your Walkman during your daily walks, a spiffy workout suit, or a semiextravagant night out with your mate or best friend. Whatever it is, let it serve as a tangible symbol of your success, and enjoy it!

Date: _____

Weight: _____

WEEK 8: SET UP A REWARD SYSTEM
Exercise goal: Walk five days, two miles per day

Remember how wonderful it felt last week to reward yourself for seven weeks' worth of care and attention to your food and fitness program? Well, that delightful little thank-you to yourself for a job well done needn't be a sporadic thing. In fact, a reward system should be built into Your Perfect Weight 52-Week Plan.

Sure, a slim body that comes from a sane and sensible weight-loss program is its own reward—and an excellent one. But even though you have a great reward awaiting you at the end of Your Perfect Weight 52-Week Plan, 52 weeks is frankly too long to wait to collect! We're human beings who crave instant gratification. And so while we learn to live without the immediate (but short-lived) pleasure of a hot fudge sundae, there ought to be something to take its place.

We need small but regular rewards to continually remind us of our success and to keep us motivated to achieve each minigoal along the way to our maxigoal of reaching our desired weight.

Giving Yourself a Boost

We've already established that weight loss is harder to control than behavior, so a reward system should be based on positive behavioral changes, not pounds lost. Therefore, start by making a list of good food and fitness habits you are adding to your life. In order to make them the basis of your reward system, they must be specific and measurable, such as:

- Keeping up your walking program for the next four weeks

- Avoiding all cakes, cookies and pastries for three weeks

- Drinking eight glasses of water daily for two weeks

- Signing up for a low-impact aerobics class and attending the first four sessions

- Not putting butter on bread or rolls for a full month

- Keeping Your Perfect Weight Success Diary up-to-date for three weeks

Now the fun part comes with making a list of rewards—small yet meaningful gifts you give yourself with the completion of each minigoal. Depending on your own personal preferences, these rewards might include:

- A bouquet of flowers

- A new CD

- Two uninterrupted hours spent reading a novel

- A manicure

- A day at the beach with your favorite person

- A long-distance phone call to your best friend in Arkansas

- A $25 splurge at the store of your choice

- An afternoon locked in the bedroom watching rented videos

- A 90-minute scented bubble bath

- A concert ticket

Remember you can always add to this list—and should, for variety's sake. Rewarding yourself periodically is a tried-and-true way to keep you going to the weight-loss finish line.

Date: _____

Weight: _____

WEEK 9: GO VERY, VERY VEGGIE
Exercise goal: Walk five days, 2½ miles per day

We've been urging you right along to eat your vegetables, just as your mom might. That's because veggies are healthy, delicious, filling and the basis of a lifelong weight-control program.

 Current government nutritional guidelines recommend that you have three to five servings per day, and if you've been hitting that mark, great! But you may be one of those folks who finds it hard to squeeze in all the vegetables you should be getting. Maybe that's because you still think of veggies as little more than boring old steamed broccoli or green salad. These quick, creative tricks will give you some new ideas for how to slip extra produce into your program.

Turn on the juice. Drink low-sodium vegetable juice. It's quick, easy, and a four-ounce glass equals one vegetable serving.

Be a cut-up. Keep a supply of cut-up raw veggies in the fridge, so they're always available for snacking. Go beyond the ho-hum carrot and celery sticks. Experiment with raw broccoli, cauliflower, green beans, green and red peppers, even snow peas or fresh peas.

Brown-bag it. Prepare a little extra salad at dinnertime, and pack up the leftovers for lunch the next day.

Sneak in the veggies. Fortify your omelets, pasta dishes, stews, soups and casseroles with your favorite vegetables. Add shredded carrots or zucchini to low-fat muffin, pancake or quick-bread batter. And use pureed, cooked carrots as a soup thickener.

Play 'em up. Have a vegetarian main dish at least once a week. Try a veggie enchilada, lasagna or stir-fry.

Spruce up your spuds. Make your potato special by dressing it up with a steamed or stir-fried veggie combination. Or make a "pizza-potato"—top it with nonfat cottage cheese or nonfat mozzarella and tomato sauce. (One-half cup of tomato sauce is one vegetable serving.)

Is your family starting to enjoy vegetables more than before? Good! Remember, the earlier you get your kids following healthy eating habits, the more it'll become second nature to them and they'll never have to worry about their weight.

And note that you're now up to an impressive 2½ miles a day. This will be your new walking goal for the next four weeks.

Date: _____

Weight: _____

WEEK 10: CREATE AN AT-HOME GYM FOR UNDER $150
Exercise goal: Walk five days, 2½ miles per day

Finding your extra half-mile-per-day walk challenging? That's the way it ought to be. Always keep in mind that you shouldn't push yourself beyond what's fairly comfortable—huffing, puffing and pain are out.

Once again, the key is to simply exercise as regularly as you can manage. And if you occasionally have a tough time getting your body up and out to walk because of bad weather or just a case of the blahs, we have the perfect solution: Stay in and exercise, with an inexpensive, at-home gym you create yourself.

"A home gym is an excellent idea," says Dr. Mollen. "It's so convenient, and it motivates people who live in environments that are not always conducive to outdoor exercise. And it's one way to prevent yourself from coming up with excuses to not exercise!"

If you're thinking you've got to re-create a flashy health club atmosphere in the corner of your bedroom, think again. You can put together a few simple yet extraordinarily effective items for well under $200.

"The first piece of essential equipment is a jump rope, the kind with ball bearings in the handles," says Dr. Mollen. (Cost: $10 to $20.) "I like jump ropes because, in a five- to eight-minute period, you burn up 100 calories—the equivalent of running almost one mile. It's a good way to warm up and get started with your daily exercise routine."

Dr. Mollen calls the stationary bike his favorite piece of home gym equipment. Sure, you can pay up to $2,000 for a model with pulse monitors and other fancy attachments, but he suggests you check out your local newspaper for a perfectly good used stationary bike instead.

"A lot of people have their bikes sitting as coat hangers, so someone might want to sell it and be happy to get $50 for it," he suggests.

Dr. Mollen particularly likes stationary bikes because people tend to stick with them—the fact that you can pedal while you read, watch TV or chat on the phone is a tremendous plus. And, he adds, four miles on your exercise bike burns a solid 100 calories.

You'll also need some gear to help you do your resistance-training work. During Week 5 you were asked to invest in an exercise band. If you haven't already, they're generally under $5. Free weights can cost you little or nothing. You can use anything from a couple of cans of tomatoes or soup already sitting in your kitchen cabinet, to bricks to inexpensive iron weights. (A pair of five-pound weights from the sporting-goods store should run anywhere from $10 to $25.)

If you still haven't bought a good pair of athletic shoes, do it now! They'll set you back $50 to $75. (These can be a lot more expensive.)

Plus, you'll want an exercise mat, which you can get for under $15. Total cost: $140 or less.

Of course, you don't have to purchase these things all at once. It's just that having several pieces of exercise gear readily available serves as a reminder and a motivator. Once you find yourself really getting into your home gym, you can always add new fitness toys to your collection, such as a step platform, a treadmill, a couple of workout videos or a rowing machine.

Enjoying Your Home Gym

Here are a few additional tips for making your home gym even more effective.

Pick a proper place. Set up your equipment in an area of the house that can ideally be used exclusively for your exercise—a small spare bedroom, say, or a den. And be sure it's well ventilated. Give yourself plenty of room to move around, and keep breakables or furniture with sharp edges out of the room. Soft-wood floors are best, but if you've got a floor covered with rugs or carpeting, make sure they won't slip and slide while you bend and stretch.

Time out to work out. Your exercise time is yours. Try to schedule your workouts when few or no people are at home, to avoid distractions. Unless you're on your stationary bike, leave your phone off the hook or keep your answering machine on.

Pamper yourself. For an added incentive to use your at-home gym, follow up each workout with 20 to 30 minutes of pampering in your at-home spa (translation: bathroom). Enjoy a scented bath or a long, bracing shower while your favorite music plays in the background. After drying off, slather yourself with body lotion or talc, then have a cool glass of water or iced herbal tea.

While some at-home gym equipment is a jim-dandy idea, it's still meant to be a back-up for your regular walking regimen. By the way, ten weeks into the program, you're probably wondering how you ever let entire weeks go by without a brisk walk!

Date: _____

Weight: _____

WEEK 11: PREPARE FOR A SNACK ATTACK!
Exercise goal: Walk five days, 2½ miles per day

Ever get an uncontrollable urge to snack? We all have. Whether it comes from the pungent aroma of hot buttered popcorn at your local six-plex movie theater or the desire to do *anything* but the work on your desk, the siren call of food can be seductive, all right.

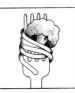
By now you've probably headed off many of these urges successfully because week by week Your Perfect Weight 52-Week Plan is teaching you smart tricks for getting through those tough, should-I-or-shouldn't-I-have-that-delicious-looking-Big-Mac moments. Along with the muscles you're building via resistance training, you're *also* building your resistance to impulse eating.

But everyone can use a few extra tips on fighting those powerful snack attacks. Now's the time to reread the list of eating alternatives found in "Change Your Ways, Change Your Weight," on page 89. You need to remind yourself of the many options available to you *besides* mindless snacking, which is often the result of nothing more than boredom. Just as the best way to deal with a baby's whining or crying is by distracting him with a rattle or some other toy, the best way to deal with your own snack attack is through distraction.

Here's a hit list of distractions to choose from.

• Make a phone call.

• Go for your daily walk.

• Do some mending.

• Wash your hair.

• Record your feelings in Your Perfect Weight Success Diary to determine why you think you want to eat.

- Read the next chapter in the book you're currently reading.

- Play with your kid(s).

- Groom the dog.

- Write a letter to someone you've been meaning to contact.

- Clean out a closet.

- Give yourself a manicure (use *slow*-drying polish so you can't pick up food!).

This week think of ways to add to this list. It's handy to have as many strategies as possible to fend off a snack attack.

If all else fails, remember that it's *okay* to have an occasional snack that fits into your food plan. A healthy snack like a glass of skim milk or a bunch of grapes or some fat-free yogurt is perfectly fine and will help you stick to your sensible eating program. But here's another secret: It's *also* okay to sometimes have a snack that doesn't fit into your food plan. Deprivation is out.

If a chocolate mint chip ice-cream cone or a slice of pepperoni pizza should enter your life once in a while, and you're following the program to the T otherwise, you're not going to see any real weight gain.

Go ahead. Have that snack, and *enjoy* it, knowing that you'll immediately return to your normal eating plan. Be sure to jot it down and work it off with a smidgen of additional exercise. You'll be fine. And guilt-free.

Perhaps the best way to avoid unplanned snacking is to give all high-fat, high-calorie foods in your house their eviction notice. This would be a good time to do another kitchen patrol. Toss out all the offending foods that have somehow sneaked back into your home when your back was turned.

Make a list of worry-free snack foods—fresh fruit, sugarless hard candies, rice cakes, frozen-fruit bars—for your next supermarket expedition, to help you ward off future temptation.

And if you haven't done so in a while, go back to your original list of goals from Day 1 to see how you're doing.

Date: _____

Weight: _____

WEEK 12: LEARN HOW TO BROWN-BAG IT
Exercise goal: Walk five days, 2½ miles per day

How do you spell brown-bag lunch?

B-O-R-I-N-G, or so many of us believe. "When people think of brown-bag lunches, they think of a balogna sandwich on white bread, a Coke, and dessert like a commercially made cupcake," says registered dietitian Anita Hirsch, nutritionist for Rodale Press. Not exactly low-cal fare, nor particularly good-tasting. But there's no reason why your carry-along meals can't be as delicious and creative as those you whip up to eat at home.

For instance, check out our Catalina Shrimp in Pita Pockets recipe, on page 316, for a terrific example of a brown-bag meal that'll have you tickled pink. In fact, Hirsch is a big pita fan.

"You can use it as the basis for sandwiches with interesting combinations," she explains. (Shrimp and coleslaw is anything but boring.) "Or stuff a pita with cut-up vegetables—then it's like a salad in a pita. You can also make some bean dip, or you can buy ready-made hummus, and pack it in a plastic container. Wrap the pita separately, to dip in the hummus."

Soup is also a super brown-bag item, whether it's the dried kind you fix on the job, or prepared at home and carried in a Thermos.

Round out the meal with some bread or fat-free crackers, and some fruit for dessert. There are apples and bananas, of course, but Hirsch says: Think exotic.

"Try kiwi or other kinds of less familiar fruits," she suggests. "Or cut up different kinds and make fruit salad."

Look Forward to Lunch

To save morning prep time, use something from dinner the night before. "For instance," says cookbook author Marie Simmons, whose syndicated column "Fresh and Fast" appears in approximately 90 newspapers, "if you're making chicken breasts or salmon steaks, throw in an extra one." You can then brown-bag it the next day for lunch.

"I pack lunch for my husband every day, and he doesn't want to eat junk food," says Simmons. "Today, for example, he took a salad of cooked potatoes, some leftover salmon steak and cucumber slices drizzled with a little lemon juice and olive oil."

In fact, Simmons rejects the notion that take-along food must be bread-based. "I always think it's nicer to eat with a fork, even a brown-bag lunch," she says. "Sandwiches can be hard to handle, and the real good ones don't store that well. So I think in terms of salads and other room-temperature food—pasta, beans, chili, potatoes, raw vegetables and even cooked vegetables are all good at room temperature."

But if prep time's short, your midday meal can be as simple as a chunk of low-fat hard cheese and a couple of breadsticks, with some cut-up veggies on the side. If you love yogurt, Hirsch suggests keeping a container of fat-free or low-fat vanilla or plain yogurt in your freezer. Take it to work with you frozen, and by lunchtime it will be ready to eat.

And there's no reason you can't have a totally nontraditional brown-bag lunch. How about a single-serving box of your favorite whole-grain cereal topped with fat-free yogurt or skim milk, along with some cut-up fruit?

What to drink? Sure, there's always coffee or diet soda that you can buy from the coffee wagon or vending machine. But consider carrying along some bottled water or an herbal tea bag and making a cup of hot tea during your lunch break.

Be as wild and crazy with your brown-bag lunch as you dare, and the more fun it'll be sticking to low-fat fare. "Whatever you do," urges Hirsch, "maybe the best thing to do is to tell yourself, no more bologna."

Keep On Trucking

Hope you've been keeping up your three miles a day of walking. Remember that those three miles are burning off a couple of hundred calories! And if you're having trouble squeezing in your fitness walk each day, why not plan to pack a lunch for work one day this week and spend part of your lunch hour walking through a nearby park or working out at your company fitness center? Keep an extra pair of shorts and walking shoes in your desk drawer or locker, and it will make it easier for you to get up and go!

Date: _____

Weight: _____

WEEK 13: BOOST YOUR MOTIVATION

Exercise goal: Walk five days, three miles per day

Why is it that the best of intentions get so easily sidetracked? The going was great back in Weeks 1 and 2, maybe even in Weeks 8 and 9. Remember?

If you're like most people, you're starting to feel like your get-up-and-go just got up and went. Slicing and dicing those veggies isn't *nearly* as much fun as it looks on those 2:00 A.M. TV commercials. And when you tie up those walking shoes, sometimes it feels like you're tying on lead boots.

Sure, you still have every intention of reaching your goal weight . . . someday. But now, despite your many successes to date, that day seems lost in a haze, far, far off on the horizon. And that chocolate layer cake is oh, so *close*.

What happened to that gung-ho diet spirit you used to bound out of bed with every morning? The explanation is simple, says Peter McWilliams, co-author of *DO IT! Let's Get Off Our Buts*. It's the law of reversibilty. "That's when everything reverses on itself, and it's a standard pattern with any addiction, like overeating or smoking," he says. "The law of reversibility happens after three days, then again after three weeks, then three months, then six months, one year, two years and seven years. It's at those intervals after starting a new regimen when the desire to go back to way things were becomes very strong, when you find yourself saying, 'I'm tired of doing this' or 'I'm tired of the struggle.'"

And look, here you are at Week 13—three months after you began Your Perfect Weight 52-Week Plan. Luckily, says McWilliams, your what-the-heck attitude shouldn't last too long—just a day or two. But as you well know, that's all it takes to send your eating and exercise program into a tailspin. So the solution is to just hang in there, monitor your behavior extra carefully, and know this attitude should pass within 24 or 48 hours.

There may be other causes of your diet lethargy right now, McWilliams points out. He compares an ongoing weight-loss program to a long marriage. "When you're married for years and years, sometimes the eye starts to wander—it's the old grass-is-greener syndrome," he says. "You may not even *want* someone else, really. You simply want a change from what's become so familiar."

What you need, then, is to give your lifestyle changes a shot in the arm. Try out a new walking path or a whole new *type* of exercise you've been curious about.

If you normally work out in the morning, have an early evening session instead. Buy a low-fat cookbook and vow to whip up three new recipes this week. Start saving now for a trip to a nearby spa where you can continue your good diet habits and be pampered all in the same weekend—it'll give you something special to look forward to.

Perhaps the best motivation booster of all, says McWilliams, is to simply remind yourself why you're losing weight to begin with. He suggests you begin keeping a "good book" of all the positive things that have happened to you since launching your diet program. Your book might include everything from "fitting into that red dress again" to "going to the beach and not feeling self-conscious" to "climbing the steps to the attic and, for the first time, not getting winded" to "getting the best check-up in a long time from the doctor."

"Sometimes we focus on the bad and forget all the good," he says. "But if you keep a book listing your positive experiences, it'll keep you motivated and help you avoid food temptations."

Date: _____

Weight: _____

QUARTERLY INVENTORY

Hip, hip, hooray! You've completed one quarter—a full 13 weeks—of Your Perfect Weight 52-Week Plan! And speaking of hips, yours must be looking pretty good by now, not to mention your tummy, thighs and derriere.

Low-Fat Living Progress Report

	Yes!	Usually	I was afraid you'd ask that
1. I review my list of long-term goals regularly.	❑	❑	❑
2. I keep the kitchen as fat-free as possible.	❑	❑	❑
3. I meet my weekly exercise goal.	❑	❑	❑
4. I weigh myself once a week.	❑	❑	❑
5. I keep my success diary up-to-date.	❑	❑	❑
6. I eat a good breakfast every morning.	❑	❑	❑
7. I stick to low-fat items when I snack.	❑	❑	❑
8. I do de-stressing exercises to head off my urges to overeat.	❑	❑	❑
9. I drink eight glasses of water a day.	❑	❑	❑
10. I reward myself for meeting my minigoals.	❑	❑	❑
11. I do strength training two or three times per week.	❑	❑	❑
12. I stick to reasonable-size portions.	❑	❑	❑
13. I eat five servings of fruits and vegetables a day.	❑	❑	❑
14. I review my success diary whenever I need to give my program a boost.	❑	❑	❑

If the compliments and admiring looks are rolling in, enjoy them! You've worked hard for them.

To help you keep track of your ever-improving habits as well as to keep you going full steam ahead for the next 39 weeks, fill out the checklist on the page 212. There'll be a new one every quarter. If you've checked "Yes!" or "Usually" fewer than ten times, it's time to review this section and see where your weight-loss behavior needs a boost.

Oh, we almost forgot the *good* news: A positive quarterly "report card"—ten or more "Yes!" or "Usually" answers—should bring with them a fairly major reward, just as you've been rewarding yourself all along. What shall it be for your 13 weeks of diligent dieting? A new head-to-toe outfit? A vacation you've been constantly postponing? A new bike?

Whatever it is, make it something absolutely *wonderful*. And start now to plan for your next quarterly reward, so you have something special to look forward to. Write it on your calendar. That 13-week mark will be here before you know it!

WEEK 14: BETTER CHOICES FOR DINING OUT
Exercise goal: Walk five days, three miles per day

There you are in the kitchen, about to prepare your umpteenth meal for the week, when somebody with a credit card announces, "Hey, let's go *out* for dinner tonight!"

Once you would've been the first one at the door, like a puppy with a leash in his mouth, ready to bolt to that diner or deli. But now that your weight-loss program has been going so well, you're worried that you might blow it.

Not likely—not with all the weeks of healthy meals and hearty exercise under your belt. But if it feels like it's been forever since you've gone out to eat and you are concerned about how to handle restaurant dining, rest easy. You can use the handy guide on page 216 to help you meet the challenge of dining out head on.

Date: _____

Weight: _____

Restaurant Survival Guide

This week, make a special point of dining out a couple of times. And instead of partaking of the fattening foods and behaviors you might have in the past (column A), try some alternatives (column B). They will add to your dining experience while subtracting from the scale.

Always remember that if you've got a special restaurant meal coming up, plan ahead so you can enjoy it to the fullest. That means starting each day with a good breakfast, maybe going a bit easy on the calories at lunch, and squeezing in a tad more exercise over the weekend.

Speaking of exercise, how's that going? It might be time for a mileage check of your walking shoes. They may need to be replaced.

Column A	Column B
You leave the house famished. You could eat a horse!	Drink a glass of water or club soda and have a celery stalk or a carrot at home to take the edge off your hunger.
Your dining companion says, "How about French food (or pizza or ribs) tonight?" You say, "Fine—anything."	You say, "Hmmm, how about seafood (or vegetarian or Thai) instead?"
The moment you're seated, you attack the bread basket. (And don't forget the butter!)	You drink the water poured for you and, with your companion's okay, ask the waiter to remove the bread and butter.
You order an alcoholic beverage to start.	You continue to drink the water or order tomato juice or mineral water.

WEEK 15: USE POSITIVE SELF-TALK
Exercise goal: Walk five days, three miles per day

Nobody's perfect! Every now and then we need to remind ourselves of that trite but true saying.

Throughout this period of weight loss and establishing new health habits, you've got to be your own best friend, supportive of your efforts and

Column A	Column B
Somebody orders something that sounds good, and although you hadn't intended to order it yourself, you do.	You ignore what everyone else is ordering and just focus on your own meal. In fact, you don't even open the menu— you know what you can eat.
You recite your order to the waiter, no questions asked.	You're unsure about how a dish is prepared. You ask the waiter about it and possibly ask to have it changed—say, from fried to baked, or with sauce on the side.
You eat and eat and eat and eat.	You eat and talk and eat and talk.
You finish everything on your plate.	You leave about half of your meat or fish (and ask to have it wrapped so you can take it home).
You ask the waiter to bring more rolls.	You ask the waiter to refill your water glass.
You order a slab of cheesecake for dessert.	You order some sorbet (and maybe have a forkful of a friend's cake).
You get in the car and lean against the door, moaning, "I'm so full!" (The seat belt's feeling a *mite* snug all of a sudden.)	You stroll home, or if it's not too late once you get home, you take a brisk walk.
You feel guilty.	You feel great!

forgiving of your mistakes. So says Kelly D. Brownell, Ph.D., professor of psychology and co-director of the Yale University Eating and Weight Disorders Clinic and co-author of *Weight Maintenance Survival Guide*. And there *will* be mistakes and setbacks—no doubt about it. Chances are you've already experienced one or two.

But you have to be kind to yourself and focus on your achievements, not your slip-ups. To do this, you have to pay attention to your self-talk. If you ever catch yourself saying or even thinking the words *stupid, bad* or *cheat,*

Switch On the Positive

Get into the habit of switching "pain words" to "power words," suggests psychologist Susan Jeffers, Ph.D., author of *Feel the Fear and Do It Anyway.* "It's important that you monitor your words, using phrases that empower rather than weaken you," she insists. "So eliminate the 'can'ts,' 'shoulds,' 'problems' and 'struggles' from your vocabulary, and replace them with power words."

Here are some word-swaps she recommends.

Instead of . . .	Say . . .
I can't	I won't
I should	I could
It's a problem	It's an opportunity
Life's a struggle	Life's an adventure
I hope	I know
If only	Next time
What will I do?	I know I can handle it

take a minute to change them to positive ones. Instead of telling yourself, "I was bad to have that piece of cake," say, "I did eat that cake, and I will be more careful at my next meal."

If you think you've been too harsh on yourself, jot down some notes to that effect in Your Perfect Weight Success Diary, so you can review them in days and weeks to come. Remind yourself that you're up to future eating challenges, and give yourself regular, much-deserved pats on the back for your awesome accomplishments.

Date: _____

Weight: _____

WEEK 16: COLD-WEATHER WALKING
Exercise goal: Walk five days, three miles per day

You've been doing a bang-up job with your walking program so far; don't let cold weather stop you! You can still keep up your outdoor workout, as long as you know what to expect from exercising in lower temperatures and you take the necessary precautions. This week, concentrate on getting your act together for cold-weather walking. Here are a few tips from the pros to help you keep up the good work. (If your Week 16 falls during warmer weather, please read the "Warm-Weather Workout," on page 265, instead.)

Take it easy. Be sure to warm up more slowly than usual, and do so indoors. "Give your cardiovascular system a chance to get going before you hit the cold air," says Ronald Lawrence, M.D., president of the American Medical Athletic Association. "You'll feel better about going outside, and you'll create less stress on your heart."

Dress for the chill. Less is more in the world of high-tech textiles. New fabrics insulate, block the wind and wick away moisture without bulk or heaviness, and they do their job more effectively than wool or cotton. Start with a layer of synthetic fabric like polypropylene or hollow-core fibers to wick away perspiration. Next you need an insulating layer for warmth, such as down. And last, you'll need an outer layer, or shell, to protect you from the wind—something that's waterproof and breathable.

Treat your feet. As you warm up by exercising, your feet stay warm with you, and so you may not need any footwear other than your usual walking shoes. But as temperatures drop or as road conditions get icy, wet or slushy, you might consider a pair of hiking shoes. The type of hiking shoes that are appropriate for dirt trails should be flexible enough for a fitness walk.

As for socks, Douglas Richie, D.P.M., associate clinical professor, California College of Podiatric Medicine in Seal Beach, recommends a light trekking sock for cold-weather walking. A combination of wool and acrylic is the way to go. "Wool absorbs moisture and stays stiff, which allows it to hold air, and air is what keeps you warm," says Dr. Richie. "And the acrylic makes the sock more comfortable and moves the moisture out."

Protect your skin. Your face and hands generally suffer the most from exposure during the winter. To protect your hands most effectively, use two types of gloves: first a thick, insulated glove for warm-up, and then, as your body and hands warm up, switch to a lighter glove. To protect your face, a thin, silk ski mask is best. But if you'd rather not wear one, be sure to apply plenty of sunscreen—ideally one that's water-resistant and with a sun protection factor (SPF) of 15. Allow it to dry, then follow up with an application of moisturizer or petroleum jelly.

Know when to chill out. While you may be eager to keep up your walking program, despite severe weather conditions, you should be reasonable. On very bitter days, switch to an indoor workout—use a stationary bike, swim laps in an indoor pool, skate (roller or ice) at an indoor rink or walk around a mall.

Pick the right fuel. Cold days demand hearty, tummy-warming foods. Choose a hot breakfast featuring oatmeal and a warm drink, hot soups and stews for lunches and dinners and a postexercise mug of cinnamon-spiked tea or sugar-free cocoa.

Date: _____

Weight: _____

WEEK 17: LEARN HOW TO GRAZE
Exercise goal: Walk six days, three miles per day

How has your eating been going? Concentrating on getting fruit, veggies, grains and pastas into your day, every day? Exercising portion control? Keeping track of snacks? Good.

Now, while you (and your family) may be accustomed to your three squares a day, switching to several small meals throughout the day instead may actually be better for fat burning, according to some experts. If you're hoping to see better numbers on the scale during your weekly weigh-ins, this might be something worth trying.

What's wrong with three meals a day, you wonder? Well, after you eat, your body releases the hormone insulin, and the larger the meal and the higher it is in fat and sugar the more insulin your body releases in response.

"Insulin causes your body to save fat and burn carbohydrates," explains registered dietitian James Kenney, Ph.D., nutrition research specialist at the Pritikin Longevity Center in Santa Monica, California. "Things that tend to pump insulin levels higher tend to promote weight gain."

Insulin helps prevent your fat cells from breaking down fat and releasing it into the bloodstream, where it could be burned as fuel. And it also helps turn your fat cells into magnets for the dietary fat that's been absorbed into your bloodstream.

But smaller meals, eaten more frequently during the day, keep insulin levels lower and more stable. "If you have less insulin in your blood, you store less fat and burn more fat," Dr. Kenney explains. "And because you burn more fat, you have less of an appetite because you're using calories instead of storing them."

But grazing only prevents insulin surges if you choose the right kinds of foods. Stick to high-complex-carbohydrate, low-fat foods like baked potatoes (with vegetable or nonfat cheese toppers), whole-grain pretzels, bagels and breads, legumes and vegetables. A typical grazing menu might go something like this.

Breakfast: oatmeal; skim milk

Midmorning snack: half a bagel with all-fruit jam; herbal tea

Late-morning snack: small banana

Lunch: sandwich of low-fat ham and low-fat Swiss cheese with lettuce and tomato slices on wheat bread; cucumber slices

Midafternoon snack: pretzels

Late-afternoon snack: tomato juice with nonfat crackers

Dinner: broiled fish with rice or pasta; two servings steamed vegetables; small green salad

After-dinner snack: nonfat yogurt

You should also be continuing to drink your six to eight glasses of water throughout the day.

If you do try this way of eating this week, it's especially crucial for you to keep your food diary up-to-date, so you don't "forget" about that half sandwich here or that container of yogurt there. The meals may be smaller, but the calories and fat grams still add up.

Check out your new walking goal: six days a week at three miles per day. Remember, the closer you come to daily exercise, the easier it'll be to keep those pounds away . . . for good!

Date: _____

Weight: _____

WEEK 18: RESISTANCE TRAINING REVISITED
Exercise goal: Walk six days, three miles per day

Week 18: You're over a third of the way through the 52-week plan, and you're stronger and more toned than you ever thought possible! Good work!

There was a time not long ago that you never dreamed you'd be pumping iron. Now, if a week goes by without some resistance training under your belt, you don't feel as vigorous or as energized. Like the other good-for-you habits you've been cultivating for the past four-plus months, once you start 'em, it's hard to kick 'em!

This week we offer you a new assortment of five exercises involving free weights and a chair. If you haven't purchased a set of free weights yet, remember you can always use five- or seven-pound weights you might have at home—large cans of food, bags of sugar or what have you. Plastic detergent jugs have convenient handles and can be filled with water or sand.

Repeat each of the movements 8 to 12 times to make up one set. If possible, do three sets of each exercise. And as always, remember to warm up, cool down and start off slowly, especially if you haven't been doing resistance training all along for the recommended two- or three-times-a-week sessions.

Lateral raises. Using a hand weight, raise one arm away from your side until it's parallel to the floor. Lower and repeat. Alternate arms.

Triceps presses. Hold a hand weight behind your head with both hands. Extend your arms up overhead, keeping your elbows close to your ears. Return. Repeat.

Biceps curls. Hold the weight in one hand. Start with your arm at your side, palm foreward. Slowly curl your fist up toward your shoulder. Lower, and repeat.

Crunches. You won't be using weights for the next two exercises. Lie flat on your back, with your knees bent and your feet flat on the floor. Look up at the ceiling. Now lift your head, shoulders and upper back from the floor. Don't tuck your chin and keep the movement slow. (No jerky movements allowed.) Hold the position for two seconds, then return. Remember to breathe. Repeat.

Chair push-ups. Place a sturdy chair against the wall, with the front of the chair facing you. Kneel in front of it. Grip the chair seat and do a push-up against the chair. Remember to keep your back straight. Repeat.

Keeping up your motivation so you can keep up your resistance training isn't always easy, we admit. But before boredom can set in, try these ideas.

S-l-o-w down. To add a bit of variety and challenge to your workout routine, do your exercises twice as slowly as you normally do, suggests Wayne L. Westcott, Ph.D., strength-training consultant to the National Academy of Sports Medicine and the American Council on Exercise. Another way to make things more interesting is to strap on ankle or wrist weights.

Find a friend. "Do your training with someone else," urges Dr. Westcott. "It can be a friend or a spouse, or work with someone at your local Y or fitness center. Then you'll feel confident that you're doing the exercises properly, so that you can then do them on your own much better." What's more, having a pal to pump up with is just plain fun.

Spice it up. When you feel the tedium creeping in on you, change the workout around, or find new exercises to do that work a different set of muscles. Mix walking or jogging into the exercises. A little music with the muscle can't hurt either.

Keep track. "A logbook will help you see your improvement, and will motivate you to see greater success," says Dr. Westcott. You can use Your Perfect Weight Success Diary for this purpose. By keeping an accurate record, you'll know exactly how you're progressing in terms of the number of reps you do and the increased weight you can lift. "It's very helpful if you can be accountable to yourself through a logbook," says Dr. Wescott.

Date: _____

Weight: _____

WEEK 19: DO SEVEN DAYS OF SIMPLE SWAPS
Exercise goal: Walk six days, three miles per day

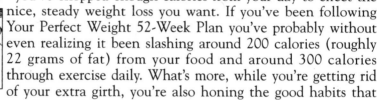

As you've seen, week in and week out for nearly five months now, losing a pound or so a week is simply a matter of making small, daily changes in your eating and exercise routine. A bit less fat here, a bit more activity there and—presto!—you've chopped enough calories from your day to effect the nice, steady weight loss you want. If you've been following Your Perfect Weight 52-Week Plan you've probably without even realizing it been slashing around 200 calories (roughly 22 grams of fat) from your food and around 300 calories through exercise daily. What's more, while you're getting rid of your extra girth, you're also honing the good habits that will keep your weight off forever—without your ever having to diet again!

Here, we offer a week's worth of simple little tricks for shaving up to 500 calories each day. Some are activities we hope you've already built into your lifestyle, but chances are many of these things are new ones for you to try. The nice thing is, they're so painless you won't even know they're helping you lose weight.

Day 1—Sunday

- Walk one mile to church (save 100 calories).

- Mow the front lawn for one hour (save 240 calories).

- Quench your thirst with seltzer and a squeeze of lemon instead of soda (save 152 calories).

Total Calories Saved: 492

Day 2—Monday

- Revamp your breakfast: Grab a fat-free bran muffin and 1 percent milk instead of a cinnamon Danish and whole milk (save 305 calories).

- Swear off the office elevator: Use the stairs instead (save 100 calories).

Total Calories Saved: 405

Day 3—Tuesday

- Catch the bus at a different stop a mile away, and get off at that stop after work, too (save 200 calories).

- Dress down your lunchtime salad with nonfat Italian dressing (save 129 calories).

- Forgo an afternoon candy bar—have a crisp apple instead (save 169 calories).

Total Calories Saved: 498

Day 4—Wednesday

- Take the dog for a two-mile stroll (save 200 calories).

- Instead of two slices of pepperoni pizza for lunch, have one slice of cheese pizza and nonfat frozen yogurt (save 122 calories).

- For dinner, have vegetarian fat-free chili and fat-free whole-wheat crackers instead of beef chili and tortilla chips (save 84 calories).

Total Calories Saved: 406

Day 5—Thursday

- Use nonfat cream cheese on your breakfast bagel instead of regular cream cheese (save 68 calories).

- Snack on light microwave popcorn instead of potato chips (save 140 calories).

- Play Ping-Pong with the kids for 20 minutes (save 90 calories).

- Jitterbug your way through an hourlong dance class (save 180 calories).

Total Calories Saved: 478

Day 6—Friday

- Sweat it out during a low-impact aerobics class (save 395 calories).

- Switch to light beer during happy hour—two beers (save 98 calories).

Total Calories Saved: 493

Day 7—Saturday

• Take a family bike ride for an hour at ten miles per hour (save 370 calories).

• Lunch on tuna sandwiches with nonfat instead of regular mayo (save 87 calories).

• Drive past the drive-through car wash—bathe the Chevy yourself (save 70 calories).

Total Calories Saved: 527

Date: _____

Weight: _____

WEEK 20: DEALING WITH A WEIGHT-LOSS PLATEAU

Exercise goal: Walk six days, three miles per day

You've been doing your diet thing wonderfully well for the past five months. The compliments are still trickling in, your stretch pants don't have to stretch quite as much as they once did, and you're generally feeling pretty terrific.

Then it happens: The weight that was dropping off at a nice one- to two-pound-a-week clip stays on like glue, day after day, week after week.

This is exactly what makes a dieter want to head for the cold cuts (lots of mayo, thank you). What's going on?

It's a pretty basic phenomenon: You've hit a weight-loss plateau, and the first thing to understand about it is that it's perfectly normal. If you haven't deviated from your basic low-fat, high-exercise program (and that's a big if—more on that in a minute), then your body is simply taking a rest. You may be losing weight in a completely healthful way, but your body is still going through a lot of changes and the plateau is just its way of saying, "Hey, pal, give me a week or two to catch my breath!"

Remember that your weight is going to level off from time to time and that the situation isn't permanent. "When people hit a plateau, they often fall into a thinking trap of 'I can't lose weight! It's all over!' But your body has an internal wisdom," explains Ronna Kabatznick, Ph.D., psychological consultant to Weight Watchers International. "Just keep following your food and exercise plan, and you'll eventually lose the rest of the weight."

Make certain, she adds, that you're not contributing, consciously or unconsciously, to the plateau. How?

"Take an inventory to see if there's been any change," urges Dr. Kabatznick. "Have you been eating a lot of salty or fatty Chinese food lately, or consuming more alcohol or other high-calorie foods that might account for the plateau? It's also important to take an inventory of exercise. Have you been doing less, or reduced the intensity? Usually that inventory will give you some clues as to where to clean up your efforts."

Now's the Time to Fight

On the other hand, you may well be experiencing a different kind of plateau—a psychological plateau, where you just don't feel like making the effort and pushing forward, says Dr. Kabatznick.

"It usually happens when a person has lost enough weight where she feels different but hasn't yet reached her goal—for example, she wants to lose 30 pounds and after a 20-pound loss, her motivation may begin to wobble," she explains. This is the phase in your diet when your desire to continue to lose weight and your desire to eat more fattening food are about equal. "That's a vulnerable time for many people," says Dr. Kabatznick.

Her advice: Change something. "A lot of times, plateaus come from being bored. Do something new and exciting so you can renew your commitment. If you haven't had Indian or Italian food for a while, have some. Find a new cookbook or a new spice. Don't bring the same brown-bag lunch every day. Get out of your rut."

Last week's suggestions for simple food and activity swaps should give you some additional ideas for perking up your routine.

Pretty soon now, your newfound motivation to keep going will kick in. We promise.

Date: _____

Weight: _____

Week 21: Fine-tune
Your Walking Program
Exercise goal: Walk seven days, three miles per day in 45 minutes

Over the past five months you've become an exercise champ—no question! You should be feeling slimmer and more fit than you have in a long time. If you've diligently followed Your Perfect Weight 52-Week Plan walking program on a daily basis, you can rightfully feel a surge of pride and accomplishment.

By the way, we recognize that there have undoubtedly been days when you couldn't get out for your walk. We hope you've done your walk most of the time and have substituted an indoor workout whenever necessary. If you are sticking with this program, you deserve a reward! You should be keeping up your own personal reward system for meeting your minigoals, including your walking goals.

This is the week, though, when we separate the men walkers from the boys, the women walkers from the girls. Because now you have an option: to either continue your very impressive walking routine (seven days, three miles per day in 45 minutes) or step up the pace even more.

We will continue to give the above numbers as the weekly exercise goal through the end of the 52-week plan. However, as Casey Meyers, our walking expert, notes, you'll get even greater weight-loss benefits if you shave more time off your daily three-mile walk or if you walk farther each day.

Meyers, at age 66, generally does seven days a week, covering anywhere from three to five miles per day at about 12 minutes per mile. "I vary it, depending on the weather, the amount of time I have and my desire," he says. "You don't have to walk the same distance or at the same pace every day. But if you have no time constraints, add as many miles at a half mile per week as your schedule permits, up to five miles a day."

Alternatively, if you don't have an hour-plus to devote to exercise, you can work on cutting your three-mile time down to 36 minutes (doing 12-minute miles) by reducing your daily time by a minute or half a minute per week. So, let's say you decide to go from your present 15-minute mile to a 12-minute mile, three miles a day. If you reduce your walking time in a slow and steady way by a minute per week, you can expect to be down to a 12-minute mile by Week 26, the program's halfway mark.

Need an incentive to go for the walking gold? Listen to Meyers: "Do three 12-minute miles a day, combined with a low-fat diet, and you'll have your weight-loss program nailed!"

And while we've built the 52-week plan on a walking-for-weight-loss foundation because of walking's ease and accessibility, always keep in mind that exercise can take many forms. If boredom with walking is setting in, switch to something else you might like—swimming, tennis, cross-country skiing, biking. Whatever exercise option you choose, the key has got to be consistency. Permanent weight loss, remember, means being active for life.

Date: _____

Weight: _____

WEEK 22: COOK UP A
LOW-FAT FAMILY FAVORITE
Exercise goal: Walk seven days, three miles
per day in 45 minutes

Getting your family to learn to love healthy, low-fat fare makes your losing weight and keeping it off much simpler. After all, how can you hope to slim down when your dining room becomes a nightly battleground between the fat eaters versus the fat fighters?

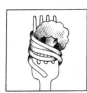
So this is an excellent time to focus on retraining your family's taste buds, for their sake as well as yours. The Shortcut Chili recipe on page 298 is a great addition to your low-fat repertoire. The palate-pleasing spiciness is sure to win raves at home. The spouse and kids will never know something so delicious is also good for them, and why bother telling them? The worst thing you can do is apologize for the food.

"You shouldn't present the meal saying, 'This is low-fat. I hope you like it.' It might turn the family off," says registered dietitian Anita Hirsch, nutritionist for Rodale Press. "Just serve it, without saying anything."

And try a new twist when you're asked that age-old question, "Hey, Mom, what's for dinner?"

"It used to be that when people asked 'What's for dinner?' the meat would always be mentioned first, or else the response would be, 'Roast beef,' as if there were nothing else on the menu. That's not good," says Hirsch. This perpetuates the idea that high-fat protein should still be the cornerstone of a meal, she says. You're probably not eating this way anymore, so why cling to old language that suggests you are? Instead, suggests Hirsch, "If the kids ask 'What's for dinner?' say 'Salad and corn,' even if you're serving some steak. Don't even mention the steak."

Recruit the Whole Family

Getting the family involved in meal planning and preparation is a good way to get them to understand why fried chicken and potatoes au gratin seldom appear on the dinner table these days. Hirsch says that, when her daughter was in junior high school, she'd be given simple, healthy recipes she could make as part of the family meal. Even younger kids can get in on the culinary act, as long as you're around to supervise.

Happily, serving food low in fat and high in taste is easier than ever before, says Hirsch. "Those recipes are everywhere. Everybody's looking for them now," she says. "It's true for commercially prepared food as well." It's just as well that it's becoming easier to eat low-fat fare, because, as you've known for months now, eating right is a lifelong proposition.

"You want your family to eat healthier from now on, not simply think that once Mom or Dad loses weight, they'll then go back to their old ways," says Hirsch. "As long as the food tastes good, they'll eat it."

And speaking of fine food, check out the other low-fat, high-taste recipes both in this book as well as in some of the newer low-fat cookbooks. Most recipes you'll see nowadays include nutrition information, including calories and fat grams per serving. While you don't need to keep a written record of these in order to lose weight, you should by now be able to eyeball a recipe's nutrition info and tell whether it fits into your diet.

Date: _____

Weight: _____

WEEK 23: HELP YOUR FAMILY BECOME MORE ACTIVE

Exercise goal: Walk seven days, three miles per day in 45 minutes

You were never thrilled about your kid's devotion to Beavis and Butt-Head. Now the word is out that television may be doing even worse things to your youngster's metabolism than to his brain. Research suggests that just 30 minutes of watching the tube can cause your child's metabolism—his calorie-burning engine—to plummet by 14 percent, a level lower than if he or she were doing nothing at all!

"That 14 percent drop is dramatic and can add up if the child watches a lot of TV," says study researcher Robert C. Klesges, Ph.D., associate professor of psychology at Memphis State University. "If a child goes from watching an hour a night to six-plus during summer vacation, for example, you may be talking about a five- to seven-pound weight gain." And that doesn't even count the snacks your kid may be gobbling while in his TV-induced trance.

Because you're now in the midst of your own serious weight-loss program, you can help yourself at the same time you encourage your youngsters to watch less TV—by organizing active family activities.

"It's best to get involved with your child and a new activity, rather than expect her to be suddenly inspired to go do something on her own," suggests human development specialist Susan K. Perry, author of *Playing Smart: A Parent's Guide to Enriching, Offbeat Learning Activities for Ages 4 to 14* and *Together Time: The Disney Book of Family Activities, Celebrations and Fun.*

You all might be in for a bit of a jolt when you first turn off the tube. "The silence can be uncomfortable," admits Perry, the mother of two sons. But the rewards of swapping sedentary time for calorie-burning time are well worth it. Here are a few activities to share with your children.

Go for a walk. "One of my favorite things to do with children is to take a walk," says Perry. "It's such a simple thing, and there are lots of ways to make it interesting. For example, try a cat-counting walk, where you and your young child look for and count cats together. You may have to look sharply—for example, a cat may be up on a roof—so it trains the child's eye. Another walk is called Who Lives Here? where you look for clues around a person's house for his occupation or hobby—say, a car parked in front with a business logo painted on it, or an open garage filled with lots of carpentry tools."

Pump up the pulse. Another game that combines physical activity and learning about the body involves teaching your child to measure her pulse. "You show her how to take her pulse first at rest and then after various activities—for example, before and after jumping rope for 30 seconds, or before and after walking around the room three times," says Perry. "It makes her aware of how the heartbeat increases as you become more active," she explains.

Hit the beach. If your usual M.O. at the shore is to slather on the sun protection factor (SPF) 15, open up your spy novel and remind the kids to be back before nightfall, try something new: a family beach workout. There's swimming, of course, but also volleyball, jogging and Frisbee throwing. Running around at the beach seldom feels like exercise, and yet it's great for calorie burning.

Plan an active vacation. Pick a vacation with your weight-loss program and your family's health in mind. Instead of the usual theme park weekends or car-bound sightseeing trips, select an active holiday. Depending on the time of year and your destination, pick a vacation centered on nature walks, cycling through one or more states or backpacking. Or check into a tennis clinic to learn the game or improve your skills. You'll all come home feeling invigorated instead of feeling like you have to go on a diet.

A combination of stepped-up activity and a steady diet of low-fat meals such as the one described last week will ensure a better shape for everyone in your family. And remember that any physical activity you do counts toward your daily and weekly totals. You don't have to necessarily walk as much as you usually do if your walks are being supplemented by, say, a family bike trip or backyard basketball game.

Date: _____

Weight: _____

WEEK 24: FIGHT BACK AGAINST SNACK ATTACK

Exercise goal: Walk seven days, three miles per day in 45 minutes

What makes a winner, whether fighting the Battle of Bull Run or the battle of the bulge? One simple secret: preparing for war in time of peace.

What do we mean? That it's simple for any of us to eat smart and exercise daily, even eagerly, when we're feeling good, when our lives are going well, when the weight is falling off, when we're happy—in other words, during peacetime.

But what happens when something rotten happens—the family car has finally given up the ghost or you just had a rip-roaring fight with your sister or your weight hasn't budged for the past three weeks? You are not a happy warrior, and just about any kind of food (the fattier the better) will quickly make you forget that you're trying to lose weight and why.

"When it comes to ingrained habits, it's foolish to think that they'll be gone forever," says Ronette Kolotkin, Ph.D., who heads the behavioral program at the Duke University Diet and Fitness Center in Durham, North Carolina. "Most people are capable of sticking to their diet plan when they feel motivated and do well. The thinking is, 'I feel so good, I'll never go back to my old, bad habits.' But that's unrealistic. Circumstances will cause some bad habits to come back, so you need to know which ones they are. If you can analyze your high-risk situations, you can plan for them because they're always just around the corner."

If you've been pretty much in control of your eating right along, good for you! By now you may have already learned to head off certain binges— for instance, by recognizing your so-called red-light foods and keeping them out of the house, or by getting into the habit of going out for a ten-minute walk so you can chill out whenever you're angry or upset. Jotting down your feelings and how you've dealt with problem emotions is another smart solution you've probably used often.

Yet there are still going to be times when you'll be caught with your guard down, and you'll want to eat to satisfy some urge other than hunger. While negative emotions, including anger, depression, loneliness, boredom and frustration, are among the most common eating triggers, there are other things that can trigger eating, says clinical psychologist Joyce D. Nash, Ph.D., weight-loss expert based in the San Francisco Bay area and author of *Now That You've Lost It: How to Maintain Your Best Weight*. These are more insidious.

"You may be walking along, and suddenly you encounter a bakery and smell the most wonderful cookies," says Dr. Nash. "The next thing you know, you wander in and end up eating something inappropriate."

At other times, says Dr. Nash, certain demands placed on us will act as eating triggers. "A mother may be fixing lunch for her children or providing cookies and other snacks, so she might eat inappropriately," she says. "Or if you're having to entertain for business, you might say to yourself, 'If I don't have a cocktail, my customer won't feel comfortable doing it, so I'd better join him,' even if you didn't plan to drink."

Prepare a Battle Plan

So how do you prepare for war in times of peace? Here are some strategies that would even have impressed General MacArthur.

Study your past. It sounds pretty basic, but how quickly we forget. What exactly caused you to go haywire in the past? "Ask yourself, 'How am I going to handle it the next time I'm angry, or tired, or sick?'" says Dr. Kolotkin. Those emotional triggers are going to reappear sooner than you think. You can't dodge them, but you can cope without overeating, through careful planning.

Take a peek at your week. What challenges do you anticipate in the next few days? Do you have a deadline for completing an important report? Is your mother-in-law due for a visit? How will you handle the stress food-lessly? Consult the alternative-activity lists in "Change Your Ways, Change Your Weight," on page 89, whenever you catch yourself sleepwalking to the refrigerator or candy counter.

Keep good munchies handy. "Simultaneously with solving your problems directly, keep the right kinds of foods around," urges Dr. Kolotkin. "Then, if you're thinking, 'I'm going to want to eat because I'll be tense,' at least you can munch without doing a lot of damage." She recommends low-fat, grab-able foods, such as cut-up veggies and air-popped popcorn.

Leave your money at home. It may seem extreme, but it's one way to make sure that your fitness walk doesn't terminate at KFC.

Anticipate lifestyle changes. Dr. Kolotkin recalls one dieting couple who was remodeling their house. But they failed to take into account that during that period of time they couldn't get access to their kitchen (so they couldn't prepare their usual low-fat meals) and that there was a lot of construction chaos (which meant their exercise routine went on the back burner). Guess what? The couple gained weight. Says Dr. Kolotkin, "If they had thought about all this ahead of time, they could have made adjustments."

Ask for help. If troublesome times are ahead, recruit the assistance of friends and loved ones. If you feel a cold or the flu coming on, ask the family to fend for themselves a bit more so you can tend to your own needs. If getting ready for moving day is overwhelming you, divvy up the packing chores among the whole gang, and be sure to build in some rest time for yourself each day when you can put up your feet and have a cup of tea.

Be gentle with yourself if you blow it. Every dieter goes off the deep end sometimes. Try to figure out where and why you went out of control, then resume your usual eating and exercise diligence. It will be rewarded.

Date: _____

Weight: _____

WEEK 25: CHOOSE THE BEST AND YOU'LL EAT LESS

Exercise goal: Walk seven days, three miles per day in 45 minutes

How are you doing this week? If you've been having some hard dieting times lately—and just barely making it through some days without caving in to your cravings—were last week's words of wisdom helpful?

The answer to any doubts about your program—whether it's because your weight has been coming off more slowly than you'd like, or because you've binged once or twice—is to keep on going. Keep drinking your water. Keep eating your low-fat foods. Keep up your daily workouts. Whatever psychological or scale-related plateau you may have hit, you'll get over it in time. Stick to the program and you'll see results.

Perhaps part of what you're experiencing now is the wish that you could somehow eat differently and still lose weight. You're not quite sure what you're craving, you just know that you need to light some kind of fire under your food plan. Well, maybe what you need to do is to perk up your palate and eat better.

After all, gourmets as well as weight-loss experts are in agreement on this subtle yet important point: Fine-quality, well-prepared food is much more pleasing to us than bad food. As a result, you're generally more satisfied with less when the food is first-rate. And if you think we're just talking champagne wishes and caviar dreams, you're wrong.

"If I decided I wanted to spend some calories on, say, a hot dog because I had a craving for it, I couldn't imagine eating a cheap, fatty hot dog—I'd want the best one I could find. And then one would be enough to satisfy that craving," says Jim Fobel, the author of seven books including *Jim Fobel's Diet Feasts*. Fobel has lost 100 pounds following his own advice. "After you get accustomed to eating the best, you wouldn't think of going back," he says.

"It seems to me that one has less desire to eat in quantity if one is concentrating on quality," adds Edward Behr, editor of the newsletter *The Art of Eating*. Good food often means the freshest food, certainly when it comes to things like produce or baked goods. And yet, Behr notes, "Few people or stores understand the importance of freshness."

Still, the reality is, lots of us settle for lots of not-very-good stuff, and that's the key right there: how to reeducate your taste buds to appreciate and hold out for truly fine food so you'll be perfectly content eating less. How do you start to treat your palate like a king? A few suggestions from the pros:

Do it yourself. If you have room for a vegetable patch or a couple of fruit trees, grow your own for the freshest flavor. Or bake your own bread. Behr makes a three-day white bread that's very slow to rise and very delicious.

Be a local yokel. "It's generally better to buy locally raised meat—it has more character," says Behr, who gets his lamb, beef and chicken close to home. "The area in Vermont where I live has lots of good pasture, and good pasture produces good meat."

Go organic. Behr says it's a "fair generalization" that organic foods are superior. He acknowledges that the first interest of people who raise organic food isn't quality but to avoid chemicals. But there's a plus. "I think that the same variety of vegetables raised under the same conditions will almost always taste better if raised organically," he says.

Skip dessert; drink wine! You may not be a wine drinker, but Behr has discovered that at dinnertime a bit of good wine, which he says can be had for just $8 to $10 a bottle, undercuts the need to eat desserts. Try this and you'll find a very nice calorie savings, since most wines are only about 100 calories per four-ounce glass and fat-free.

Teach your taste buds new tricks. "It takes work to retrain your taste buds. Most people need help with it," admits Fobel. One way is by treating yourself every now and then to a meal at a really fine restaurant. Adds Fobel, "If you know someone who knows and appreciates fine food, that person can help show the way. I do that with my friends. Once good food is pointed out and presented to you, you'll find that your taste memory is magnificent."

Date: _____

Weight: _____

WEEK 26: SEE YOURSELF THIN

Exercise goal: Walk seven days, three miles per day in 45 minutes

How do you see yourself at Week 26? As an attractive person at (or close to) a healthy weight? Or someone who's about as trim and graceful as Barney the dinosaur?

The funny thing is, the image you have of your body may have little or nothing to do with the number that comes up on your bathroom scale, your body-fat composition, the way your clothes fit or any other common measuring techniques. "Fat," "thin" and everything in between often has far more to do with what's in your head than what's on your hips. Think of how often you've said to someone, "I feel fat!" only to hear, "What are you talking about? You look fine."

In very extreme cases, this inability to accurately judge body size and an obsession with being "thin enough" can lead to the eating disorder anorexia nervosa, which is gradual starvation. More typically, an out-of-kilter mental picture of yourself can keep you from reaching and sustaining your goal weight.

Your feelings about yourself can actually distort what you see in the mirror. That's why it's so important to get an accurate sense of your body and not let your feelings about it interfere with your weight-loss program.

How do you do that? A number of ways. You can ask a relative or friend you trust for an honest evaluation, and at this stage of the weight-loss game, you're bound to hear that you're looking better than ever. Also pay attention to unsolicited comments, especially compliments about yourself. And keep accurate records of your weight and measurements in "Your Perfect Weight Success Diary," on page 275.

Even with all this proof of your improving dimensions, distortions can still occur. Weight loss experts note that it's common for dieters to continue to "see" themselves as heavy, even as the weight drops off. It's a familiar, comfortable version of yourself that can often be hard to part with, even as you say you want nothing more than to be thin.

If you continue to think of yourself as overweight you may, on some unconscious level, slip back into the old behaviors—snacking when you're not especially hungry, overeating at mealtimes, not exercising. And these behaviors will keep you at a higher weight. Guaranteed.

Getting the Right Picture

"Whenever you catch yourself wondering, Should I eat this? it's good to step back and reflect on where you are in your weight-loss plan and where you want to be," says registered dietitian Judy E. Marshel, director of Health Resources of Great Neck, New York. "Keep that mental picture of yourself at your desired weight in the forefront of your mind, and keep retrieving it. That will help you make the decision about whether to eat just a small piece of that food you crave, or not eat it at all."

You can make that mental picture real by tacking a photo—of someone whose figure you admire, or of yourself at the lower weight you aspire to—in a prominent place, such as on the refrigerator door. Or carry a smaller version of the picture with you in your handbag or wallet, and sneak a peek at it whenever you're tempted to overeat. Be sure the image you choose is realistic for who you are. A 5'1", 49-year-old woman aiming for the figure of a 5'11", 22-year-old model is silly and will only frustrate you in your efforts.

Want more help? Here are some other ways to "see" yourself straight to your goal weight.

Visualize creatively. Visualization is a technique that involves using your imagination to create positive changes in your life. Are people always telling you that you have an active imagination? Then here's your chance to put it to good use! As frequently as possible, conjure up a mental picture of your soon-to-be-thin self. "See" yourself wearing the kinds of body-hugging outfits and doing the kinds of things—proudly walking across a crowded beach, for instance—that might not feel comfortable for you quite yet. Keep forming these pleasant mental pictures, and you'll find yourself motivated to make them a reality.

Say goodbye to your unrealistic body image. Sometimes people get "stuck" at a point in their diet because they cling to an impossible-to-attain body image. They don't look like the women they see in *Vogue* or turning letters on game shows, and their frustration turns into a binge. But not until you accept what is reasonable for your body can you expect to reach a comfortable goal, one you can be happy with long-term.

Do a body image spot-check. Your body, like the rest of you, will just naturally change over time, due to things like a slowing metabolism and shifts in body composition. So, periodically you may have to adjust your expectations for your body. What was realistic for you ten years ago may not be realistic for you today.

Date: _____

Weight: _____

QUARTERLY INVENTORY

Twenty-six weeks down, 26 to go! How does it feel to be more in control of your weight and your health than ever before? If there was ever a time to pat yourself on the back, this is it!

And it's time again to review the good habits you've learned and incorporated into your daily life. As you did before, fill out the checklist below.

Aim for 14 or more "Yes!" or "Usually" answers out of 18, and don't forget about your reward!

Low-Fat Living Progress Report

	Yes!	Usually	I was afraid you'd ask that
1. I review my list of long-term goals regularly.	❏	❏	❏
2. I keep the kitchen as fat-free as possible.	❏	❏	❏
3. I meet my weekly exercise goal.	❏	❏	❏
4. I weigh myself once a week.	❏	❏	❏
5. I keep my success diary up-to-date.	❏	❏	❏
6. I eat a good breakfast every morning.	❏	❏	❏
7. I stick to low-fat items when I snack.	❏	❏	❏
8. I do de-stressing exercises to head off my urges to overeat.	❏	❏	❏
9. I drink eight glasses of water a day.	❏	❏	❏
10. I reward myself for meeting my minigoals.	❏	❏	❏
11. I do strength training two or three times per week.	❏	❏	❏
12. I stick to reasonable-size portions.	❏	❏	❏
13. I eat five servings of fruits and vegetables a day.	❏	❏	❏
14. I review my success diary when ever I need to give my program a boost.	❏	❏	❏
15. I don't overdo it in restaurants.	❏	❏	❏
16. I use positive self-talk to keep myself motivated.	❏	❏	❏
17. I try one new low-fat recipe a week.	❏	❏	❏
18. I find alternatives to outdoor walking when the weather's bad.	❏	❏	❏

WEEK 27: SWAP YOUR HIGH-FAT FAVORITES FOR SLIM TREATS

Exercise goal: Walk seven days, three miles per day in 45 minutes

By now you're slashing fat from your diet like a skilled swordsman! If you've been using the "Fat Budget," on page 23, as a guide, you know precisely what your fat-gram limit is so you can keep fat to no more than 25 percent of your daily calories. (If you haven't been using this handy guide, this week is a good time to familiarize yourself with it.)

Did you know that there are even more ways to reduce the fat in your diet while still letting you splurge every now and again on goodies like pizza, brownies and oatmeal cookies?

While you're paying close attention to your fat intake, be sure to also write down your meals and snacks in Your Perfect Weight Suc-

Think Light

Remember, we told you from the beginning that there is no room in Your Perfect Weight 52-Week Plan for denial and deprivation. Enjoying your food is in! So this week work with the list below to see how you can have your cake, eat it, too . . . and lose weight to boot! Amounts in column two are the same as those in column one, unless noted otherwise.

Instead of . . .	Have . . .	And Save (g. fat)
Brownie, from mix (1)	Light brownie, from mix	5.0
Caramel-corn snack mix (1 oz.)	Nonfat caramel-corn puffs	4.0
Cheese pizza, frozen (1 slice)	Low-fat frozen cheese pizza	4.0
Chocolate-covered vanilla ice-cream bar (1 bar; 2½ oz.)	Low-fat chocolate/vanilla ice-milk bar	4.0
Chocolate cupcake (1)	Light chocolate cupcake	4.0
Chocolate pudding, instant (½ cup)	Nonfat chocolate pudding, instant	3.0

cess Diary every day. Don't neglect your water intake, either. Those eight glasses a day keep you feeling satisfied.

Date: _____

Weight: _____

WEEK 28: VARY YOUR WORKOUT PACE

Exercise goal: Walk seven days, three miles per day in 45 minutes

Want to really maximize your fitness and give your weight loss—and your commitment level—a boost? Then introduce the concept of interval training to your walking (or running or cycling) workout. That means alternating higher-intensity spurts with low-intensity cool-down intervals.

Instead of . . .	Have . . .	And Save (g. fat)
Corn tortilla chips (about 10; 1 oz.)	Low-fat tortilla chips (22–28)	6.6
Fruit Danish (1 piece; 3⅓ oz.)	Nonfat fruit-filled breakfast pastry	15.9
Granola bar (1 bar; ¾ oz.)	Low-fat granola bar	2.2
Lasagna with meat, frozen (10¼ oz.)	Low-fat frozen lasagna with meat	7.0
Microwave popcorn (3 cups)	Light microwave popcorn	3.0
Oatmeal-raisin cookies (about 4; 2 oz.)	Nonfat oatmeal-raisin cookies	8.0
Potato chips (about 7; ½ oz.)	Nonfat pretzel chips (about 8)	4.7
Pound cake (1 slice; 1 oz.)	Nonfat pound cake	3.6
Tortilla chips, nacho-flavored (1 oz.)	Nacho-flavored rice cake (1)	6.5
Vanilla ice cream (½ cup)	Vanilla nonfat frozen yogurt	7.2
Wheat crackers (½ oz.)	Nonfat crackers	3.0

"Interval training means you're burning more calories per minute, and you're going to maintain a higher metabolic rate throughout the exercise," says Wayne L. Westcott, Ph.D., YMCA national strength-training consultant, and strength consultant to the National Academy of Sports Medicine. And it's going to ignite the afterburn effect, too. That means you'll continue to burn fat at a higher rate even after you stop exercising.

"The more intense the exercise, the greater the afterburn effect," says Bryant Stamford, Ph.D., exercise physiologist and director of the Health Promotion Center at the University of Louisville in Kentucky. With moderate exercise like walking, the afterburn bonus is minimal. But upping the intensity with interval training or engaging in other intense aerobic activities can make the afterburn linger for hours after your workout. (And preliminary research suggests that resistance training might produce a slight afterburn effect, too.)

Here's how interval training works: Let's say you're doing your daily walk. First warm up for ten minutes by walking at a moderate rate. Then pick up the pace till you're breathing harder (but not all out), for about a minute, or however long you feel comfortable. Slow down to a speed that lets you catch your breath—probably slower than your warm-up speed—for another minute. Then pick up the pace again, for another minute. Continue to alternate as long as you can, leaving time for a five-minute cooldown. (Make sure the time you allow for recovery is equal to the time you spent at higher intensity.)

Try this every now and then to give an added punch to your usual walk. But you still want to make sure that your bigger goal is to slowly improve your walking time each week until you reach your three-mile, 45-minute goal.

Date: _____

Weight: _____

WEEK 29: DRESS THIN UNTIL YOU GET THIN

Exercise goal: Walk seven days, three miles per day in 45 minutes

You'll hear a lot of dieters insisting, "I'm not going to buy any new clothes until I'm thin!" Maybe you're even one of them. Why, you wonder, should I shell out good money for a size-X dress when I can have the thrill of buying one a couple of sizes smaller in a few weeks?

That kind of thinking is a real mistake, on two counts insists Beryl Meyer, former *Harper's Bazaar* fashion writer and co-author of *Style: Developing the Real You.* "Buying some clothes to create a 'transitional wardrobe' will not only help you look your best right now but will also keep you motivated to keep going until you reach your goal weight," she says.

Meyer points out that "transitional" dressing usually refers to clothes that can be worn from one season to the next, but it can just as well refer to changing from one size to another. Buy one or two key pieces that will look good now and as you slim down even further in weeks to come, she urges.

Her own favorite transitional item: stirrup pants. "I love them because they're more comfortable than jeans, they bend and stretch with me and they make me look thinner than jeans, which have a tendency of standing away from the body and adding bulk." In fact, she says, although jeans are found in most people's wardrobes, they frequently end up being a fashion "don't."

"Overweight people think they have to squeeze into either very tight jeans, which emphasize every bump and lump and make you look like a stuffed sausage and are painful to wear, or baggy jeans, which make you look heavier," says Meyers. "But stirrup pants are flattering to most figures."

Here are a few more of Meyer's do's and don'ts for selecting clothes to make you look slimmer and more svelte right now.

Wear dark colors. Black, charcoal gray, navy, chocolate brown and hunter green are great for areas you wish to play down; wear bright tones in areas where you're already slim. So, if hips and thighs are trouble spots but you're fine above the waist, stick to deeper shades for pants and skirts and more vibrant hues for blouses, shirts, sweaters and vests.

Consider monochromatic dressing. This is another great way to look like you're thinner than you are. A top and bottom in the same or similar tone create a single slimming line of color, which tends to make you look taller and skinnier.

Watch that silhouette. Choose clothes that help give your body definition. It's a common misconception among overweight people that loose-fitting, baggy clothes disguise pounds, but visually they can tack on even more weight. So, opt for leggings or stirrup pants, which skim the trouble spots of your lower body while showing that you do have legs under there. Or, if you want to wear, say, a long, loose skirt in spring or summer, pair it with a waist-nipping jacket—again, to give some hint of definition to your body.

Don't pad yourself. Avoid clothes with unnecessary bulk—thick knitted sweaters, very nubby fabrics, or anything quilted or with popcorn or cable stitching. All that heavy material will only make you look heavier.

Indulge in a little syn. Synthetics, that is. Unlike the tacky polyester you probably remember from the *Saturday Night Fever* disco era, many of the clothes made from modern "miracle" fabrics boast the kinds of finishes you'll also see in luxury fabrics. As a result, they look expensive while retaining polyester's big plus: easy care. A big advantage of the new synthetics is control power. The new stretch fabrics have the controlling power of a traditional girdle, but are much more comfortable to wear. More and more top designers are using these fabrics to create clothes that are chic, sleek and often very slimming.

Focus on the vertical. Look for clothes that help create a visual vertical line. Good choices include pants with pleats (for men and women), slits in skirts (for women with great legs), V-neck blouses or sweaters, shoes with a bit of a heel and subtle vertical stripes. "You don't want to look like a barber pole," warns Meyer.

Accessorize wisely. Avoid details and accessories that call attention to trouble spots. If you've got an ample derriere, for example, what you don't want to wear are pants with back pockets (and certainly none with a designer's name on them). Nor would you choose a wide, chunky belt or one with a Frisbee-size buckle if it's going to encircle a wide, chunky waist. Use accessories to play up your best features—big, bold earrings, for instance, if you have a long, lovely neck, or eye-catching rings and bracelets if you've got pretty hands and arms.

Dressing well while you're still losing weight isn't mere vanity. It will go a very long way in keeping you motivated to the weight-loss finish line.

Date: _____

Weight: _____

WEEK 30: BOUNCING BACK FROM A BINGE

Exercise goal: Walk seven days, three miles
per day in 45 minutes

It's hard to keep up your discipline week after week. An occasional slip-up is inevitable. Now is a good time to look at how to handle it when you goof. You know the scene (probably all too well). Your cravings, or your emotions, get the best of you, and before you know it you're polishing off an entire _____(fill in the blank) of that incredibly fattening _____(fill in the blank).

Okay, these things happen—that's the first rule to keep in mind. You're only human, not a weight-loss machine, and every now and then you're going to overdo it. But if you think this is the beginning of the end, think again.

You're not on a diet anymore. You've got a whole new lifestyle, and lifestyles accommodate blips and binges in a way ordinary diets can't. So accept what you did, and move on by following this simple, step-by-step plan for bouncing back from a binge.

Stop eating! Quit while you're behind. Don't compound the problem by continuing to eat. One brief episode of bingeing probably won't do much harm to your weight-loss program, but letting it go on for hours or days will.

Forgive yourself. Errors in judgment happen. You can't eat perfectly at every meal, every day of your life. Be gentle with yourself when you slip up. Watch your self-talk. Avoid thoughts like, "How could I have been so stupid?" and, "I blew it; I'm awful." And certainly, don't punish yourself further by getting on the scale immediately. The gain, if any, probably won't have registered by then, but if it has, it won't make you feel better about yourself.

Have a glass of water. Or brush and floss your teeth. Rinsing the taste of the food from your mouth sort of says "Okay, now, playtime's over" to your brain.

Record what happened. This is one entry you're not going to enjoy making in Your Perfect Weight Success Diary, but make it you must. Not only will writing about your slip-up discourage you from doing it again but it also will help put things into perspective. You may not have binged as badly as you initially thought.

Reread past diary entries. How did you handle eating urges during other stressful moments? What were the strategies that worked for you then? What made this time different? Make a vow to review these passages before your next binge. (Maybe you can head it off at the pass.)

Immediately resume normal eating. Don't try to compensate by skipping the next meal or two, or by having just a celery stalk and black coffee for dinner. You'll only get hungry and may overeat again. Instead, have a normal meal and maybe go a bit easier than usual on portions. Your meals and your appetite will be back on track in no time.

Exercise. Here's one good way to compensate for the binge—with a little extra fat busting. If you've only walked six days this week, walk a seventh, or add 30 minutes on your stationary bike or in the pool. You'll be helping to burn a couple of hundred of those unwanted calories.

Reward yourself. Rewards aren't just for doing good things, they're also for avoiding bad things, like uncontrolled eating. Every time you successfully avoid a major binge by doing those tried-and-true activities—drinking water, doing de-stressing exercises, jotting down your feelings, going for a walk, calling a friend—you deserve a little extra reward for your efforts. Pretty soon, binge busting will be second nature to you.

Date: _____

Weight: _____

WEEK 31: CHOOSE A WALKING BUDDY

Exercise goal: Walk seven days, three miles per day in 45 minutes

One of the beauties of walking is that it gives you precious time to think and to be alone. But let's face it. Sometimes it's better not to be alone, especially when your motivation starts to slip.

You're now seven months into your new low-fat eating and fitness program. And while you're undoubtedly seeing results from your steady efforts, that daily discipline can sometimes be a drag. At such times, there's no better way to boost your flagging motivation than with a walking buddy. And because you know by now that exercise should be a daily (or almost daily) goal to produce the best weight-loss results, it's wise to stay close to home when seeking a partner.

See if you can enlist your spouse, child, parent, a close neighbor, even the family dog. That way, every time you exercise you're also strengthening the most important relationships in your life.

Some days you choose your walking partners, and some days they choose you! Be open and flexible to whomever happens to stroll your way. You may not find someone who shares your enthusiasm for walking every day, but you may find two or three different people to keep you company throughout the week.

Here are a few ways to keep yourself in walking partners.

Pair up with a pooch. Although we're not saying you should get a pet just to have a walking companion, there's a reason a dog is called man's best friend—Rover may be the most reliable walking buddy you can find.

Dogs always want to go for a walk and tend to be very happy about the idea. They remind you when it's time to go out (in case you've forgotten or gotten too comfortable in front of the TV). They make good company— they rarely complain and are great listeners if you want to talk. And when you decide to slip on your headphones and listen to music, a dog won't feel slighted.

Enjoy young company. Children can be great walking partners, provided you're walking toward some destination that appeals to them. Good examples: video arcades and baseball card or comic book stores. The distance never seems to be daunting if the goal is enticing enough and you can have lots of fun and exercise along the way.

When walking with young kids, remember: You're the adult, the one with the ability to adapt. Walk slowly enough to match their pace. Don't walk so far or so fast that they'll never want to go out with you again. And don't take this as an opportunity to lecture to a captive audience. Relax, let them talk and enjoy your company.

Walk at work. Your workplace can be fertile ground for finding walking partners. A 15-minute walk break during lunchtime or instead of a coffee-and-doughnut break is a terrific stress-reducer and rejuvenator.

Seek out various kinds of partners. On days you're not up to working up a sweat, find somebody who likes to stroll, and someone else for those half-hour uphill strides. Keep an extra pair of walking shoes and socks at work so you can be ready at a moment's notice.

Form a mutual motivation society. To keep motivation high, find a walking buddy with the same agenda as yours: weight loss and overall fitness. This might be a good opportunity to discuss low-fat recipes you've tried or swap information about which local restaurants cater to your healthy-eating needs. Your common goals will help bring you together again and again for fat burning and for friendship.

And speaking of recipes, you should always be on the lookout for new, yummy dishes to try at home. This book is loaded with some great ones, but during one of your daily walks you might want to meander your way to a bookstore to check out the low-fat cookbooks. A new one every so often will help give your meals, and your motivation, a much-needed boost.

Date: _____

Weight: _____

WEEK 32: LEARN TO LOVE THOSE LABELS

Exercise goal: Walk seven days, three miles
per day in 45 minutes

Are you sticking to high-energy, low-fat breakfasts to get your day off on the right foot? As you may know by now, a good breakfast and a vigorous walk is a dynamite combination for keeping weight off and spirits high! Paying attention to these basics will pay off for the rest of your life.

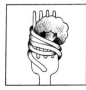
And speaking of basics, have you learned how to take advantage of all the information available on your favorite packaged food labels? A little over a year ago, our friends at the U.S. Department of Agriculture saw to it that the labels—now called Nutrition Facts—are easier to read and understand, more accurate and, ultimately, more useful.

"They're better because they provide more relevant information," says registered dietitian Donna Dispas-Gebert, director of nutrition services at the Benjamin Franklin Weight Management and Metabolism Center in Allentown, Pennsylvania. "The new label emphasizes nutrients that are most important for today's consumers, who worry about getting too much of things like fat and saturated fat, cholesterol and sodium. Even the larger size of the label is nice."

The biggest single change you'll notice is the introduction of a section called Percent Daily Values, for all the nutrients contained in that food. Sure, there were nutrients listed on the old labels. But now you'll see that, in addition to the amount of nutrients found per serving, they've also been broken down into percentages, to show you how the food fits into a 2,000-calorie-a-day diet.

For example, if you eat ½ cup (dry) of oatmeal for breakfast, the Nutrition Facts label tells you that you've consumed 5 percent of the fat, 0 percent of the sodium and 15 percent of the fiber you need for the day. Naturally, if you're eating fewer than 2,000 calories a day—as you probably will if you're a dieting woman—you'll make adjustments accordingly. "Using the Daily Values, you can build a healthful diet based on your personal nutrient goals," advises Dispas-Gebert.

What she particularly likes about the new labeling is the truth and consistency now found in portion listings. "Before, manufacturers were allowed to state portions in a way that made their products look more attractive. The people who've been most guilty of taking advantage were juice manufacturers. For example, a 12-ounce bottle of a certain juice might have said '90 calories,' so at first glance you'd think there were 90 calories in the whole bottle. Then if you looked closer, you'd see there were 90 calories in just 3 ounces of juice. This kind of labeling was done by a lot of manufacturers of soft drinks and carbonated beverages, too. But with the new USDA mandate, you have a much better sense of what you're getting."

Now, all products within the same basic category are evaluated in terms of equal-size portions, portions that are realistic for the average adult. (No more 3-ounce servings of juice.)

In short, the new labels are a boon to everyone, but to no one more than the dieter. "From a weight-control standpoint," says Dispas-Gebert, "the labels help you juggle your food and plan your whole day."

This week pay particular attention to the labels on all the prepared foods that you eat or prepare for your family. Try to see how many ways you can come up with to make this useful information a part of your regular eating plan.

Date: _____

Weight: _____

WEEK 33: TICKLE YOUR TASTE BUDS!

Exercise Goal: Walk seven days, three miles per day in 45 minutes

By now you know firsthand that low-fat eating doesn't have to mean bored-to-death taste buds. But you have to be vigilant!

It's all too easy to return to the same three or four dishes over and over again simply because they're quick or convenient. That's a one-way trip to dull eating. Not only that, dull repetition can sabotage your resolve. "You're not going to last, and you'll go back to the full-fat stuff," warns nutritionist and registered dietitian Evelyn Tribole, author of *Eating on the Run* and spokesperson for the American Dietetic Association.

Finding new ways to keep your eating interesting is an on-going challenge. But it's a challenge that you have to meet in order to get slim and stay slim. This week spend some time thinking of new ways to spark your interest in healthy eating. Here are a few tips to get you started.

Buy the freshest vegetables you can find. "Vegetables right out of the ground are incredible," says food consultant Aliza Green, a chef with 15 years' experience in Philadelphia. But that heavenly flavor vanishes when veggies sit around. To get the most intense flavor, look for vegetables in season. Go to farmers' markets or to roadside stands, or find the supermarkets in your area known for the best produce.

Check out today's newfangled foods. Ever had a plumcot—a sweet, tangy cross between a plum and an apricot? Or yellow fingers—rich, buttery-tasting potatoes the size of your fingers? Dazzle your family and your palate with one or more of these new varieties of produce.

Spice up your life. Many wonderful seasonings, such as cilantro, coriander seed and cumin are acquired tastes. You need repeated exposures—and then you love them! Green's gentle-but-firm advice for trying a new herb or spice? "Don't be afraid! Have a little bit, and give it a chance."

Bet on basil. Green calls basil the "number-one, most-important, don't-live-without-it herb." She also says it's best when fresh: "It's practically worthless when it's dried." Look for fresh basil in farmers' markets or the produce section of your supermarket. To store it, cut the fresh stems and place the "bouquet" in a glass of water, then cover it with a plastic bag and refrigerate. If stored properly, it'll keep about a week. (Make sure your refrigerator isn't too cold; basil freezes easily.)

Expand your condiment collection. Perk up bland meals with fat-free condiments from the gourmet aisle of your supermarket. Try mango chutney with a plain baked chicken breast. Or how about swapping the usual mayo for some coarse-grained mustard on a turkey breast sandwich? You and your family will love the tangy difference.

Date: _____

Weight: _____

WEEK 34: ADD NEW STRENGTH TO YOUR STRENGTH TRAINING

Exercise goal: Walk seven days, three miles per day in 45 minutes

It's Week 34 and Your Perfect Weight 52-Week Plan is in superhigh gear! By now you should be a convert to the low-fat way of life. And your walking program is helping to burn calories nearly as fast as you take them in. And now's the week to try (if you haven't already) some strength-training work with free weights and machines.

Weeks ago we suggested you check out a local fitness facility so you could start to feel at home in the weight room. While you may have some strength-training gear in your bedroom or basement, you'll probably get even better results and jolt your fat-burning metabolism up a notch once you start putting in time with the professional equipment at the Y or health club.

Here are five exercises to try. Remember, the closer you come to two or three strength-training sessions per week, the better the results you'll see on the scale. One set of each exercise consists of 8 to 12 repetitions. Try to do three sets of each exercise. If you haven't worked with weights or machines before, ask for help in selecting the amount of weight appropriate for you and for instruction in proper form.

Bench press. Lie back on an exercise bench with your feet flat on the floor. Grasp dumbbells or a barbell with your hands slightly more than just shoulder-width apart. Start with your arms extended straight up. Slowly lower the weight to your chest. Then press it back up until your arms are fully extended. Don't lock your elbows. Repeat.

Leg press. Sit in a leg-press machine, place your feet on the foot pads, and press out until your legs are straight. Slowly return the weights to the original starting point. Repeat.

Seated pulley row. Sit on the machine with your knees slightly flexed. (Your feet should be resting against an object to help you maintain stability.) Keep your upper torso erect and your lower back flexed. Grab hold of the handle and pull it slowly and smoothly to your chest, just below your chest muscles. Try not to use your torso to pull the weight. Return to the starting position, with the weights going back down. Repeat.

Seated quadriceps extension. Sit with your feet under pads. Straighten your legs, then slowly lower your feet back down. If your knees hurt or it's too difficult to go to the full extension, just do a partial repetition, shortening the path.

Hamstring curl. Lie face down, with your heels under pads, holding on to the front of the leg-curl machine. Curl your legs up until your calves touch the backs of your thighs. Return to the down position and repeat.

Date: _____

Weight: _____

WEEK 35: MAKE SOME NEW WEEK'S RESOLUTIONS

Exercise goal: Walk seven days, three miles per day in 45 minutes

New Year's resolutions—in theory, they're wonderful. They give all of us a chance to start fresh by reviewing those things about ourselves that could use a little fine-tuning, and then doing something about it. And for most people, a set of New Year's resolutions wouldn't be complete without some mention of weight loss—dropping a few pounds, doing a few push-ups or some combination of both.

But the truth is, New Year's resolutions have become a joke. Most folks know almost as they announce their resolutions that it's just a matter of time before their pound-shedding plans will go awry. In fact, one popular survey revealed that more than 25 percent quit their diet within a month, while another 25 percent managed to hang in for another couple of months before throwing in the towel. No wonder losing weight crops up as a resolution year after new year.

Yet that's just the point: The time frame is out of whack. As we've said all along, goals need to be broken down into small, reachable ones. Yearlong goals, no matter how admirable, don't work, particularly when it comes to dieting. Most of us think about eating (or not eating) several times a day, so who can wait 365 days to measure weight-loss successes?

So it's time to finally dump the idea of New Year's resolutions and switch to new week resolutions, which is exactly what Your Perfect Weight 52-Week Plan is all about. What we've been doing for the past 35 weeks is, in effect, giving you a new resolution to adopt each week, along with a weekly walking goal.

Some of these weekly resolutions will be more challenging for you than others. For instance, you may already be pretty smart about fat cutting but need to work on your strength training. Each week, from now on, you should focus on those specific areas you'd like to improve, and turn them into your own personal resolutions. And feel free to come up with a few others you may not have seen in these pages.

Personalizing Your Program

We've also made it easier to stick to your resolutions by giving you three important tracking tools: the Date/Weight lines at the end of every week, the quarterly inventories and Your Perfect Weight Success Diary. Whenever you find you're not happy with some of your eating or exercise behaviors, you can make a few quick changes and then check out how you've done immediately. (No more waiting till December 31 to do a final inventory!)

Spend a little time this week reviewing these three items, and make some notes about individual goals you'd like to work on in the coming weeks.

This is the beauty of weekly resolutions. And when you make and monitor your own personal resolutions each week, on January 1 you can sit back and smile about how far your resolutions have already brought you while other people struggle to make theirs stick for the next 52.

Date: _____

Weight: _____

WEEK 36: LEARN HOW TO BANK YOUR FOOD
Exercise goal: Walk seven days, three miles
per day in 45 minutes

If you haven't hit your weight-loss goal by now, you must be getting closer to it. Feels great, doesn't it? But with that excitement comes the sobering reality that soon you must face the looming specter of possible weight regain.

If you're like most folks, you've been on and off diets . . . and on and off . . . and on and off. It's time for you to say goodbye to that on again, off again merry-go-round. Your near-daily walking should be doing its bit to help you keep those pounds far, far away. But equally vital to successful weight loss and maintenance is *trading off*.

What do we mean? All of life is trading off—giving up this so we can get that. You've been living that principle for the past 36 weeks, yet every now and then you may have slipped a little, and maybe even seen your weight inch up a bit.

But if you continually practice the fine art of trading off, your weight will come off and stay off. Just ask Carole Livingston, author of *I'll Never Be Fat Again!* who has maintained a 40-pound weight loss for more than two decades.

"Let's say today is Monday, and there's a wedding coming up Saturday night," says Livingston. "Bank your food, eating very cautiously during the week so you can eat more, but not pig out, at the wedding. Or, if I know I'll be going out to eat this evening, then I'll eat a little bit less at breakfast and lunch. It's just common sense, but most people don't think about it."

Livingston is not advocating skipping meals. "The most dangerous thing for any dieter is being hungry. That's when you lose control," she says. "You may not even realize you're hungry; it may come out in crankiness or irritability, and you unconsciously start reaching for whatever you think will satisfy that hunger. But if you let yourself eat during the day, you won't have that uncontrollable hunger."

After a while, the whole routine becomes second nature. "So, if I want one chocolate chip cookie tonight with a cup of tea, I know I can't also have dessert for dinner. Or if I have a larger-than-usual business lunch, I may skip my after-dinner snack," she explains. "It's contantly trading one thing off against another. I don't believe you should miss out on something you enjoy, though, as long as it's within reason. For example, if you're going to a dinner party at the home of a wonderful cook, that's not the time to pass up dessert if you think you'll feel deprived. But what you can do to trade off is at lunchtime to cut your sandwich in half instead of eating the whole sandwich."

Simple? Absolutely. And yet it's a trick that successful weight maintainers like Livingston swear by. And it's also a nifty, calorie-saving habit to develop.

"The ultimate trade-off," adds Livingston, "is giving up some food now so you can slim down later."

Trading off, by the way, also applies to things like exercise. Walking for nearly an hour a day translates into an hour a day less of TV. Oh, but what a terrific body you're getting in return!

Date: _____

Weight: _____

WEEK 37: TRY AN EXERCISE VIDEO

Exercise goal: Walk seven days, three miles
per day in 45 minutes

Your walking program is great, but for those days you feel like switching to some indoor exercise, nothing could be simpler than to roll out the exercise mat and pop a workout video in the VCR. But which video?

Everyone from Oscar-winner Jane Fonda to country singer Tanya Tucker to Golden Girl Estelle Getty wants to help get you in shape these days via their own personalized workout tapes. And there's no question about it: Exercise videos are a boon to those of us who have neither the time nor the inclination to expose our spandex-clad bodies to the harsh glare of an aerobics class. A workout tape helps you get your heart rate up and your body toned—at your own pace, at your own place.

But with literally thousands of exercise videos to choose from, how do you choose? After all, why plunk down $20 or $25 for a tape you might play once and never use again because it's too easy, too difficult, too boring—or because the instructor's voice just drives you crazy?

These tips from Liz George, former new-products editor at *Weight Watchers Magazine*, will help you get the most from an exercise video.

Borrow before you buy. Before you invest in a particular video, borrow several from the public library or rent a few from your local video store. It's a low- to no-cost way to preview a range of workout styles and instructors.

Get the right tape for your level. "If you're just starting out, the best thing is to look for something that incorporates both an aerobic workout and toning exercises," advises George. "By combining both, you'll see results quicker and you'll also get a better overall workout. If you're more experienced—let's say you're in pretty good shape and want to improve one particular area of your body—then you'll want a video that focuses on that. Look for buzzwords like *beginners* or *advanced* on the box."

The best videos include about ten minutes of warming up and cooling down, says George. If they're not on the tape, be sure to include them in your workout sessions anyway.

Check out the credentials. Someone might be a terrific actress, but does that make her a good workout instructor? Maybe . . . and maybe not. George suggests looking for a seal on the video box that indicates that the instructor is properly certified.

"Is she just the celebrity of the month or does she have a real background in fitness? Look for some kind of accreditation," she says. "Then you can trust the instructor."

Go slow. Some videos give guidelines for frequency, but regardless of the recommendation on the box, you should start out slow. "If you try to use it every day, you'll end up getting burned out," warns George. "If you're in good shape, it may be okay to do it every day, but if not it may discourage you. Instead, try for three times a week, 20 to 30 minutes per session. If you find you're getting too tired, don't push yourself. Find your level of comfort and try to build on it instead of trying to keep up with Jane Fonda right off the bat."

And don't ignore the video if it has stopping points along the way. Says George: "They're for you to check your pulse and to see how you're feeling. If it seems as though you're going beyond what you're comfortably capable of doing, these will remind you to assess the workout and maybe slow down."

Date: _____

Weight: _____

WEEK 38: GET A GRIP ON THOSE FANTASIES
Exercise goal: Walk seven days three miles
per day in 45 minutes

Will weight loss change your life? What a silly question. You've been on Your Perfect Weight 52-Week Plan long enough to know that the answer is a resounding "Yes!" Surely you've seen lots of changes—everything from the way the scale seems to moan a bit less when you get on it now to the thrilling bagginess of your clothes, from your extra energy to the compliments you've been hearing.

Why, then, with all that's different since launching your new eating and exercise plan, do you sometimes feel like nothing's changed? Can it be that, despite your trimmer body, you and your life are really very much the same as before?

Another resounding "Yes."

What happened, you may be wondering, to all those fantasies you had about your future once you were finally slim and svelte? You might be very close to your goal weight right now, and yet that pot of gold or that loving mate or that better job seems as elusive as ever.

"One of the things that happens with weight loss is that you lose a lot of your old fantasies," says Ronette Kolotkin, Ph.D., director of the behavioral program at Duke University Diet and Fitness Center in Durham, North

Carolina. "People have fantasies like: 'When I'm thin, my partner will treat me better,' or 'My sex life will improve,' or 'I'll make money because my weight won't hold me back any longer,' or 'I won't be shy anymore'—that's a common one. They run the gamut."

Checking In to Reality

The reality is that while being slim will probably make you happier, it's certainly no guarantee of a perfect, hassle-free existence. Getting what you want out of life takes action, whether you're fat, thin or in between, and who better than you knows the terrific rewards of taking action? It's what you've been doing for most of the past year!

Sure, you may be more confident going on a job interview today without that belly bulge, but your job skills probably aren't all that different now that you're slimmer.

"I always remind people of that old saying, 'Watch what you wish for— you might get it,'" says Dr. Kolotkin. "One woman I worked with wished that she'd have so many dates that the men would be breaking down her door. After she lost weight, it happened—she's very attractive. But suddenly she started wondering about these guys: 'Are they sincere? Do they like me just for my looks? Why weren't they here before, when I was the same person?' She isn't just dating now; now she has to deal with the challenges of dating, figuring out who's decent, how far she should go sexually. All the normal things everyone has to deal with, she was protected from before. So she traded one problem for another."

Get Ready for Action

Which isn't to say that you should abandon your weight-loss program—not at all. But now's an ideal time to start thinking ahead realistically to what you want your life to be like, now and when you're as thin as you want to be.

Itemize your expectations. Make a list of the changes you hope will happen once you reach your goal weight. One way of outlining those changes is to write a page or two describing "My Life Six Months (or one year, or whatever) from Now." What kind of work would you like to be doing? Where would you like to be living? What kind of relationship do you want to be in, or how would you like to see your current relationship change? Would you like to be pregnant by then, or growing roses, or traveling in the Orient? Whatever you hope to see happen, write it down.

Stop putting your life on hold. The longer you postpone making those wished-for changes and the more you attach them to a particular goal weight, the less your chances of seeing them happen. Ask yourself what you can do right now to start making your dreams reality.

If you want to switch careers, for example, begin by ordering some appropriate college catalogs and talking to people in the field you're considering. Tired of being so shy? Take an adult education course in public speaking, or make a lunch date with a friendly co-worker within the next couple of weeks. You don't have to wait till you reach your perfect weight to start improving your life.

Expect gradual, not radical, changes. Just as it's foolish to expect to lose weight overnight, it's equally silly to believe that a smaller number on the scale will instantly bring you a whole new personality or an exciting new life. All worthwhile change takes time.

Date: _____

Weight: _____

WEEK 39: INDULGE IN A MASSAGE
Exercise goal: Walk seven days, three miles per day in 45 minutes

For many months now you've been treating your body with nothing but TLC. You've been feeding it the most healthful foods, taking it for walks just about every day, and making it strong through strength training. Want to do something extra special for it? Indulge in a soothing, spirit-lifting massage.

"Massage is important for everyone's well-being, both physical and emotional," says Betsy Bickel, a certified massage therapist and director of the massage therapy department at the Duke University Diet and Fitness Center in Durham, North Carolina. It connects you to your body in ways that other activities don't. It makes you more conscious of where you're holding tension. If you're in deep stress, it can help you relax. It helps prevent injury by letting you know whether the amount of tension in your body is about to throw you over the pain threshold. It increases the blood flow and lymph flow, it stretches and relaxes muscles and releases toxins from muscles."

As if all that weren't enough, says Bickel, massage has all these benefits and more for dieters. "Massage is doubly important for people in the process of trying to change their weight and physical habits because it can help you get a truer body image," she says. "A lot of people have a distorted image. They see themselves as either much heavier or much thinner, and massage helps give you a reality check. My clients tell me that the tactile stimulation gives them a sense of coming back into their body. Many of us live so much in our head that having your skin touched draws you back into living in your body."

People who are starting to delight in seeing their body grow slimmer and stronger simply love having it pampered with soothing strokes and fragrant oils, says Bickel. And a massage is a terrific reward for following a sensible eating and exercise program, as well as a motivator to keep it going.

Not only does massage feel great after exercising, but for some people, massage has enabled them to exercise for the first time in a long time. "If you're in pain, you're not going to want to run or bicycle or lift your arm to throw a baseball," says Bickel. "But massage often relieves pain, and so it can free people up to do the physical activities they want to do." Keep this in mind if you haven't been exercising as much as you'd like to.

Massage also has the remarkable power to put you in greater touch with your feelings and emotions, says Bickel. "One thing I've been aware of is that people may overeat because they're not getting certain needs met," she says. "It's like with any addiction: If you can't have what you want, you try to use something else to fill that need.

"One basic need that often goes unfulfilled is human touch. We have to be touched to be healthy. For overweight people, that might be one of the needs they're trying to fill through eating, but massage may reduce their desire to eat. It can give them a deep sense of nourishment not related to food."

Reach Out and Touch

Nothing beats an hourlong massage at the hands of a trained massage therapist. But just because you don't have the time or the money to indulge on a regular basis doesn't mean you have to neglect the satisfaction that comes from a quick and simple at-home massage.

"I encourage people to work on each other. It's easy to give someone a nice touch and relieve their stress," says Bickel. "Family members can rub each other's shoulders or work on each other's neck, head and feet while watching TV at night. It's a way to connect with one another."

You can also give and get mini massages at work. Instead of eating a sugary snack during your coffee break, how much better to have your neck and shoulders rubbed for five or ten minutes!

In a pinch, you can even massage yourself, says Bickel. "I work on my shoulders all the time. It's good to combine massage with stretching; you'll find out what's tight as soon as you start stretching," she says. "You can work down your arms and legs, do your feet, your stomach. You can even do your own back! Place a couple of tennis balls on the floor. Then lie down on your back, with the balls on either side of your spine, and roll slowly against them."

Date: _____

Weight: _____

QUARTERLY INVENTORY

It's that time again. Here's your chance to review the progress you've made in the past four months. Your habits are no doubt in tip-top shape by now, but here's your chance to see where they might need a bit of sprucing up.

Low-Fat Living Progress Report

	Yes!	Usually	I was afraid you'd ask that
1. I review my list of long-term goals regularly.	❑	❑	❑
2. I keep the kitchen as fat-free as possible.	❑	❑	❑
3. I meet my weekly exercise goal.	❑	❑	❑
4. I weigh myself once a week.			
5. I keep my success diary up-to-date.	❑	❑	❑
6. I eat a good breakfast every morning.	❑	❑	❑
7. I stick to low-fat items when I snack.	❑	❑	❑
8. I do de-stressing exercises to head off my urges to overeat.	❑	❑	❑
9. I drink eight glasses of water a day.	❑	❑	❑
10. I reward myself for meeting my minigoals.	❑	❑	❑
11. I do strength training two or three times per week.	❑	❑	❑
12. I stick to reasonable-size portions.	❑	❑	❑
13. I eat five servings of fruits and vegetables a day.	❑	❑	❑
14. I review my success diary whenever I need to give my program a boost.	❑	❑	❑
15. I don't overdo it in restaurants.	❑	❑	❑
16. I use positive self-talk to keep myself motivated.	❑	❑	❑
17. I try one new low-fat recipe a week.	❑	❑	❑
18. I find alternatives to outdoor walking when the weather's bad.	❑	❑	❑
19. I use binge-busting techniques when I'm on the verge of overdoing it.	❑	❑	❑
20. I trade off food at one meal when I'm anticipating a bigger meal later on.	❑	❑	❑

How'd you do? Did you get at least 16 "Yes!" or "Usually" answers? We hope you've been continuing to give yourself rewards as you've reached your minigoals over the past 13 weeks. By now, you're probably due for a fairly major reward! Don't deny yourself: It's a bigger motivation booster than you'll ever know. You've just read about the joys of massage, why not sign up for an hourlong soothing massage now? You'll love it. And, again, start thinking about what you'll plan for yourself during your next, and final, inventory just a short 13 weeks from today.

WEEK 40: MAKE A FEW MORE LITTLE CHANGES

Exercise goal: Walk seven days, three miles per day in 45 minutes

By this time in the 52-week plan, you've learned and experienced the true secret of diet success: that tiny lifestyle changes can lead to big results.

"Permanent weight loss means making small, manageable changes and sticking with them for life," says Michael Hamilton, M.D., director of the Duke University Diet and Fitness Center in Durham, North Carolina. Now you want to keep building on those small eating and exercise improvements you've been making all along, and find a few more nonthreatening changes you can make to keep the weight heading downward and the motivation steady.

For instance? When Steve Purser, with the San Francisco public health department, felt ready to lose weight, he made only two changes: "I cut out alcohol, and instead of diving into sweets after dinner, I took a walk. If I still wanted dessert after my walk, I'd have it. But usually, when I got home, I felt fine going without it."

"To keep weight off, make small changes over time, and make them at your own pace," urges Joan Price, author of *The Honest Truth about Losing Weight and Keeping It Off*.

When you're pondering possible changes, registered dietitian Trish Ratto, associate director of health promotion at the University of California, Berkeley, advises, "Be honest with yourself. Don't even consider a change you're unwilling to stick to. If you can't live with it, it won't become permanent."

Right now, make a list of all the additional things you're truly willing to do. Looking back at some of the changes you've already made will show you if, for example, you tend to be more amenable to making exercise rather than dietary changes. Perhaps you've gotten into the daily walking groove. Maybe now's the time to consider giving up the office elevator and walking the three flights of stairs to your office every day. Or, you might have easily made the switch from ice cream to frozen yogurt, but what if you now limited your weekly frozen-dessert intake to twice a week instead of your usual three or four?

Again, list—and attempt—only those adjustments you know you'll make comfortably and permanently. Notes Ronette Kolotkin, Ph.D., director of the behavioral program at the Duke University Diet and Fitness Center, "It's the small changes that become permanent, and permanence is crucial. I applaud switching from cheeseburgers to hamburgers, if it's for life."

Date: _____

Weight: _____

WEEK 41: GET SOME SUPPORT
Exercise goal: Walk seven days, three miles per day in 45 minutes

---

Here you are, having successfully completed ten-plus months on the program, and you may still find it tough to stay on track every now and then. It's perfectly normal; life is packed with ups and downs, and it's typical for people who've had weight problems to try to handle their emotions with food.

Even though you've undoubtedly learned a number of ways to cope, the time inevitably comes when you feel like you simply can't do it alone. That's when you may need to ask for help, which is perfectly fine. No man is an island, and no dieter has to be one, either. Indeed, seeking weight-loss support is not only okay, but may also actually be the best thing you can do for yourself right now.

"If you look at the factors that predict successful, permanent weight loss, social support ranks near the top of the list," says John Foreyt, Ph.D., co-author of *Living without Dieting* and director of the Nutrition Research Clinic at Baylor College School of Medicine in Houston, Texas. "I'd go so far as to say it is absolutely critical."

If you haven't already, you should make a public commitment to your new, slimmer lifestyle, says Dr. Foreyt. "It's not that you want to force yourself into a situation you can't back down from because everyone knows about it," he says. "What you are actually doing is making an assertive ap-peal for help and understanding."

Dr. Foreyt outlines four levels of support, each with its own special pur-pose and benefit.

First there's your family. By now they've surely gotten used to your new lifestyle. But you may have to periodically remind them that certain foods have to be kept out of the house.

"Compromises on family time may have to be made when your exercise or other activities conflict with family plans," says Dr. Foreyt. But recruiting your family's support in your weight-loss and weight-maintenance efforts means always having a willing ear nearby when you need someone to talk to. It also means that you may get to spend more time together doing family fitness activities.

The second level is composed of close friends. "Everyone should have someone they can call at three in the morning when temptation rears its ugly head," insists Dr. Foreyt. "Even one really good friend can make the dif-ference in a crisis."

If you haven't yet established a strong relationship with a diet buddy, now's the time to do so. That bond will hold you in good stead throughout your weight-maintenance efforts.

The third and fourth levels involve support groups and your doctor. "Support groups are the perfect place to get advice and encouragement from people experiencing the same thing you are," notes Dr. Foreyt. "And your doctor gives you information and knowledgeable feedback, and helps you monitor your progress."

If you find yourself experiencing a weight-loss plateau, for example, your physician will probably be glad to look over your food and exercise diary and offer some suggestions for getting unstuck.

Support groups range from reasonably priced, diet and behavior modifi-cation organizations like Weight Watchers to no-cost, more spiritually ori-ented groups such as Overeaters Anonymous. You might want to sample several before committing your time (and money) to any one in particular. You might also form your own support group of friends who are in the process of making the same kinds of lifestyle changes that you are.

Family and friends usually make the best all-around cheerleaders, but they have to know that you need to be cheered on! Don't be shy. Remind them of your accomplishments. Have a friend or family member join you on one of your daily walks whenever you want somebody to chat with. And periodically invite a pal—somebody who's dieting or not—to share one of the low-fat meals that have become the cornerstone of your slim, new way of life.

Date: _____

Weight: _____

Week 42: Go for the Walking Gold

Exercise goal: Walk seven days, three miles per day in 45 minutes (or less)

If you haven't yet hit the walking goal we set for you in Week 26—that is, three miles in 45 minutes or three 15-minute miles—don't worry. In time you probably will. Your primary aim is to improve your own habits, at your own pace. Whatever your walking speed may be at the moment, you've surely come a long way from where you started way back on Week 1. So, good for you! And keep it up.

And if you're a superwalker who did reach that 15-minute-mile mark, a big pat on the back is in order! This week, and through the end of the 52-week plan, you have the option to either continue at this pace or try to do a tad better. "For most people," says our walking expert, Casey Meyers, "three miles a day in 45 minutes will be all they need to do. But you might be feeling so fit and good now that you may want to aim for a higher fitness level."

If you're in that hearty group, Meyers recommends you aim to walk faster, not farther. Shave a little more time off your daily three-mile walk, at the modest rate of 30 seconds less per week, until you're down to a 13-minute mile. To make your fitness walking more of a challenge, your walking goal this week will be three miles in 44½ minutes, then 44 minutes next week, 43½ minutes the following week, until the end of the 52-week plan, when you may be able to do your three daily miles in an aerobic 39 minutes.

Again, a big reminder: Don't push yourself beyond reasonable limits. "Always err on the side of conservatism," insists Meyers who, at age 66, generally walks seven days a week, covering three to five miles per day in anywhere from 12 to 15 minutes per mile.

"I vary it, depending on the weather, the amount of time I have and my desire," he says. "You don't have to walk the same distance or at the same pace every day." But if you need an incentive to go for the walking gold, listen to Meyers: "Do three 13-minute miles a day, combined with a low-fat diet, and you'll have your weight-loss program nailed!"

And speaking of diet, are you still monitoring your snacks and portion sizes? It's those little extras that can so often undo all your exercise efforts. Keep a watchful eye, now more than ever, as you get closer and closer to your goal. Don't let unexpected food find its way to your mouth, and it won't end up on your hips.

Date: _____

Weight: _____

WEEK 43: LEARN 21
QUICK SLIMMING TRICKS
Exercise goal: Walk seven days, three miles per day in 45 minutes (or less)

This week, as you head into the home stretch of the 52-week plan, we offer a list of 21 more smart ways to cut fat and keep your tummy satisfied, all week long. Try as many as you like, and don't be surprised if they help give your weight loss a nice, extra boost.

1. For a quick, sweet snack, eat ten jelly beans. They're fat-free and have just 100 calories.

2. Turn in your membership card in the Clean Plate Club. Get in the habit (if you're not already) of leaving a little food on your plate, particularly the higher-fat, higher-calorie items.

3. Never buy Girl Scout cookies! It may sound un-American, but there are other ways to support our girls in green without gaining weight in the process.

4. Say a little prayer before meals, even if you're not especially religious. It will make you feel good, appreciate what you have and put you back in touch with the true purpose of eating: to give nourishment to your body.

5. Buy yourself a new kitchen gadget. (A garlic press? An automatic rice cooker?) It'll make cooking that new low-fat recipe more fun.

6. Eliminate from your life forever one food favorite that has little or no nutritional value. Whether your choice is cherry cheesecake or cheese in an aerosol can, making the commitment to keep it out of your diet, and succeeding, month after month, will give you a greater sense of mastery over your weight-loss program and yourself. (If you're even more ambitious, you might try this with a different item each month.)

7. Every time you go food shopping, select something low-fat you've never tried before. One week, it might be jícama, the next it could be a fat-free granola bar. The more you try new tastes, the less you'll be bored with your diet.

8. If you usually read while you eat, stop. The longer the article or book, the longer you'll want to keep eating!

9. Get "known" for eating certain healthy foods, whether it's broiled fish or brown rice or whole-wheat pita sandwiches. Then your friends and relatives will make a greater effort to have these items on the menu when they invite you over.

10. Ask yourself, "Am I really hungry?" before you pop any food into your mouth. It's a surprisingly simple technique for avoiding the unconscious eating that packs on pounds.

11. On a cold or rainy day, prepare several low-fat, freeze-ahead meals, and save yourself cooking time later in the week.

12. Don't get fooled by foods labeled "no cholesterol." They still might be high in calories.

13. Shift your mealtimes to 30 or 60 minutes later than usual. It will help you get out of the habit of eating whether or not you're hungry just because the clock says it's 8:00 A.M. or 6:30 P.M.

14. Change your attitude about vacation eating. Instead of thinking, "This is my vacation and I'm going to eat as much as I like!" tell yourself, "This is my vacation and I'm going to eat the best healthy foods I can find." It's hard to feel deprived when you're dining on succulent lobster, broiled jumbo shrimp, plump figs or sugar sweet fresh pineapple.

15. Ask your mother or grandmother to give you the recipe for one of your favorite dishes from childhood. Then adapt it to the new, low-fat way you're eating these days.

16. Don't arrive at the party too early, or else you'll just be tempted to eat more.

17. If you should happen to overeat (or suffer an out-and-out binge), nip the behavior in the bud and resume your normal eating at your very next meal. Don't keep bingeing or skip the next meal to try to compensate, just eat as you usually would. Remember, one episode of overeating seldom does much harm.

18. Skip the salt. Each day we only need 250 to 375 milligrams of salt, roughly a small pinch. You're probably already taking in this amount from the foods you eat without shaking on more. And stay away from such high-sodium foods as regular soy sauce, luncheon meats, pickles and certain frozen entrées and canned soups. Read nutrition labels to see just how much sodium you're getting.

19. Buy a large (64-ounce) plastic bottle with built-in straw for your on-the-job water consumption.

20. When you spy some vending machines, keep walking. They rarely have selections that will do your diet any good.

21. Don't let a day go by without having a bit of some food you love.

Date: _____

Weight: _____

WEEK 44: MUSCLE UP WITH SOME MACHINES
Exercise goal: Walk seven days, three miles per day in 45 minutes (or less)

Along with your walking and your low-fat eating, we do hope you've been keeping up your two- or three-time-a-week strength-training sessions! If so, you're well on the way to transforming yourself into a lean, mean, calorie-burning machine! This week, for your workout pleasure, we offer you five more ways to pump up and bump up your metabolism rate. First, a few strength-training reminders.

- Space out your sessions. Give yourself a day off between workouts.

- Don't neglect your warm-ups and cooldowns.

- Periodically ask a pro at the gym or health club to spot-check you to make sure you're using the machines and weights properly.

- Vary your exercises. Aim to work on several different muscles and muscle groups during each session.

- Don't push yourself beyond your limits.

And now, the exercises. Each set consists of 8 to 12 repetitions. Try to do three sets of each.

Overhead press. Sit with your feet firmly on the floor. Raise the weight to shoulder height. Keeping your back straight, press the bar to arm's length overhead, pause, then lower. Repeat. (This can be done with free weights or on a machine.)

Biceps curl. Hold a barbell with both hands, palms facing up. Stand with your back straight, with the bar at arm's length against your upper thighs. Curl the bar up in a semicircular motion until your forearms touch your biceps. Keep your upper arms close to the sides of your body. Lower the bar slowly to starting position using the same path. Repeat.

Triceps extension. While sitting with your feet firmly on the floor, hold a dumbbell, with both hands overhead at arm's length. Lower the weight behind your head in a semicircular motion until your forearms touch your biceps. Return using the same path. Repeat.

Lower back. Position the front of your upper body over the end of a waist-high bench. Bend over with your head down and your hands placed lightly behind your ears. Slowly raise your torso until you're level with the bench. Repeat.

Abdominal curl. Lie on your back with your knees bent, fingers lightly touching your ears. (You can place your hands behind your head as long as you don't use them to pull your head forward.) Slowly curl your upper torso up until just your shoulders leave the floor. Hold for a few seconds, go down and repeat, inhaling as you go down. (If this is too difficult, keep your arms at your sides.)

Date: _____

Weight: _____

WEEK 45: TAME YOUR STRESS AND LOSE YOUR BELLY

Exercise goal: Walk seven days, three miles per day in 45 minutes (or less)

Those pounds of stress weighing on your shoulders. You feel them, even though you can't actually see them. But maybe you're looking at the wrong place. It could be they've migrated south, down to your potbelly. You've done a lot of work these past months on changing your exercise and eating habits. But if you haven't yet banished those last unwanted pounds (and any remaining belly bulge) it's time to take another look at the role that stress plays in weight gain.

This unexpected notion that stress affects your weight comes from researchers at Yale University's Department of Psychology. And it could help explain why some people have more trouble with their midsections than they apparently deserve.

What could well be happening, the Yale team believes, is that uncontrolled stress triggers the release of a hormone called cortisol, which in turn causes fat to be preferentially deposited around your middle.

Now what exactly is "uncontrolled" stress? It's not knowing what dreadful thing is going to happen to you next, or why. Or else it's feeling as though you're not in control, that no matter what you do, you just can't get on top of the situation. This is the kind of stress that's purely negative. What's more, it's been found that the inability to handle stress is just as bad for the size of your belly as having stress in the first place.

Banish Stress, Banish Your Belly

Now, a potbelly isn't simply unsightly but it's a health problem, too. Excess fat carried in the abdominal area has been tied to increased risk of heart disease, stroke and diabetes, so there are lots of good reasons to try to tame your stress besides wanting to look good in that new two-piece bathing suit you've got your eye on.

Marielle Rebuffe-Scrive, Ph.D., and colleague Judith Rodin, Ph.D., have been investigating the relationship between stress and abdominal fat for some time. Eliminating stress won't mean an automatic end to belly bulge, but dealing with stress is an important component of banishing a pot-belly, says Dr. Rebuffe-Scrive. Here are a few tips to get you started.

Ask yourself why. "Try to think: Why am I under stress? Why is this happening?" says Dr. Rebuffe-Scrive. Understanding the source of your stress is the first step in dealing with it.

Take a walk. Many people report that the quickest, easiest and most pleasant way to calm down and de-stress is by going for a walk. This can be your regular daily workout walk or a slow saunter around the block. Plus, walking, like any other exercise you may prefer, tends to burn belly flab for energy, so this is a two-way health and shape improver.

Don't hesitate to meditate. Redford B. Williams, M.D., director of the Behavioral Medicine Research Center at Duke University Medical Center in Durham, North Carolina, says that research shows that cortisol levels go down through transcendental meditation (TM). To learn how, you can read a book on TM or take a local course. Or try this quick meditation. "Just pay attention to your breathing," suggests Dr. Williams. "Every time you breathe in and out, notice it. Each time you breathe out, say a word or phrase to yourself that conjures up the mental image you're trying to achieve, like 'Calm down' or 'Cool it.' When your mind starts to wander back to what-ever was bugging you, just say to yourself, 'Oh well' and come back to paying attention to your breathing and saying the word or phrase." About ten min-utes a day of practice, and soon you'll be able to call on your skill in any stressful situation.

Record it. Don't forget about the stress-busting benefits of writing things down! Your success diary can be your best ally in fighting stress, if you use it.

Date: _____

Weight: _____

WEEK 46: WARM-WEATHER WORKOUT

Exercise goal: Walk seven days, three miles per day in 45 minutes (or less)

Maybe it's summertime, or maybe you're planning a vacation at some warm-weather resort. (And after 46 weeks on the 52-week plan, you must be looking pretty terrific in those shorts or swim togs!) But if you're concerned that it might be too hot to exercise as usual, you needn't be. You can keep up your walking routine by keeping cool: Head for the air-conditioned comfort of a mall, or to a treadmill in the hotel gym or your own climate-controlled bedroom.

Even if you prefer the great outdoors, you can probably continue your fitness walking as long as you take a few extra precautions. (If your Week 46 falls during cold weather, see "Cold-Weather Walking," on page 216, instead.)

Acclimate. If you're already walking every day, you'll tend to acclimate naturally to the hot weather. But on really hot days, back off a little on your speed or distance. Avoid the midday sun; try to take your walks in the morning or early evening. And if you can find a shady trail, use it!

Hydrate. Drink six to eight ounces of fluid for every 15 minutes of exercise in the heat. Carry a water bottle and take sips along the way.

Evaporate. On a really hot day, dampen your clothing; use a misting bottle, or get your shirt wet and then wring it out. As the water evaporates, it will act like a portable air conditioner. Short sleeves are better than going sleeveless: You'll be covering more surface area with wetness and protecting yourself from sunburn.

Slather on protection. Always wear a sunscreen of at least sun protection factor (SPF) 15 when you're outdoors. And spread petroleum jelly on your toes and the bottoms of your feet to keep feet from blistering.

Do a switcheroo. Two pairs are better than one. By alternating your walking shoes, you give them a chance to dry out between workouts.

Warm weather, for most people, also means eating light, and you'll probably want to stick to simple fare: crisp greens, cold pasta salads or maybe a fresh-fruit salad accompanied by some low-fat cheese or nonfat yogurt. And if you're bullish on barbeque, there's nothing more wonderful than skewers of fresh vegetables like zucchini, mushrooms, peppers and cherry tomatoes, alternating with chunks of fish (try tuna or swordfish) or lean meat, all grilled to perfection. Who said watching your weight has to be depressing?

Date: _____

Weight: _____

WEEK 47: HANDLING THOSE DEVILISH DIET SABOTEURS

Exercise goal: Walk seven days, three miles per day in 45 minutes (or less)

Everybody loves a winner! That's what they say, don't they? And heaven knows, by Week 47, after all your hard weight-loss work, you're definitely a winner! So, why do the people who care about you give you such a hard time about your diet? If you didn't know any better, you'd almost think they wanted you to go back to your pudgy days. That's nonsense . . . or is it?

Not really, says Ronette Kolotkin, Ph.D., who heads the behavioral program at the Duke University Diet and Fitness Center in Durham, North Carolina. "When you change and become successful, the very people who wanted you to change may suddenly start saying things like, 'I hate the way you're cooking now,' or 'All you do is go to the gym!' You have to realize that there may be negative consequences to weight loss. You feel great about it, but perhaps others won't."

How maddening! Just when you may be looking to your friends, family and co-workers to give you support and a pat on the back for your weight-loss efforts, they turn into diet saboteurs. Now you're hearing little wisecracks about how you've sworn off double-bacon cheeseburgers, for example, or they keep insisting you have one teeny weeny taste of that key lime pie when you really don't want it.

Change is always hard, and when people see you changing in ways that affect them directly or cause them to question their own behavior, they may consciously or unconsciously try to get you to resume your old, familiar ways. "They may feel threatened or jealous, and they may try to make you feel inadequate," says Dr. Kolotkin.

The solution? "Just hang in and deal with it, rather than get frightened by their reactions," she advises. And the best way to deal with it: Assert yourself when others try to make you feel bad or silly about your weight-loss program, or encourage you to deviate from it. You may find these responses to the food pushers in your life helpful.

- "Thanks, but that cake doesn't fit into my program."

- "Thanks, but I don't want any right now—maybe later" (and, of course, don't eat it later either!).

- "Thanks, but I'm allergic to chocolate" (or peanuts or milk products or whatever).

- (with someone who's especially persistent) "Fine, just put some on my plate" (and don't eat it!).

Remember, you need not get angry. In fact, the calmer you stay, the more likely you are to succeed in getting them off the subject and on to something more interesting.

Remember, too, that no one need become your diet saboteur unless you allow him to be. As long as you're completely in control of your own behavior, nobody can sway you from your slim-down mission. It's easy to blame your weight-loss setbacks on your kids' junk food or on your co-worker's birthday cake or on your spouse's frequent business dinners. But you can handle all these situations and more if you choose to. After all you've done to lose weight, you don't want to undo it. Watch out that you don't allow yourself to become the biggest diet saboteur in your life.

Date: _____

Weight: _____

WEEK 48: MAKE YOUR STATIONARY BIKE MORE FUN

Exercise goal: Walk seven days, three miles per day in 45 minutes (or less)

Week 48! Can you feel the excitement? The programs's coming to a close, and you've never felt better in your life! You're eating well and feeling anything but deprived. And when you look in the mirror, you love what you see!

As your weight-loss program gradually turns into a weight-maintenance program, you've got to be continually on the lookout for ways to keep your meals interesting, your workouts fun, and your motivation up. And as we've said before, there will be days when whatever you've been doing all along seems dull, dull, dull. Don't let that happen! Shake things up! Change something—anything.

For instance, instead of walking this week, think about giving that old stationary bike buried under that load of laundry a whirl. And why not? Riding a stationary bike is a superb way to shed fat fast and build lean muscle. In fact, in a recent Tufts University study, a group of stationary cyclists, burning only 360 calories a day over 12 weeks, were able to lose a whopping 19 pounds of fat and gain 3 pounds of lean muscle, all with-out dieting!

If your bike has bored you in the past, here are some snappy suggestions to make it more fun and more productive.

Do intervals. Once you've been cycling at a steady pace for a while, kick up the speed and spin faster for a half minute or even a minute. Then return to your original pace. This'll help break the monotony and burn extra calories.

Take a stand. Get an attachable reading stand so you can peruse the morning paper or a thick paperback as you burn fat.

Use big words. Try finding big-print books and magazines, so you don't have to bend forward to read, risking a backache.

Listen up. If reading on a bike makes you dizzy, listen to books on tape. You can program your workout by chapters, or "reread" the steamy parts to work up a better sweat.

Keep moving with movies. Rent some of your favorite videos, or finally catch up with soap opera episodes you've been taping for weeks. There are even videos available that provide tours through beautiful terrain or let you race against other riders. Just position the bike near the TV set.

Make it scenic. If you have a window with a nice view of a busy street, park your bike facing it and people watch, dog watch or bird watch.

Tune in. A personal headphone stereo can help keep the mental beat flowing. Keep the volume low enough, though, to hear the phone, doorbell or comments from your envious, inactive relatives.

Get a speaker phone. While sweating away, call your friends, your accountant, the Home Shopping Network, anyone who'll listen to you.

Sing! Sing! What's more fun than riding a stationary bicycle? How about doing it as you bellow off-key renditions of Broadway show tunes?

"Perspirate" and dictate. A handheld Dictaphone is great for letters, random thoughts, shopping lists or awful poetry you'd share with no one else.

Don't forget to give yourself credit for your time on the bike! Jot down your cycling time in your success diary. It'll allow you to knock a day or two off your weekly walking goal. And why not polish up that old bike sitting in the garage or reward yourself with a spiffy new one so you can remind yourself of the pleasures of outdoor cycling?

Date: _____

Weight: _____

WEEK 49: COME TO THE AID OF YOUR PARTY

Exercise goal: Walk seven days, three miles per day in 45 minutes (or less)

One of the main lessons we have been trying to teach is that it's possible to lose weight and still live in the real world. That means taking vacations, celebrating birthdays, going on picnics, dining in restaurants—you name it. Yes, by Week 49 you're well aware that enjoyable events and eating your way are not mutually exclusive.

But maybe parties still throw you a bit. After all, there you are surrounded by friends, high spirits, and all that fabulous finger food! The potential for overeating is there, no question. But skip a party because you fear you might overdo it? We wouldn't hear of it! Spend a little time this week planning how you'll get through your next party without putting back on a couple of pounds. Here are some tips to help you party hearty without becoming heavy.

Eat before you greet. Have a light snack or a couple of glasses of water before you leave the house. That way you won't be tempted to dive into the first trayful of canapés you see at the shindig.

Take the cake. If you're planning to bring the hostess a gift, why not make it something you'd like, too? Whether it's a small basket of fruit or an assortment of fat-free cookies, you'll be assured of something you can eat guiltlessly.

Wait it out. Don't dash to the buffet (or bar) the moment your hostess takes your coat. Look at your watch and delay your eating and drinking for 15 minutes. If someone tries to ply you with food during that time, just smile and politely answer, "Not right this minute, thanks."

Check it out. What's on the menu? Don't grab the first thing that you see, or assume that there's "nothing I can eat" because you haven't bothered to really look. Case the place: You just might discover a platter of crudités and yogurt dip in the kitchen or some sliced roast turkey and veggies on a sideboard.

Don't sit near the fattening food. Need we say more?

Skip the intro. Invited to a sit-down dinner party? Then go easy on, or avoid completely, the hors d'oeuvres. That way you can save your appetite (and calories) for the main meal.

Bottoms up. Keep a glass filled with diet soda, mineral water or tomato juice nearby at all times. If your host sees you drinking, he won't push liquor or other high-calorie beverages on you.

Mix it up. Remember, parties aren't just about eating—they're also about schmoozing and socializing. Eat less and talk more. (If you spend more time mingling, you're also likely to hear more compliments about your weight loss!)

Be sure to record your party eating in your success diary when you get home, or first thing the next morning. Your notes may reveal that you had a bit more than you'd planned, but as you learned in previous weeks, you can always compensate by eating a smidgen less at your next meal and exercising a smidgen more.

Date: _____

Weight: _____

WEEK 50: DANCE OFF THE POUNDS
Exercise goal: Walk seven days, three miles per day in 45 minutes (or less)

Whoever thought up the expression "No pain, no gain" was full of hot air! It's official: Working out can be fun. And there are few calorie-burning techniques that are more fun and more effective than dancing.

This week you should make arrangements to give this marvelous form of exercise a try. (And if you're already a regular, make sure you get out on the dance floor at least once.)

"Today we know that exercising at a lower intensity, like walking for fitness, produces better long-range fat-burning benefits than running or other excessive exercise. And what is social dancing but walking to music?" says Cal Pozo, an exercise physiologist, former professional dancer and instructor on Parade Videos' *Learn to Dance* video series.

In fact, depending on the kind of dancing you do, you can get an even better aerobic workout than you would just walking. "The music dictates the speed and intensity at which you're moving," Pozo points out, adding that while dancing you can expend 250 to 300 calories per hour. Even though most dances last just two or three minutes, over the course of an evening you're burning calories like crazy. "And because you're following different patterns of movement," says Pozo, "you're using your whole body, which adds to your caloric output."

Not the least of dancing's pluses is that it's pleasant and relaxing. "With social dancing, there's the mind/body connection," says Pozo. "While you're dancing your mind is engaged—you're listening to the music and coordinating your movements with your partner—so it actually helps reduce stress. It's a very complete exercise."

Most folks who like to dance socially tend to focus on four basic dances.

- Swing, which has become very popular again

- Latin, including the cha-cha—dances that take some practice to perfect

- Country/western, especially line dancing, where you don't need a partner and so you're freer to interpret the music your way

- Low-impact dance/exercise, such as Jazzercise

Another plus: Unlike other forms of exercise, no real warm-up is needed with dancing. As Pozo says: "A warm-up should be specific to the movement you're going to do. For example, if you're going to jog, you should do some slow running first for two or three minutes. But with social dancing, as you get into the dance, your body automatically starts warming up, so you don't really have to do any stretching exercise. Just get up and dance!"

You can find dance classes listed in your Yellow Pages, as part of adult education programs or at your local Y. You can also rent a dance video and practice in the privacy of your living room until you're ready to sweep onto a dance floor with your partner.

Music, maestro!

Date: _____

Weight: _____

WEEK 51: GET READY FOR MAINTENANCE!

Exercise goal: Walk seven days, three miles per day in 45 minutes (or less)

What can we say? You're one week from the finale of the 52-week plan, and you've become your own finest role model! You're not just slimmer but, better still, wiser. You've learned so much about making your body stronger, leaner, healthier. You've discovered firsthand how crucial exercise is to being trim and fit. And you've also become an expert at dealing with your moods and setbacks foodlessly.

You've reached your goal weight, or else you're well on the way. And now you're at a crossroads. Yes, this is the time when either you will mentally turn a corner for good, leaving your overweight lifestyle behind you forever, or you might find yourself lured by external influences to waver from the good habits you've been honing over the past year.

We understand the temptations, and we also realize that weight maintenance is tough. The glory and gratification that come with seeing an ever-shrinking number on the scale just aren't there anymore once you reach your goal.

The weight-loss experts agree it's all very challenging. But the good news: It's all very doable.

This is the week to get psyched for maintenance. Start by rereading "Keeping It Off Forever," on page 168. Really study it and take its message to heart.

You truly want this to be the last time you ever have to lose weight—you've worked too hard for it not to be. Continue to weigh yourself weekly so you can keep a watchful (but not fanatical) eye on your situation. And be ready to sound the "three-pound alarm" whenever your weight goes up by that much. Taking off a little weight is so much easier than taking off a lot.

Let this also be the week to renew your vow to continue for life the exercise program you've been following so impressively. The experts have said it time and time again: The successful weight maintainers keep exercising, the yo-yo dieters stop.

Vow, too, to vary your menus, so food boredom doesn't become an excuse to binge. Keep recording what you eat and how you exercise in your success diary—it's even more vital to weight maintenance, when habits often start getting sloppy.

Keep up your reward system throughout your maintenance just as you did during weight loss. Give yourself a gift, say, for every month you maintain your weight within your three- to five-pound range. And promise yourself that no matter how tough things might get sometimes, you'll be kind to yourself and not try to stuff your problems with food, as you might've done a year ago.

Weight maintenance isn't easy. But if anyone can do it, you can.

Date: _____

Weight: _____

WEEK 52: TAKE A FINAL INVENTORY . . . AND TAKE A BOW!

Exercise goal: Walk seven days, three miles per day in 45 minutes (or less)

Hooray!
Yippee!
Great job!
Mazel tov!
Right on!
Congrats!
A year full of achievement! We're proud of you but, most of all, you should feel extremely proud of yourself. We're hoping that you're not only enjoying your slim new body but also the realization that a slim way of life can actually be fun. After all, as you now know, being thin also means:

- Eating delicious foods in nonstarvation quantities

- Having snacks and alcohol in moderation

- Exercising in ways you find enjoyable

- Looking good and feeling comfortable in your clothes

- Participating in all life has to offer, without worrying about how you look or feel

Take this final inventory, on page 274, and if you have 18 or more "Yes!" or "Usually" answers, take a bow—a deep bow! Just think: You've successfully completed the 52-week plan with barely a hitch! This is the time for a major reward: Whatever you choose for yourself, make it extra special. And if you're wondering what lies ahead for you in Week 53, Week 54 and beyond, it's this: You can look forward to a better, happier life than you could ever have imagined. And, frankly, we can't think of anyone who deserves it more.

Low-Fat Living Progress Report

	Yes!	Usually	I was afraid you'd ask that
1. I review my list of long-term goals regularly.	❏	❏	❏
2. I keep the kitchen as fat-free as possible.	❏	❏	❏
3. I meet my weekly exercise goal.	❏	❏	❏
4. I weigh myself once a week.	❏	❏	❏
5. I keep my success diary up-to-date.	❏	❏	❏
6. I eat a good breakfast every morning.	❏	❏	❏
7. I stick to low-fat items when I snack.	❏	❏	❏
8. I do de-stressing exercises to head off my urges to overeat.	❏	❏	❏
9. I drink eight glasses of water a day.	❏	❏	❏
10. I reward myself for meeting my minigoals.	❏	❏	❏
11. I do strength training two or three times per week.	❏	❏	❏
12. I stick to reasonable-size portions.	❏	❏	❏
13. I eat five servings of fruits and vegetables a day.	❏	❏	❏
14. I review my success diary whenever I need to give my program a boost.	❏	❏	❏
15. I don't overdo it in restaurants.	❏	❏	❏
16. I use positive self-talk to keep myself motivated.	❏	❏	❏
17. I try one new low-fat recipe a week.	❏	❏	❏
18. I find alternatives to outdoor walking when the weather's bad.	❏	❏	❏
19. I use binge-busting techniques when I'm on the verge of overdoing it.	❏	❏	❏
20. I trade off food at one meal when I'm anticipating a bigger meal later on.	❏	❏	❏
21. I seek support from others when I need it.	❏	❏	❏
22. I know how to deal with diet saboteurs.	❏	❏	❏

YOUR PERFECT WEIGHT SUCCESS DIARY

Need to remind yourself to pick up some cereal and tomatoes at the store? Simple: You write it down. The grandson's birthday is coming up and a pitstop at the local toy store is in your future? You jot down some gift ideas. Heard some interesting medical news on a talk show that you want to discuss with your doctor? You write it down.

In this busy life we all lead, it's impossible to remember everything that's crucial, and luckily it's unnecessary to keep all that stuff in your head. Writing things down helps us remember what we need to, focus on what's important and then get on with the rest of our lives. And now that you've decided that losing weight and keeping the extra pounds off is a priority for you, there's no better way to help you meet your goals than with a food and exercise diary.

If you're a bit intimidated by the idea of maintaining a written record of everything you eat and drink and how much exercise you do (and don't!) get each day, fear not. The point of this diary is to help you keep your mind on your short- and long-term health and fitness goals.

Was it three pieces of toast you had yesterday, or only two? Did you walk for 20 minutes, or was it actually more like 45? Did you drink two quarts of water you'd planned on, or just a couple of glasses at lunchtime? Knowing what you've done can help you better plan what you want to do the next time around.

What's more, keeping a written record of your progress and your step-by-step successes—whether that means dropping a pound and a half last week or comfortably boosting your walking program from 30 to 40 minutes per session—gives you a continuous pat on the back for a job well done, all of which tends to lead to a very positive spiral.

Over the next 15 pages you'll see a week's worth of diary pages to help you get started. You'll note that the first day's diary (one for a woman, one for a man) has already been filled in and commented on. That's to help you see how you might use and work with your own diary entries.

We suggest that for the first few days you not attempt to change your usual eating and exercise pattern: Just write down whatever you've been doing all along. (Don't forget that under the category "Type of Exercise" come such lifestyle workouts as vacuuming the carpets, raking the leaves and those brisk, twice-daily walks with your collie, Samson.)

As you review what you've written, start to look for patterns. Do you always join the guys for beers and high-fat snacks during Friday night happy hour? Do you invariably wind up eating those cookies you bake with your granddaughter whenever she comes to visit? Do you eat especially carefully when you go out to lunch with your slim, fashionable cousin?

The food and exercise sections are fairly self-explanatory. As for the "Mood" sections, the notes you jot down here will help you begin to get a better idea of why, for example, you grabbed that chicken leg on the way to the car on Tuesday even though you'd eaten a substantial dinner and you weren't even particularly hungry at the time. The diary aims to help you grow in awareness of your habits. And you'll also notice spaces provided so you can record how your changing eating and exercise patterns are affecting your sleep and medication requirements.

You should also be aware of those items you're not being asked to fill in on these diary pages—things like "Calories Consumed" or "Total Daily Fat Grams." Surprised? It's simply that we believe that as long as you're making a concerted effort to increase your level of exercise and decrease your intake of fat, particularly saturated fat, you needn't count calories or grams or anything else—that effort is certain to be rewarded with a slimmer, healthier body.

As for checking and recording your weight and body measurements, we recommend that you do so no more than once a week. (You'll see there's only one space provided each week for those numbers.) Anything more frequent may lead to inaccuracies about how much fat you're really losing and may cause you to fixate needlessly on the scale rather than your improving health and fitness levels.

Plan on reviewing your diary entries each evening before bed (it'll help ward off midnight snacks!) or the next morning, and jot down your own comments, more or less as we have. Do that, and you'll soon begin to find new and clever ways to cut back on fat, increase your fiber and get more out of your exercise.

When you see that you're coming to the end of the sample diary pages in this book, simply photocopy them to use in future days and weeks. Or just get a notebook (a spiral-bound type is probably easiest to use) and keep track of the same information there.

Good luck! Actually, the success you're sure to see won't be a matter of luck but of your decision and determination to take charge of your weight and your health, now and forever.

SAMPLE DIARY FOR WOMEN

YOUR PERFECT WEIGHT
SUCCESS DIARY

TODAY'S DATE

Oct. 7

BREAKFAST

Food (include all foods and amounts):

1 cup mini raisin-filled shredded wheat

Great! Good source of fiber.

1 cup 2% milk

Try 1% low-fat or skim milk to cut fat even more.

1 cup coffee with 2% milk

Could use some fresh fruit—how about an orange?

and 1 packet artificial sweetener

MOOD

Great! A busy day ahead, but I feel good.

LUNCH

Food (include all foods and amounts)

Next time, make it whole-grain instead of white.

Tuna fish salad on roll (approximately 4 oz.

Turkey would've been a better choice.

tuna mixed with 2 Tbsp. mayonnaise),

If preparing at home, substitute low-fat mayo.

lettuce and tomato

1 apple

Filling and good source of fiber.

MOOD

Fine. Work is hectic, but lunch with

Judy was fun.

DINNER

Food (include all foods and amounts)

4 oz. grilled chicken

Chicken's a great choice, provided you don't eat the skin.

1 cup steamed green beans

Terrific. Steaming is a great way to retain vitamins and minerals.

2 cups salad with 2 Tbsp. Russian dressing

Next time, choose the low-fat or fat-free kind.

1 baked potato with 3 Tbsp. sour cream

Potato is a good source of fiber and vitamin C, but swap the sour cream for the low-fat kind or fresh herbs.

MOOD

Peter and I "discussed" the remodeling

costs over dinner.

SNACKS

Food (include all foods and amounts)

3 cups light microwave popcorn

Check out the amount of fat—light may not necessarily mean low in fat.

1 cup vanilla swirl ice cream

Try ice milk or sorbet instead.

MOOD

Tired, but fine.

Number of glasses water consumed __4__ ⟵————Try for 6 to 8.

Number of minutes aerobic exercise __0__ ⟵——— A 20-minute walk would've
been good.

Type of exercise _____

Number of minutes strength training __0__⟵   Shoot for two sessions
per week.

Medication (type/quantity)__O_____

Vitamins (type/quantity) 1 Centrum multivitamin with minerals ⟵— Ok

Number of hours slept last night __7_____

HOW I DID TODAY

How well I met my food and fitness goals;
handled periods of stress, boredom and
other moods; and how I plan to cope better
next time:

Not bad, considering I was tired and

dinnertime wasn't so pleasant.

I've got to skip that 3:00 ice cream break

at work.

TOMORROW'S GOALS/SPECIAL CHALLENGES

Stressful periods I anticipate—parties,
restaurant dining and so forth—and the
ways I intend to handle them:

Tomorrow the boss is taking my

department to lunch. I have to be extra

careful with the butter and bread

basket!

OTHER NOTES TO MYSELF
Additional words of advice/encourage-
ment/praise:

I can't wait to get started on my exercise

program! I'm determined to make this my

last diet ever!

WEIGHT (record only once weekly)

147 lbs.

MEASUREMENTS (record only once weekly)

Bust/Chest: 39"

Waist: 29 ½"

Hips: 38 ½"

Thighs: 23"

SAMPLE DIARY FOR MEN

YOUR PERFECT WEIGHT SUCCESS DIARY

TODAY'S DATE

Oct. 7

BREAKFAST

Food (include all foods and amounts)

1 bagel with 2 Tbsp. butter ← — Swap the butter for a thin layer of cream cheese or, better yet, jam.

Black coffee

MOOD

Could've used another couple of hours

of sleep!

LUNCH

Food (include all foods and amounts)

Turkey club sandwich—4 oz. turkey and 2 — Hold the bacon!

slices bacon on 3 slices white bread ← — Try nutrient-rich whole-wheat bread or pita.

Handful of french fries ← — Have a baked potato instead.

1 cup coleslaw ← — Drain it to remove some of the mayo. Better yet, have some tomato or cucumber slices.

MOOD

All hell broke loose at the office;

tense all day.

DINNER

Food (include all foods and amounts)

Broiling's good; next time
cut back an ounce or two.

8-oz. broiled veal chop

Great selection!
More nutrients and
fiber than white rice.

1 cup brown rice with sautéed onions

2 cups salad with vinegar and herbs

Try to limit oil used to sauté.

Tastes great, no fat!

MOOD

First time to finally unwind!

SNACKS

Food (include all foods and amounts)

Uh-oh—loaded with fat and
sugar. What about a toasted
whole-wheat English muffin
topped with some jam?

1 bran muffin

Empty calories. Better to have a
light beer or sugar-free iced tea.

1 beer (12 oz.)

Handful of pretzels

Good snack, if they're the
unsalted kind.

MOOD

Bushed.

Terrific! You're right on target.

Number of glasses water consumed   8

Number of minutes aerobic exercise   15

Type of exercise Running up and down ← A good "lifestyle" workout. Add walking or active sports, plus a
three flights of stairs at work strength-training program.

Number of minutes strength training 0

Medication (type/quantity) 4 chewable
Try eating more slowly and in relaxed settings as much as possible.
Pepto-Bismol tablets ←

Vitamins (type/quantity)   1 Theragram

multivitamin with minerals;

1 tablet (500 mg.) vitamin C

Number of hours slept last night 5 ½ ← Need to get more rest.

HOW I DID TODAY

How well I met my food and fitness goals; handled periods of stress, boredom and other moods; and how I plan to cope better next time:

I probably ate too much, but the stress

has been unbelievable lately.

TOMORROW'S GOALS/SPECIAL CHALLENGES

Stressful periods I anticipate—parties, restaurant dining and so forth—and the ways I intend to handle them:

Big presentation at 8:00. I'll have a good

breakfast first (and I'll skip the conference

room Danish).

OTHER NOTES TO MYSELF

Additional words of advice/encourage-
ment/praise:

I should've done this before, but better late

than never! Jane's going to be a real help to

my diet.

WEIGHT (record only once weekly)

188 lbs.

MEASUREMENTS (record only once weekly)

Bust/Chest: 48"

Waist: 38"

YOUR PERFECT WEIGHT
SUCCESS DIARY

TODAY'S DATE

_____

BREAKFAST

Food (include all foods and amounts)

_____

_____

_____

_____

_____

MOOD

_____

_____

_____

_____

_____

LUNCH

Food (include all foods and amounts)

_____

_____

_____

_____

_____

_____

MOOD

_____

_____

_____

_____

_____

_____

DINNER

Food (include all foods and amounts)

_____

_____

_____

_____

_____

_____

MOOD

_____

_____

_____

_____

_____

_____

SNACKS

Food (include all foods and amounts)

_____

_____

_____

_____

_____

_____

MOOD

_____

_____

_____

_____

_____

_____

Number of glasses water consumed_____

Number of minutes aerobic exercise_____

Type of exercise_____

Number of minutes strength training_____

Medication (type/quantity)_____

Vitamins (type/quantity)_____

Number of hours slept last night _____

HOW I DID TODAY

How well I met my food and fitness goals;
handled periods of stress, boredom and
other moods; and how I plan to cope
better next time:

_____

_____

_____

_____

_____

_____

_____

TOMORROW'S GOALS/SPECIAL CHALLENGES

Stressful periods I anticipate—parties,
restaurant dining and so forth—and the
ways I intend to handle them:

_____

_____

_____

_____

OTHER NOTES TO MYSELF

Additional words of advice/encourage-
ment/praise:

_____

_____

_____

_____

WEIGHT_____ (record only once weekly)

MEASUREMENTS (record only once weekly)

Bust/Chest:_____

Waist:_____

Hips:_____

Thighs:_____

Part Four

RECIPES
FOR LOW-FAT LIVING

QUICK AND EASY LOW-FAT RECIPES

Welcome to a wonderful new world of healthful eating that will keep you trim, energized and satisfied. Gone are the days when "diet food" meant a well-done burger with no bun and a scoop of cottage cheese on a bed of lettuce.

These days there's no reason that paying attention to your weight should leave you feeling deprived. Today's low-fat fare is easy to prepare and flavorful. Here are several recipes for low-fat breakfasts, brown-bag lunches, dinners and party fare to help get you started.

BREAKFAST

MAPLE-ALMOND OATMEAL

Oatmeal is a filling breakfast choice for those watching their weight. This recipe elevates plain oatmeal above the ordinary. To make it even more special, sprinkle it with some raspberries or blueberries.

3	cups water
1⅓	cups rolled oats
¼	cup chopped dates
2	tablespoons ground almonds
2	tablespoons honey
1	large banana, thinly sliced
1–2	cups skim milk

In a 2-quart saucepan over medium heat, bring the water, oats, dates, almonds and honey to a boil. Simmer for 5 minutes, or until thick.

Serve with the bananas and milk.

Makes 4 servings.

Per serving: 229 calories, 3.3 g. fat (12% of calories), 2.9 g. dietary fiber, 1 mg. cholesterol, 39 mg. sodium.

FRUITED FRENCH TOAST

French toast has a reputation for being really high in fat, but it doesn't have to be like that. Using egg substitute and skim milk for the soaking mixture removes some of the fat. Sizzling the pieces in a no-stick frying pan takes out more. And serving the french toast with a syrup and fruit topping instead of butter lightens this dish even further.

    ¾   cup fat-free egg substitute
    ½   cup skim milk
    ½   teaspoon ground cinnamon
    ½   teaspoon vanilla
    8   slices Italian bread
    2   cups raspberries or other berries
    ¼   cup maple syrup

In a large shallow bowl, whisk together the egg substitute, milk, cinnamon and vanilla. One by one, dip the bread slices in the batter, turning to coat both sides.

Coat a large no-stick frying pan or griddle with no-stick spray. Place over medium heat until warm. Working in batches, add the slices in a single layer and brown on both sides. (Keep finished pieces warm in an oven set at 150° until all the pieces are done.)

Serve topped with the berries and drizzled with the syrup.

Makes 4 servings.

Per serving: 282 calories, 0.4 g. fat (1% of calories), 4.4 g. dietary fiber, 1 mg. cholesterol, 383 mg. sodium.

POTATO AND ONION FRITTATA

A frittata is an Italian version of the omelet—the difference being that the filling ingredients are mixed right in with the eggs rather than being added after the eggs cook. This frittata is great for breakfast, but it's also nice as a low-calorie brunch, lunch or dinner entrée.

    2   baking potatoes, peeled, halved lengthwise and thinly
             sliced crosswise
    1   onion, thinly sliced
    1   tablespoon olive oil
    1½   cups fat-free egg substitute
    ¼   teaspoon curry powder
    ¼   teaspoon ground ginger

Steam the potatoes for 5 minutes, or until tender.

In a large ovenproof frying pan over medium heat, sauté the onions in the oil for 5 minutes, or until transparent.

In a medium bowl, whisk together the egg substitute, curry and ginger.

Add the potatoes to the pan with the onions. Pour the egg mixture over all and cook for 5 minutes over medium heat.

Transfer to the oven and broil 6″ from the heat for 5 minutes, or until the frittata has puffy edges and is a golden color.

Makes 4 servings.

Per serving: 145 calories, 3.5 g. fat (22% of calories), 2.2 g. dietary fiber, 0 mg. cholesterol, 127 mg. sodium.

BREAKFAST MELON BOWL

*If you don't have a big appetite in the morning, try a fruit mixture
like this for breakfast. The yogurt and ricotta cheese add protein that
will help keep you satisfied until lunch.*

1	cup nonfat ricotta cheese
¾	cup nonfat vanilla yogurt
1	small cantaloupe
2	peaches, pitted and thinly sliced
½	cup sliced strawberries
½	cup blueberries
2	tablespoons toasted sunflower seeds
	Mint sprigs

In a food processor or blender, process the ricotta until very smooth. Transfer to a small bowl. Mix in the yogurt.

Halve the cantaloupe and remove the seeds. Cut into wedges, remove the rind and cut the flesh into bite-size chunks. Place in a medium bowl. Mix in the peaches and strawberries. Add the ricotta mixture and gently fold together.

Divide among 4 cereal bowls. Sprinkle with the blueberries and sunflower seeds. Garnish with the mint sprigs.

Makes 4 servings.

Per serving: 190 calories, 2.8 g. fat (13% of calories), 3 g. dietary fiber, 1 mg. cholesterol, 110 mg. sodium.

HERBED SAUSAGE MUFFINS

These muffins have great sausage taste without delivering the hefty amount of fat that generally accompanies sausage. The muffins are best warm, so either serve them straight from the oven or reheat them in a toaster oven or microwave (to microwave, wrap one muffin in a damp paper towel and cook on high power for about 30 seconds).

6	ounces turkey sausage, casings removed
½	teaspoon onion powder
¼	teaspoon dried sage
⅛	teaspoon ground black pepper
1	cup unbleached flour
½	cup whole-wheat flour
1½	teaspoons baking powder
¾	cup skim milk
3	tablespoons maple syrup
1	egg white, lightly beaten
2	tablespoons canola oil

Coat 10 muffin cups with no-stick spray. Set aside.

Crumble the sausage into a large no-stick frying pan set over medium heat. Cook, breaking up the pieces with a wooden spoon for 5 minutes, or until browned. Transfer to a plate lined with a triple thickness of paper towels to drain. Blot the top with more towels to remove all excess fat.

Place the meat in a small bowl and stir in the onion powder, sage and pepper.

In a medium bowl, stir together the unbleached flour, whole-wheat flour and baking powder.

In a small bowl, combine the milk, maple syrup, egg white and oil. Add the maple mixture to the flour mixture and stir just until combined. Then gently fold in the meat mixture.

Spoon the mixture into the muffin cups, filling each cup about ¾ full. Bake at 400° about 20 minutes, or until golden brown and a toothpick inserted near the center of a muffin comes out clean. Remove from the muffin pan.

Makes 10 muffins.

Per muffin: 128 calories, 2.8 g. fat (20% of calories), 1.1 g. dietary fiber, 11 mg. cholesterol, 206 mg. sodium.

DINNER

Pork Chops with Apricots

Of course there's room for pork in a low-fat diet. Just make sure you choose a lean cut, like a loin chop, and trim all the fat you can from it before cooking. Tenderloin would also work very well in this recipe.

4	pork chops (about 4 ounces each), trimmed of all visible fat
1	teaspoon ground cinnamon
½	teaspoon ground black pepper
1	onion, thinly sliced crosswise and separated into rings
1	tablespoon grated fresh ginger
	Pinch of grated nutmeg
¾	cup apple juice, divided
½	cup coarsely chopped fresh or drained canned apricot halves
2	cups hot cooked bulgur
1	tablespoon sliced almonds

Sprinkle the pork chops on both sides with the cinnamon and pepper. Rub the spices into the meat.

In a large no-stick frying pan over medium heat, cook the onions, ginger and nutmeg in 2 tablespoons of the apple juice for 5 minutes, or until the onions are tender and the juice has cooked away. Transfer to a plate.

Coat the pan with no-stick spray and heat for 1 minute. Add the pork. Cook for 3 minutes per side.

Return the onion mixture to the pan. Add the apricots and the remaining apple juice. Reduce the heat to low. Cover and simmer for 10 minutes, or until the pork is cooked through and the sauce thickens slightly.

Place the bulgur on a large platter. Top with the pork and onions. Spoon on the sauce. Sprinkle with the almonds.

Makes 4 servings.

Per serving: 204 calories, 4.6 g. fat (20% of calories), 4.7 g. dietary fiber, 23 mg. cholesterol, 29 mg. sodium.

SHORTCUT CHILI

It's not always necessary to buy the very leanest ground beef that your market has to offer. When you're preparing a dish like this, in which you brown the meat and then very thoroughly drain off the accumulated fat, a slightly fattier product gives excellent results at a cheaper price.

8   ounces lean ground beef
2   cans (16 ounces each) low-sodium tomatoes,
        well drained and coarsely chopped
1   jar (8 ounces) salsa
1   can (16 ounces) kidney beans, rinsed and drained
1   cup water
1   teaspoon chili powder

Crumble the beef into a large no-stick frying pan set over medium-high heat. Cook, breaking up the pieces with a wooden spoon for 5 minutes, or until browned. Transfer to a plate lined with a triple thickness of paper towels to drain. Blot the top with more towels to remove all excess fat.

Return the beef to the pan. Stir in the tomatoes, salsa, beans, water and chili powder. Cover and bring to a boil, then reduce the heat. Simmer for 10 minutes, stirring frequently.

Makes 4 servings.

Per serving: 357 calories, 10.5 g. fat (25% of calories), 11.7 g. dietary fiber, 38 mg. cholesterol, 455 mg. sodium.

BLACK BEAN SOUP

Here's a very filling lunch dish that's quite low in fat. Take some along to work in a Thermos or reheat a bowlful in the microwave.

2   medium onions, finely chopped
2   teaspoons olive oil
4   cups defatted chicken stock
2   cans (16 ounces each) black beans, rinsed and drained
1   cup chopped tomatoes
2   cloves garlic, minced
2   bay leaves
1   teaspoon ground cumin
2   cups cooked rice
2   tablespoons balsamic or red wine vinegar

In a 4-quart pot over medium heat, sauté the onions in the oil for 10 minutes, or until lightly browned. Add the stock, beans, tomatoes, garlic, bay leaves and cumin. Bring to a boil over medium-high heat. Cover, reduce the heat to medium and simmer for 20 minutes.

With a potato masher or the back of a wooden spoon, lightly crush some of the beans. Stir in the rice and vinegar. Simmer for 5 minutes. Remove and discard the bay leaves.

Makes 8 servings.

Per serving: 219 calories, 2.3 g. fat (9% of calories), 7.6 g. dietary fiber, 0 mg. cholesterol, 21 mg. sodium.

CREAMY CARROT SOUP

We've taken the cream out of this soup but retained the creamy texture. Part of the secret is the white rice that helps thicken the pureed carrots and part is the low-fat—not skim—milk that adds a little extra body without a lot of calories.

1	pound carrots, thinly sliced
2	cups defatted chicken stock, divided
2	tablespoons white rice
¼	teaspoon dried thyme
1	bay leaf
½	teaspoon ground black pepper
1½	cups low-fat milk
	Pinch of grated nutmeg
2	tablespoons snipped chives

In a 2-quart saucepan, combine the carrots and 1 cup of the stock. Bring to a boil over medium-high heat. Reduce the heat to medium and simmer for 5 minutes, or until the carrots are almost tender. Using a slotted spoon, remove ½ cup of the carrots and set aside.

Stir the rice, thyme, bay leaf, pepper and the remaining 1 cup of stock into the pan. Bring to a boil. Cover and simmer, stirring occasionally for 20 minutes, or until the rice is tender. Remove and discard the bay leaf.

Transfer the mixture to a blender and puree until smooth. Return to the saucepan. Simmer for 5 minutes. Stir in the milk and heat through. Add the reserved carrots and nutmeg. Serve sprinkled with the chives.

Makes 4 servings.

Per serving: 118 calories, 1.6 g. fat (12% of calories), 3.8 g. dietary fiber, 4 mg. cholesterol, 98 mg. sodium.

KIDNEY BEAN AND CHICK-PEA SALAD

Canned beans are loaded with fiber, which helps satisfy your appetite. Here we combined two different types of beans with a variety of vegetables and some nonfat commercial dressing to make a salad you can mix the night before and carry along to work.

1	cup rinsed and drained canned kidney beans
1	cup rinsed and drained canned chick-peas
1	sweet red pepper, chopped
1	cup thinly sliced carrots
½	cup thinly sliced celery
3	scallions, chopped
½	cup fat-free Italian dressing
¼	teaspoon chili powder
2	cups shredded fresh spinach
1	cup cherry tomato halves

In a large bowl, toss together the beans, chick-peas, peppers, carrots, celery and scallions. Mix in the dressing and chili powder.

Line individual plates with the spinach. Top with the salad. Arrange the tomatoes around the salad.

Makes 4 servings.

Per serving: 166 calories, 1.7 g. fat (9% of calories), 6 g. dietary fiber, 0 mg. cholesterol, 335 mg. sodium.

RATATOUILLE

Traditional recipes for this French vegetable mélange use a lot of oil. Here we avoided much of the oil by microwaving the eggplant and zucchini until tender and then sautéing in just a touch of oil. You get the same characteristic flavor with a lot fewer calories.

1	medium eggplant, peeled and cubed
1	small zucchini, cubed
1	onion, diced
1	sweet red pepper, julienned
2	teaspoons olive oil
2	cloves garlic, minced
3	tomatoes, coarsely chopped
½	teaspoon dried basil
½	teaspoon dried marjoram
¼	teaspoon dried oregano
¼	cup minced fresh parsley
8	slices French bread

Place the eggplant and zucchini in a 2-quart casserole. Cover with vented plastic wrap and microwave on high for 5 minutes, or until the pieces are soft but still hold their shape.

In a large no-stick frying pan over medium-high heat, sauté the onions and peppers in the oil until starting to brown. Add the eggplant and zucchini. Sauté for 5 minutes.

Reduce the heat to medium. Stir in the garlic and cook for 1 minute. Add the tomatoes, basil, marjoram and oregano. Cover and simmer for 15 minutes, or until the tomatoes have softened and become juicy. Stir in the parsley. Cook, uncovered, for 5 minutes. Serve accompanied by the bread.

Makes 4 servings.

Per serving: 271 calories, 5.5 g. fat (18% of calories), 4.7 g. dietary fiber, 0 mg. cholesterol, 399 mg. sodium.

MINTED CHICKEN SALAD

If you like the combination of chicken and fruit, you'll love this luncheon salad. The herbs added to the nonfat mayonnaise perk up the dressing and complement the low-calorie fruit that serves to extend the salad.

2	cups chopped cooked chicken breast
1	cup diced pineapple or drained canned pineapple tidbits
1	cup seedless grapes
¼	cup minced fresh mint
2	tablespoons minced fresh parsley
½	cup nonfat mayonnaise
1	tablespoon lemon or lime juice
	Red leaf lettuce
2	kiwifruits, halved lengthwise and thinly sliced crosswise

In a large bowl, toss together the chicken, pineapple, grapes, mint and parsley. Stir in the mayonnaise and lemon or lime juice.

Line individual plates with the lettuce. Top with the salad. Arrange the kiwi slices around the salad.

Makes 4 servings.

Per serving: 221 calories, 3.8 g. fat (15% of calories), 2.3 g. dietary fiber, 59 mg. cholesterol, 440 mg. sodium.

ALMOND-BAKED HALIBUT

Although nuts are high in calories and fat, they needn't be verboten. Here we mix a small amount of almonds into the breading for fish fillets. The result is a lot of flavor for a reasonable amount of calories. The way we did save calories is by baking the breaded fish rather than deep-frying it.

¼	cup fat-free egg substitute
2	tablespoons skim milk
⅓	cup seasoned dry bread crumbs
2	tablespoons ground almonds
2	tablespoons grated Parmesan cheese
4	halibut fillets (4–6 ounces each)
2	cups hot cooked couscous
1	tablespoon minced fresh dill
1	lemon, cut lengthwise into wedges

In a pie plate or other shallow dish, combine the egg substitute and milk. On a large plate, mix together the bread crumbs, almonds and Parmesan.

Dip the fillets into the egg mixture to coat both sides of each piece, then dredge in the crumb mixture to coat well.

Coat a no-stick baking sheet with no-stick spray. Arrange the fillets on the sheet in a single layer. Bake at 350° for 15 minutes, or until the pieces are cooked through.

Fluff the couscous with a fork. Sprinkle with the dill and very lightly mix. Divide among individual plates. Add the fish and squeeze lemon juice over all.

Makes 4 servings.

Per serving: 299 calories, 5.5 g. fat (17% of calories), 4.8 g. dietary fiber, 39 mg. cholesterol, 210 mg. sodium.

Stuffed Peppers

Combining a lot of rice with a modest amount of beef lets us make stuffed peppers with plenty of traditional taste but a lot fewer calories. Corn adds extra fiber and makes these peppers especially colorful.

4	large sweet red, green or yellow peppers
6	ounces lean ground beef
1	medium onion, diced
2	cloves garlic, minced
2	cups cooked rice
½	cup corn
½	cup fat-free egg substitute
1	teaspoon dried marjoram
¼	teaspoon ground coriander
1	cup tomato sauce

Halve the peppers lengthwise and remove the seeds, inner membranes and stems. Steam for 5 minutes, or until they begin to soften. Set aside.

Crumble the beef into a large no-stick frying pan set over medium-high heat. Cook, breaking up the pieces with a wooden spoon for 5 minutes, or until browned.

Add the onions and garlic. Sauté for 5 minutes, or until the onions are translucent. Transfer to a plate lined with a triple thickness of paper towels to drain. Blot the top with more towels to remove all excess fat.

Transfer the mixture to a large bowl. Add the rice, corn, egg substitute, marjoram and coriander. Mix well. Divide among the pepper halves.

Coat a 9″ × 13″ baking dish with no-stick spray. Pour in enough tomato sauce to just cover the bottom of the dish. Add the peppers in a single layer. Top with the remaining tomato sauce.

Bake at 350° for 30 minutes.

Makes 4 servings.

Per serving: 321 calories, 7.8 g. fat (22% of calories), 4.2 g. dietary fiber, 28 mg. cholesterol, 91 mg. sodium.

MEXICAN MEATBALLS

This is a tasty change from regular meatballs. Baking the meatballs instead of browning them in oil helps keep calories and fat under control. One note: If you're watching your sodium intake, read labels and choose a brand of salsa that's low in sodium. If your market doesn't carry a brand that's low enough, consider Mexican-spiced stewed tomatoes. Or add chopped canned chili peppers and some chili powder to plain low-sodium stewed tomatoes.

12	ounces ground turkey
⅓	cup cornmeal
¼	cup fat-free egg substitute
1	tablespoon tomato paste
1	tablespoon minced fresh parsley
½	teaspoon dried oregano
1	jar (16 ounces) medium or hot salsa
1	cup water
½	cup corn
2	cups hot cooked rice

In a medium bowl, combine the turkey, cornmeal, egg substitute, tomato paste, parsley and oregano. Form into 18 small meatballs.

Coat a large no-stick baking sheet or jelly-roll pan with no-stick spray. Add the meatballs in a single layer. Bake at 350° for 15 minutes, or until browned.

In a large frying pan, mix the salsa, water and corn. Add the meatballs. Cover and simmer over medium heat for 10 minutes, or until the meatballs are cooked through. Serve with the rice.

Makes 4 servings.

Per serving: 328 calories, 3.2 g. fat (9% of calories), 3.3 g. dietary fiber, 55 mg. cholesterol, 811 mg. sodium.

FLOUNDER WITH LEMON BROCCOLI

This dinner entrée is simple, elegant and absolutely delicious.
Flounder is always a good choice for weight watchers. It's low in fat
and mild enough to please even those who aren't overly fond of fish.

2	large broccoli stalks
	Grated peel and juice of 1 lemon
4	flounder fillets (4–6 ounces each)
2	tablespoons unbleached flour
¾	cup evaporated skim milk
½	cup shredded reduced-fat Cheddar cheese
	Paprika
2	cups hot cooked bulgur

Cut the florets (tops) of the broccoli from the stalks, saving the stalks for another use. Separate the florets. Steam about 5 minutes, or just until tender. Transfer to a colander and cool under cold running water. Shake off the excess water. Place the broccoli in a medium bowl and mix in the lemon peel and lemon juice.

Coat an 8″ × 8″ baking dish with no-stick spray. Cut each fillet in half crosswise. Arrange 4 pieces in the bottom of the dish. Divide the broccoli among the pieces and spread in an even layer. Top with the remaining fillets.

Place the flour in a 1-quart saucepan. Slowly whisk in the milk to make a smooth mixture. Cook over medium heat, whisking constantly, for 5 minutes, or until thickened. Remove from the heat and stir in the cheese.

Pour the cheese sauce over the fillets. Very lightly dust with the paprika. Bake at 350° for 25 minutes, or until the fish is cooked through. Serve with the bulgur.

Makes 4 servings.

Per serving: 308 calories, 5 g. fat (14% of calories), 6.3 g. dietary fiber, 67 mg. cholesterol, 248 mg. sodium.

ANGEL HAIR PASTA WITH CARROTS AND BASIL

You needn't reserve hot pasta dishes for dinner. This one combines angel hair pasta and finely cut carrots, so it cooks quickly. And it's elegant enough to serve when you have company for lunch. To turn this into a more hearty dinner entrée, increase the pasta to 12 ounces.

¼	cup minced shallots
2	cloves garlic, minced
1	tablespoon olive oil
1	pound carrots, julienned
½	cup defatted chicken stock
¼	teaspoon ground black pepper
	Pinch of ground red pepper
8	ounces angel hair pasta
¼	cup minced fresh basil
3	tablespoons grated Parmesan cheese

In a large no-stick frying pan over medium heat, sauté the shallots and garlic in the oil for 5 minutes, or until soft. Add the carrots, stock, black pepper and red pepper. Cover and cook for 10 minutes, or until the carrots are soft.

Uncover and cook until most of the liquid has evaporated.

Meanwhile, cook the pasta in a large pot of boiling water for 4 minutes, or until just tender. Drain and place on a large platter. Top with the carrot mixture. Sprinkle with the basil and Parmesan. Toss lightly.

Makes 4 servings.

Per serving: 323 calories, 5.9 g. fat (16% of calories), 4.4 g. dietary fiber, 4 mg. cholesterol, 136 mg. sodium.

SCALLOPS VÉRONIQUE WITH LINGUINE

"Véronique" in a recipe title indicates the presence of seedless grapes, generally light green ones. Sole is often served this way. Here we've substituted scallops for an interesting variation. If you'd like to serve this for lunch or a lighter dinner, cut the pasta back to eight ounces.

2	tablespoons finely minced onions
2	tablespoons finely minced carrots
2	tablespoons finely minced celery
2	teaspoons olive oil
1	pound small scallops
⅔	cup small seedless grapes
¼	cup minced fresh parsley
2	tablespoons defatted chicken stock
2	tablespoons white wine vinegar
¼	teaspoon dried thyme
12	ounces linguine
2	tablespoons grated Parmesan cheese

In a large no-stick frying pan over medium heat, sauté the onions, carrots and celery in the oil for 5 minutes, or until translucent.

Add the scallops and sauté for 3 minutes, or until opaque. Stir in the grapes, parsley, stock, vinegar and thyme. Cover and simmer for 5 minutes.

Meanwhile, cook the linguine in a large pot of boiling water for 8 minutes, or until just tender. Drain and place on a large platter. Top with the scallop mixture. Sprinkle with the Parmesan.

Makes 4 servings.

Per serving: 474 calories, 5.6 g. fat (11% of calories), 1.8 g. dietary fiber, 40 mg. cholesterol, 255 mg. sodium.

TURKEY CUTLETS
WITH HERBED MUSHROOM STUFFING

Turkey cutlets are readily available in supermarkets these days. They are very thin pieces of turkey breast and make a less expensive substitute for veal. This recipe also calls for cooked couscous. Prepare it according to the package directions, but without the butter that's generally called for, while the turkey is in the oven; it's ready in less than ten minutes.

4	scallions, finely chopped
1	teaspoon olive oil
1½	cups finely chopped mushrooms
½	cup dry bread crumbs
3	tablespoons minced fresh parsley
¼	teaspoon dried marjoram
4	turkey cutlets (about 3 ounces each)
¼	cup defatted chicken stock
2	cups hot cooked couscous

In a large no-stick frying pan over medium heat, sauté the scallions in the oil for 3 minutes, or until wilted. Add the mushrooms. Cook, stirring occasionally for 10 minutes, or until the mushrooms have released their liquid and it has evaporated.

Stir in the bread crumbs, parsley and marjoram.

Place the cutlets flat on a work surface. Divide the stuffing among them, mounding it in the center. Fold up the ends to enclose the filling.

Coat an 8″ × 8″ baking dish with no-stick spray. Add the cutlets, seam side down. Pour the stock into the dish. Cover with foil and bake at 350° for 20 minutes, or until the turkey is cooked through. Serve with the couscous.

Makes 4 servings.

Per serving: 267 calories, 3.5 g. fat (12% of calories), 5.2 g. dietary fiber, 49 mg. cholesterol, 151 mg. sodium.

Chicken and Garden Vegetable Stir-Fry

For variety, you could substitute other vegetables, including very thinly sliced carrots, bamboo shoots, water chestnuts or Chinese cabbage. In order to have the rice ready when the stir-fry is, start it cooking before you cut up all the other ingredients.

4	boneless, skinless chicken breast halves (about 3 ounces each), cut into bite-size cubes
1	tablespoon olive oil
1	cup snow peas, halved lengthwise
1	cup small broccoli florets
½	cup thinly sliced sweet red peppers
1	onion, thinly sliced
1	cup defatted chicken stock
2	tablespoons reduced-sodium soy sauce
1	tablespoon cornstarch
1	tablespoon minced fresh ginger
1	clove garlic, minced
2	cups hot cooked rice
2	tablespoons minced fresh coriander

In a wok or large no-stick frying pan over medium-high heat, stir-fry the chicken in the oil for 5 minutes, or until opaque throughout. Remove with a slotted spoon and set aside.

Add the peas, broccoli, peppers and onions to the pan. Stir-fry for 5 minutes, or until crisp-tender.

In a small bowl, mix the stock, soy sauce and cornstarch until the cornstarch is dissolved.

Add the ginger, garlic and chicken to the pan. Stir well. Add the stock mixture and cook, stirring, for 3 minutes, or until the sauce thickens.

Serve over the rice. Sprinkle with the coriander.

Makes 4 servings.

Per serving: 314 calories, 5.2 g. fat (15% of calories), 3.5 g. dietary fiber, 49 mg. cholesterol, 338 mg. sodium.

BUTTERFLIES AND BEANS

The butterfly-shaped pasta used here gives this dish a whimsical quality. Yet it's nice and filling—and quite low in fat.

½   cup fresh basil leaves
½   cup fresh parsley leaves
1   clove garlic, coarsely chopped
1   tablespoon snipped chives
⅛   teaspoon crushed dried rosemary
2   cups fresh spinach leaves
¼   cup defatted chicken stock
1   tablespoon olive oil
12   ounces farfalle pasta (butterflies)
12   ounces green beans, cut into 1″ pieces

In a food processor or blender, combine the basil, parsley, garlic, chives and rosemary. Process until chopped. Add the spinach, stock and oil. Process until smooth.

Cook the pasta in a large pot of boiling water for 12 minutes, or until just tender. Drain and place in a large bowl.

While the pasta is cooking, steam the beans for 5 minutes, or until tender. Add to the bowl with the pasta. Spoon on the spinach mixture and toss gently.

Makes 4 servings.

Per serving: 385 calories, 5.2 g. fat (12% of calories), 3.5 g. dietary fiber, 0 mg. cholesterol, 25 mg. sodium.

THYME TURKEY SCALLOPS

This is a very quick dinner dish that's special enough to serve to guests. Round out the meal with a colorful vegetable or two, such as steamed snap peas, broccoli florets or diagonally sliced carrots.

1   pound turkey cutlets
2   tablespoons flour
2   teaspoons olive oil
1   cup defatted chicken stock
½   cup minced onions
½   teaspoon dried thyme
8   ounces thin egg noodles
2   tablespoons grated Parmesan cheese
2   tablespoons minced fresh parsley

Dredge the cutlets in the flour. Shake off the excess.

In a large no-stick frying pan over medium heat, warm the oil. Sauté the turkey, several pieces at a time, until lightly browned on both sides. Transfer to a plate.

Add the stock and onions to the pan. Cook for 2 minutes, stirring constantly to get the browned bits off the bottom of the pan.

Return the turkey to the pan, cover and simmer for about 10 minutes, or until the turkey is very tender and the sauce has thickened slightly. Stir in the thyme and cook for 1 minute.

While the turkey is simmering, cook the noodles in a large pot of boiling water for 8 minutes, or until just tender. Drain and place on a large platter. Top with the turkey and sauce. Sprinkle with the Parmesan and parsley.

Makes 4 servings.

Per serving: 408 calories, 7.6 g. fat (17% of calories), 2.7 g. dietary fiber, 124 mg. cholesterol, 149 mg. sodium.

PARTY FOOD

Prawns with Peach Dipping Sauce

Your party will be a hit when you serve this simple hors d'oeuvre. You can prepare the shrimp ahead and keep it in the refrigerator until party time. The sauce takes but a few minutes and is practically fat-free.

2   peaches, peeled, pitted and cut into chunks
1   teaspoon honey
½   teaspoon apple cider vinegar
1   teaspoon prepared horseradish
1   pound extra-large shrimp (about 30), steamed,
     peeled and deveined

In a blender or food processor, puree the peaches until smooth. Transfer to a 1-quart saucepan. Add the honey and vinegar. Simmer for 5 minutes. Stir in the horseradish. Serve warm or at room temperature with the shrimp.

Makes 6 servings.

Per serving: 97 calories, 1.3 g. fat (13% of calories), 0.5 g. dietary fiber, 117 mg. cholesterol, 123 mg. sodium.

MOZZARELLA AND ASPARAGUS CANAPÉS

These elegant party nibbles are similar to pizza rounds, but they're much lower in fat. And they're very easy to throw together.

8   asparagus spears
4   English muffins, split in half
1   tablespoon diet tub-style margarine
8   thin tomato slices
2   teaspoons Dijon mustard
8   thin slices part-skim mozzarella cheese

Snap off and discard the tough bottoms of the asparagus spears. Cut the tender parts in half to make pieces about 4″ long. Steam just until crisp-tender, then cool under cold running water. Pat dry and set aside.

Spread the muffin halves with a thin layer of the margarine. Place on a cookie sheet and toast lightly under a broiler.

Place a tomato slice on each half and lightly coat with the mustard. Place under the broiler for 1 minute to heat through.

Arrange 2 asparagus spears on each tomato slice. Cover with the mozzarella and place under a broiler until the cheese melts. Serve at once.

Makes 8 servings.

Per serving: 90 calories, 2 g. fat (20% of calories), 1.1 g. dietary fiber, 2 mg. cholesterol, 235 mg. sodium.

BABY POTATOES FILLED WITH DILL SOUR CREAM

You could really dress up these simple hors d'oeuvres by spooning a tiny amount of an inexpensive caviar on top.

16   baby potatoes, scrubbed but unpeeled
1   cup nonfat sour cream
1   scallion, minced
1   tablespoon minced fresh dill
     Tiny dill sprigs

Steam the potatoes for 18 to 20 minutes. Let cool. Use a melon scoop to hollow out the potatoes, leaving a sturdy shell. Save the pulp and place it in a medium bowl. Mash well. Mix in the sour cream, scallions and minced dill. Spoon the mixture into the potato shells. Garnish with the dill sprigs.

Makes 8 servings.

Per serving: 76 calories, 0.1 g. fat (1% of calories), 1.5 g. dietary fiber, 0 mg. cholesterol, 26 mg. sodium.

CHEESE-TOPPED MUSHROOM CAPS WITH SPINACH

Don't be alarmed by the high percent of calories from fat in these stuffed mushrooms. The figure just seems high because there are so few calories to begin with. The actual grams of fat are quite low.

8   very large mushrooms
1   small onion, minced
¼   cup grated carrots
1   teaspoon olive oil
1   cup packed spinach leaves, finely chopped
2   tablespoons toasted sunflower seeds
1   tablespoon minced fresh parsley
¼   cup shredded reduced-fat Swiss cheese

Carefully remove the stems from the mushroom caps. Finely chop the stems and set aside.

Arrange the caps, stem side up, around the edge of a large microwave-safe plate. Cover with wax paper and microwave on high for 2 minutes. Give the plate a half turn. Microwave for another 2 minutes, or until the caps are softened. Turn the caps over to drain any liquid that has accumulated in them.

In a large no-stick frying pan over medium heat, sauté the onions, carrots and mushroom stems in the oil for 5 minutes. Add the spinach and cook for 3 minutes, or until wilted. If there is any liquid remaining in the pan, cook the mixture for a few more minutes to evaporate it. Stir in the sunflower seeds and parsley.

Divide the mixture among the mushroom caps. Sprinkle with the Swiss cheese.

Arrange in a pie plate or shallow baking dish. Bake at 350° for 15 minutes. Serve hot.

Makes 8 servings.

Per serving: 43 calories, 2.4 g. fat (47% of calories), 1 g. dietary fiber, 2 mg. cholesterol, 8 mg. sodium.

HERBED CHEESE SPREAD

This spread tastes like the expensive ultrafatty one from France.
Serve it with a variety of colorful raw vegetables or low-fat crackers.

- ⅔ cup nonfat cottage cheese
- ⅓ cup nonfat cream cheese, softened
- ¼ cup finely minced fresh chives
- 1 tablespoon grated Parmesan cheese
- 1 clove garlic, minced
- ½ teaspoon dried marjoram
- ¼ teaspoon dried basil
- ¼ teaspoon ground black pepper
- 4 tablespoons finely minced fresh parsley, divided

Place the cottage cheese in a food processor and blend until very smooth. Add the cream cheese and blend briefly to combine. Transfer to a medium bowl. Mix in the chives, Parmesan, garlic, marjoram, basil, pepper and 3 tablespoons of the parsley.

Place in a small decorative bowl and sprinkle with the remaining 1 tablespoon of parsley.

Makes 1¼ cups.

Per tablespoon: 15 calories, 0.1 g. fat (6% of calories), 0.1 g. dietary fiber, 2 mg. cholesterol, 31 mg. sodium.

BROWN-BAG LUNCHES

TUNA SHELL SALAD

Tuna salad is a dieter's staple. This version extends the tuna with vegetables and pasta (any small shape will do). Nonfat mayonnaise moistens the salad without contributing the fat of regular mayo.

- 1½ cups tiny pasta shells
- 13 ounces water-packed tuna, drained and flaked
- ½ cup diced sweet red peppers
- ½ cup thawed frozen peas
- 2 scallions, minced
- 2 tablespoons minced fresh parsley
- ½ teaspoon dried oregano
- ½ cup nonfat mayonnaise
- 1 tablespoon white wine vinegar
- 2 teaspoons Dijon mustard

Cook the pasta in a large pot of boiling water for 10 minutes, or until just tender. Pour into a colander, rinse with cold water and transfer to a large bowl.

Add the tuna, peppers, peas, scallions, parsley and oregano. Toss to combine.

In a small bowl, mix the mayonnaise, vinegar and mustard. Stir the dressing into the pasta mixture.

Makes 4 servings.

Per serving: 319 calories, 3.2 g. fat (9% of calories), 1.5 g. dietary fiber, 39 mg. cholesterol, 826 mg. sodium.

TURKEY AND CUCUMBER SANDWICHES

Seasoned with horseradish and garlic, these sandwiches have a nice bite! To carry one in a brown-bag lunch, keep the filling and bread separate so the bread doesn't become soggy. Assemble the sandwich just before eating.

    ½   cup nonfat mayonnaise
    1   tablespoon prepared horseradish
    ½   teaspoon garlic powder
    ½   teaspoon ground black pepper
    2   cups finely chopped cooked turkey breast
    ¼   cup finely chopped scallions
    8   slices rye bread
    1   seedless cucumber, very thinly sliced

In a medium bowl, toss together the mayonnaise, horseradish, garlic powder and pepper. Mix in the turkey and scallions.

Divide the mixture among 4 slices of the bread, spreading it to the edges. Overlap the cucumber slices in an even layer over the turkey. Top with the remaining 4 slices of bread.

Makes 4 servings.

Per serving: 279 calories, 4.2 g. fat (14% of calories), 4 g. dietary fiber, 49 mg. cholesterol, 816 mg. sodium.

CALIFORNIA CHICKEN SALAD SANDWICHES

This low-fat chicken salad is a little out of the ordinary—getting exotic flavor from dried coriander and ginger. Mixing yogurt with mayonnaise for a dressing gives the salad extra tang that mayo alone doesn't provide.

2	cups shredded cooked chicken breast
1	cup halved seedless grapes
½	cup finely chopped celery
¼	teaspoon ground coriander
¼	teaspoon powdered ginger
¼	teaspoon dried basil
¼	cup nonfat mayonnaise
¼	cup nonfat yogurt
4	large pita breads
16	large spinach leaves

In a medium bowl, toss together the chicken, grapes, celery, coriander, ginger and basil. Mix in the mayonnaise and yogurt.

Cut each pita in half and open the pockets. Line each half with 2 spinach leaves. Fill with the chicken mixture.

Makes 4 servings.

Per serving: 296 calories, 6.2 g. fat (19% of calories), 1.9 g. dietary fiber, 63 mg. cholesterol, 512 mg. sodium.

CATALINA SHRIMP IN PITA POCKETS

What could be easier? Buy ready-cooked and peeled shrimp, a bag of premixed coleslaw vegetables and bottled dressing. Toss them all together and stuff the low-fat mixture into a pita.

12	ounces small shrimp, peeled, deveined and cooked
2	cups preshredded coleslaw mixture
½	cup reduced-calorie Catalina dressing
4	large whole-wheat pita breads

In a medium bowl, combine the shrimp, coleslaw mixture and dressing.

Cut each pita in half and open the pockets. Fill with the shrimp mixture.

Makes 4 servings.

Per serving: 217 calories, 3.4 g. fat (14% of calories), 1.7 g. dietary fiber, 84 mg. cholesterol, 559 mg. sodium.

DESSERTS

Lemon-Glazed Coffee Cake

Who says you can't eat cake when you're counting calories? This sweet yet tart coffee cake is irresistible, and it has only 100 calories and less than two grams of fat per slice.

½   cup unbleached flour
½   cup whole-wheat flour
1   tablespoon toasted wheat germ
1   teaspoon baking powder
½   teaspoon grated lemon peel
¼   teaspoon ground cinnamon
½   cup skim milk
1   egg white, lightly beaten
1   tablespoon canola oil
4   tablespoons honey, divided
1   tablespoon lemon juice

Coat a 9″ × 5″ loaf pan with no-stick spray. Set aside.

In a medium bowl, stir together the unbleached flour, whole-wheat flour, wheat germ, baking powder, lemon peel and cinnamon.

In a small bowl, whisk together the milk, egg white, oil and 2 tablespoons of the honey. Pour into the bowl with the flour mixture and stir just until combined.

Spread the batter in the prepared pan. Bake at 350° for 30 minutes, or until the top is golden brown and a toothpick inserted near the center comes out clean. Cool the cake in its pan on a wire rack for 10 minutes.

In a 1-quart saucepan, stir together the remaining 2 tablespoons of honey and the lemon juice. Heat until warm.

Using the tines of a fork, poke holes over the surface of the cake. Spoon on the honey mixture. Let the cake cool in its pan.

To serve, remove the cake from the pan and cut into 9 slices.

Makes 9 servings.

Per serving: 101 calories, 1.8 g. fat (16% of calories), 1.1 g. dietary fiber, 0 mg. cholesterol, 49 mg. sodium.

FROZEN PEACH POPS

When the hunger pangs hit, there is nothing more convenient than having a healthy snack waiting for you in your freezer. If you want a selection of flavors to choose from, make different batches using other fruits such as apricots, strawberries or bananas.

3	medium peaches, peeled, pitted and sliced (about 1½ cups)
1	cup skim milk
¼	cup pineapple juice
2	teaspoons grated lemon peel
1	teaspoon lemon juice
1	teaspoon vanilla

In food processor or blender, process the peaches, milk, pineapple juice, lemon peel, lemon juice and vanilla until smooth.

Divide the mixture among 4 (6- to 8-ounce) paper cups. Cover with foil and place in the freezer until partially frozen. Insert a wooden Popsicle stick in the center of each and freeze at least 8 hours.

To serve, let the pops stand at room temperature for 5 minutes. Then gently peel off the paper.

Makes 4 servings.

Per serving: 62 calories, 0.2 g. fat (3% of calories), 1.1 g. dietary fiber, 1 mg. cholesterol, 32 mg. sodium.

ANGEL FOOD CAKE WITH BLUEBERRIES AND STRAWBERRY SAUCE

Angel food cake is a best bet for weight watchers because it has no fat. Dress it up with an easy low-cal fruit sauce and extra berries for a dessert you can enjoy without guilt.

3	cups sliced strawberries
⅔	cup apple juice
1	cup nonfat vanilla yogurt
1	angel food cake (12 ounces)
2	cups blueberries

In a food processor or blender, puree the strawberries with the apple juice. Transfer to a medium bowl and fold in the yogurt.

Cut the cake into 12 slices. Spoon about ½ cup of the strawberry mixture over each slice. Sprinkle with the blueberries.

Makes 12 servings.

Per serving: 122 calories, 0.3 g. fat (2% of calories), 1.6 g. dietary fiber, 0 mg. cholesterol, 90 mg. sodium.

MICROWAVE STREUSEL APPLES

When you crave a sweet snack or dessert, whip up these apples.
They're done in the microwave, so they're ready in no time.

½	cup nonfat sour cream
1	tablespoon honey
	Pinch of ground cardamom or grated nutmeg
2	large Golden Delicious or other cooking apples
1	tablespoon lemon juice
¼	cup quick-cooking rolled oats
2	tablespoons brown sugar
1	tablespoon diet tub-style margarine, softened
½	teaspoon ground cinnamon

In a small bowl, stir together the sour cream, honey and cardamom or nutmeg. Cover and refrigerate until ready to serve.

Cut the apples in half lengthwise and remove the cores with a melon scoop or grapefruit spoon. Rub the cut surfaces with the lemon juice to keep them from discoloring.

In another small bowl, combine the oats, brown sugar, margarine and cinnamon. Divide the mixture among the apples and pat into an even layer on each.

Place the apples in a 9″ glass pie plate. Microwave on high for 3 minutes. Give the plate a quarter turn. Microwave for another 3 to 4 minutes, or until the apples are easily pierced with a sharp knife. Let stand for 3 minutes to finish cooking.

Serve with the sour cream sauce.

Makes 4 servings.

Per serving: 183 calories, 2 g. fat (10% of calories), 2.8 g. dietary fiber, 0 mg. cholesterol, 46 mg. sodium.

Part Five

FOOD GUIDES
FOR LOW-FAT LIVING

LOW-FAT SURVIVAL TECHNIQUES FOR THRIVING IN A HIGH-FAT WORLD

You're laughing, watching a goofy sitcom on TV, feeling relaxed, doing what you normally do, when suddenly you hear it. That double-fudge pecan chunk ice cream is calling your name. Never mind for the moment how it got in your freezer in the first place. It now knows you're listening, and it's making a pest of itself. What do you do?

You're hot, tired, irritable, and you have to make dinner. It's the last thing you feel like doing. As you're about to begin chopping veggies for a low-fat salad, your husband walks in and says, "What do you say we go out to dinner?" The catch? He wants to bop down to the fast-food burger joint on the corner. What do you do?

You've been following "Your Perfect Weight 52-Week Plan" for six months now. Lately, you've developed these annoying late-night cravings. You don't want to binge; you know a little nibble will satisfy you, but you really would like to keep the calories down to no more than 100. What do you do?

The answer is: Grab this book and refer to the tables that follow.

When chocolate ice cream calls your name, meet it head-on. Check out the "Never Say Never" table that begins on page 325 and see exactly what it is you're dealing with. The information may help you resist or even vow never to allow it in your freezer again. And if you decide to indulge, you'll have a pretty good idea of what you'll need to do tomorrow so that all that fat won't stay with you permanently.

If you find yourself heading out the door to a burger joint, refer to "Slimmer Selections from Fast-Food Restaurants," on page 334. To satisfy that craving for late-night nibbles, turn to page 346 and check out "One Hundred 100-Calorie Snacks."

Familiarize yourself with all these tables. The handy, nifty information can help you through the rough spots in your new low-fat lifestyle.

Never Say Never

Depriving yourself while trying to lose weight can often backfire, leading to an all-out binge. Next time you get a craving for some greasy potato chips or rich chocolate cake try to ride out the crave wave. Wait 15 to 20 minutes and then decide if you really want the food. If you do, indulge but don't go overboard. Remember: Everything in moderation. Listed below are a variety of high-fat, high-calorie foods that are often the sources of cravings. Check out how much fat and calories these foods contain so when you do indulge you'll know just how much you are indulging. And maybe some of these numbers are enough to quiet your cravings.

Food	Portion	Calories	Fat (g.)	% Calories from Fat
Apple pie	1 slice	231	13.1	51
Bacon	3 slices	109	9.4	78
Beef bologna	1 slice	72	6.5	81
Boston cream pie	⅛ pie	311	9.7	28
Bread stuffing, from mix	1 cup	416	25.6	55
Brownie, with nuts, homemade	1 (3 × 1 × ⅞″)	97	6.3	58
Butter	1 Tbsp.	108	11.4	95
Cheddar cheese	1 oz.	114	9.4	74
Cheddar cheese sauce	1 oz.	39	2.9	67
Cheeseburger	1	295	14.1	43
Cheesecake	1 slice	257	16.3	57
Cheese enchilada	6 oz.	319	18.8	53
Cheesesteak	1	519	18.6	32
Chicken, fried	3 oz.	234	14.6	56
Chicken gravy, canned	½ can	95	6.5	62
Chocolate bar	1.45 oz.	207	14.0	61
Chocolate-chip cookies	2	99	4.4	40
Chocolate-covered peanuts	10 pieces	208	13.4	58

(continued)

Never Say Never—Continued

Food	Portion	Calories	Fat (g.)	% Calories from Fat
Chocolate fudge, with nuts, homemade	1 oz.	119	4.9	37
Chocolate ice cream	½ cup	143	7.3	46
Chocolate ice cream, premium	½ cup	232	14.9	58
Chocolate shake	10 oz.	360	10.5	26
Croissant	2 oz.	235	12.0	46
Danish pastry	1	161	8.8	49
Devil's food cake	1 piece	227	11.3	45
Doughnut	1 plain (2 oz.)	176	10.8	55
Eclair	1	239	13.6	51
Eggnog, nonalcoholic	8 oz.	342	19.0	50
Egg roll with pork	3 oz.	165	5.5	30
Fettuccine Alfredo, frozen	5 oz.	270	19.0	63
French fries	10	111	4.4	36
Hamburger	1 plain (3.5 oz.)	275	21.5	70
Hoagie/sub	1	456	18.6	37
Hot dog	1	242	14.5	54

Food	Portion	Calories	Fat (g.)	% Calories from Fat
Hot fudge sundae	1	284	8.6	27
Lasagna, frozen	6 oz.	244	10.8	40
Manicotti, frozen	5 oz.	229	13.5	53
Nacho chips	1 oz.	141	7.3	47
Nachos, supreme	6–8	568	30.7	49
Peanut butter, creamy	2 Tbsp.	188	16.0	77
Peanut butter cookies	1	76	3.8	45
Peanut butter cups	2 (1.8 oz.)	281	16.7	53
Pecan pie, homemade	⅛ pie	431	23.6	49
Pepperoni pizza	⅛ 12″ pie	181	7.0	35
Pork sausage	1 link	48	4.1	77
Potato chips	1 oz.	152	9.8	58
Pot roast, lean	3 oz.	184	7.1	35
Sirloin steak, choice, broiled	3.5 oz.	269	16.7	56
Steak sandwich	1	459	14.1	28
Taco salad	1½ cups	279	14.8	48

NOTE: The number of calories and fat listed above are based on averages of the various brands that are available. Be sure to read individual labels, since some products may be higher or lower than the figures listed.

Training Yourself to Make Better Choices

Every time you walk into a supermarket these days there are dozens of new low-fat and nonfat products to be found. These products can be a boon for anyone trying to lose weight. Switching to a low-fat or nonfat version of a product can save you anywhere from 1 to 22 grams of fat. That translates into 9 to 198 calories. All it takes is a little exchange know-how to use low-fat products to your advantage. If you use these products to help you reduce your dietary fat intake by just 13 grams a day (and that should be easy!), you could lose one pound of body fat in one month. That's without even trying.

Use this table to get a handle on just how much calories, fat and sodium you'll be saving. Simply look up the food you're shopping for and go for the version of each product marked with an asterisk (*). Note: Even the light and low-fat versions of many of these foods can pack a pretty hefty dose of fat and calories. You need to evaluate any foods that contain fat in terms of the rest of your diet.

There are a variety of brands on the market for the following products. All figures in this chart are based on averages of these products, so be sure to check individual labels for specific figures.

Food	Portion	Calories	Fat (g.)	Sodium
BACON				
Regular	1 slice	36	3	101
Light*	1 slice	18	1	140
BOLOGNA				
Regular	3 slices	270	24	810
Low-fat*	3 slices	60	2	590
BROWNIES, FROM MIX				
Regular	1 (2″ sq.)	150	7	90
Light*	1 (2″ sq.)	100	2	75
CAKE, YELLOW, FROM MIX				
Regular	¹⁄₁₂ cake	260	11	310
Light*	¹⁄₁₂ cake	200	4	310

Food	Portion	Calories	Fat (g.)	Sodium
CAKE FROSTING, VANILLA				
Regular	1 oz.	160	6	30
Light*	1 oz.	130	1	30
CHEESE				
Regular	1 oz.	90	7	390
Low-fat	1 oz.	58	3.5	230
Nonfat*	1 oz.	40	0	260
COOKIES				
Chocolate chip				
Regular	0.5 oz.	55	2.5	45
Low-fat*	0.5 oz.	60	1	85
Double fudge				
Regular	1 cookie	77	3.2	68
Fat-free*	1 cookie	50	0	65
Oatmeal raisin				
Regular	1 cookie	59	2	22
Low-fat*	1 cookie	60	1	65
Sandwich, chocolate/vanilla creme				
Regular	1 cookie	50	2.3	48
Low-fat*	1 cookie	50	1	65
COTTAGE CHEESE				
Regular	4 oz.	120	5	460
Low-fat	4 oz.	90	1	490
Nonfat*	4 oz.	80	0	390
CRACKERS				
Cheese				
Regular	12 (0.5 oz.)	75	4	265
Low-fat*	18 (0.5 oz.)	60	1	160
Wheat				
Regular	5 (0.5 oz.)	70	3	135
Fat-free*	5 (0.5 oz.)	50	0	160

(continued)

Training Yourself to Make Better Choices—Continued

Food	Portion	Calories	Fat (g.)	Sodium
CREAM CHEESE				
Regular	1 oz.	100	9.9	90
Light	1 oz.	70	6	115
Fat-free*	1 oz.	30	0	180
FIG BARS				
Regular	1	60	1	60
Fat-free*	1	70	0	85
FROZEN DESSERTS				
Ice cream (16% fat)	½ cup	175	11.9	54
Frozen yogurt, regular, chocolate	½ cup	140	4	65
Frozen yogurt*, nonfat, all flavors	½ cup	100	0	60
FROZEN ENTRÉES				
Chicken parmigiana dinner				
Regular	11.5 oz.	400	16	1,050
Low-fat*	11.5 oz.	290	6	340
French bread pizza				
Regular	5 oz.	350	14	630
Low-fat*	5 oz.	300	4	470
Salisbury steak dinner				
Regular	11.5 oz.	410	18	900
Low-fat*	11.5 oz.	280	7	550
Turkey dinner				
Regular	11.5 oz.	340	11	980
Low-fat*	11.5 oz.	280	4	570
GRANOLA				
Regular	1 oz.	130	6	15
Low-fat*	1 oz.	115	2	55
GRANOLA BAR				
Regular	1 (0.75 oz.)	120	4.2	80
Low-fat*	1 (0.75 oz.)	110	2	95

Food	Portion	Calories	Fat (g.)	Sodium
HOT DOGS				
Regular, beef	1	180	16	690
Low-fat, beef	1	50	1	460
Fat-free*, meatless	1	40	0	290
MARGARINE				
Regular	1 Tbsp.	90	10	90
Low-fat	1 Tbsp.	35	4	50
Nonfat*	1 Tbsp.	5	0	90
MAYONNAISE				
Regular	1 Tbsp.	100	12	75
Light	1 Tbsp.	50	5	110
Fat-free*	1 Tbsp.	10	0	105
MILK				
Regular	8 oz.	150	8	125
2%	8 oz.	120	5	125
1%	8 oz.	110	2	130
Skim*	8 oz.	90	<1	130
PANCAKES, FROM MIX				
Regular	3 (4")	230	5.7	950
Light*	3 (4")	130	2	570
PASTA SAUCE				
Regular	4 oz.	110	5	510
Low-fat	4 oz.	40	<1	350
Nonfat*	4 oz.	45	0	350
PEANUT BUTTER, CHUNKY				
Regular	2 Tbsp.	190	17	140
Reduced-fat*	2 Tbsp.	190	13	170
POPCORN, MICROWAVE				
Regular	3 cups	100	6	170
Low-fat*	3 cups	60	1	160
POTATO CHIPS				
Regular	1 oz.	150	10	190
Fat-free*	1 oz.	100	<1	160

(continued)

Training Yourself to Make Better Choices—Continued

Food	Portion	Calories	Fat (g.)	Sodium
PUDDING, CHOCOLATE				
Regular	4 oz.	160	4	130
Nonfat*	4 oz.	100	0	170
RICOTTA CHEESE				
Regular	2 oz.	90	7	125
Low-fat	2 oz.	80	5	105
Nonfat*	2 oz.	40	<1	100
SALAD DRESSING				
Blue cheese				
Regular	2 Tbsp.	154	16	298
Low-fat	2 Tbsp.	80	1.8	394
Nonfat*	2 Tbsp.	40	0	280
Creamy Italian				
Regular	2 Tbsp.	110	12	510
Light	2 Tbsp.	52	14	296
Nonfat*	2 Tbsp.	50	0	280
Italian				
Regular	2 Tbsp.	45	14.2	390
Light	2 Tbsp	32	3	236
Nonfat*	2 Tbsp.	12	0	280
Ranch				
Regular	2 Tbsp.	156	17	312
Light	2 Tbsp.	40	2	280
Nonfat*	2 Tbsp.	32	0	280
Thousand Island				
Regular	2 Tbsp.	110	16.2	310
Light	2 Tbsp.	50	4	240
Nonfat*	2 Tbsp.	32	0	260
SAUSAGE, SMOKED				
Regular, pork	2 oz.	244	18	N/A
Light*	2 oz.	130	11	N/A

Food	Portion	Calories	Fat (g.)	Sodium
SOUP				
Chicken noodle				
Regular	8 oz.	130	4	1,150
Low-fat*	8 oz.	80	2	470
Cream of mushroom				
Regular	8 oz.	100	7	800
Low-fat*	8 oz.	60	2	480
Ham and bean				
Regular	8 oz.	200	3	960
Low-fat*	8 oz.	170	2	460
Split pea				
Regular	8 oz.	210	5	950
Low-fat	8 oz.	160	2	470
Nonfat*	8 oz.	100	0	95
Tomato				
Regular	8 oz.	140	4	730
Low-fat*	8 oz.	90	2	460
Vegetable				
Regular	8 oz.	122	3.7	1,010
Low-fat	8 oz.	100	1	560
Nonfat*	8 oz.	60	0	80
SOUR CREAM				
Regular	2 Tbsp.	60	6	10
Light	2 Tbsp.	40	2	25
Nonfat*	2 Tbsp.	30	0	40
STEAK SANDWICH MEAT				
Regular	2 oz.	170	15	40
Light*	2 oz.	140	11	40
YOGURT				
Low-fat	1 cup	150	4	170
Nonfat	1 cup	120	0	170

Slimmer Selections from Fast-Food Restaurants

You avoid hamburgers, french fries and drive-through windows like the plague, but occasionally you find yourself with a group of people who insist on lunching at a fast-food restaurant. What to do?

There is now a variety of healthier choices at many fast-food restaurants. So you don't have to sacrifice your diet. Here's a listing of some of the best lower-fat, lower-calorie choices from some of the most popular fast-food restaurants. And don't forget, in addition to these options, some of these restaurants also offer bountiful salad bars—just steer clear of the fatty salad dressings.

Food	Calories	Fat (g.)	% Calories from Fat	Sodium (mg.)
ARBY'S				
Baked Potato, plain	240	1.9	7	58
Blueberry Muffin	240	7	26	200
Chocolate Chip Cookie	130	4	28	95
Chocolate Shake	451	11.6	23	341
Garden Salad	117	5.2	40	134
Jamocha Shake	368	10.5	26	262
Light Roast Beef Deluxe	294	10	31	826
Light Roast Chicken Deluxe	276	7	23	777
Light Roast Turkey Deluxe	260	6	21	1,262
Old Fashioned Chicken Noodle Soup	99	1.8	16	929
Side Salad	25	0.3	11	30
BURGER KING				
Baked Potato, plain	210	0	0	15
BK Broiler Chicken Sandwich	280	10	32	770
Chunky Chicken Salad, no dressing	142	4	25	443

Food	Calories	Fat (g.)	% Calories from Fat	Sodium (mg.)
Dinner Roll	80	2	23	140
Dinner/Side Salad, no dressing	20	0	0	10
Carl's Jr.				
Bran Muffin	310	7	20	370
Charbroiled BBQ Chicken Sandwich	310	6	17	680
Chicken Salad to-Go	200	8	36	300
English Muffin with margarine	190	5	24	280
Garden Salad-to-Go	50	3	54	75
Hamburger	320	14	39	590
Lite Potato	290	1	3	60
Scrambled Eggs	120	9	67	105
Dairy Queen				
BBQ Beef Sandwich	225	4	16	700
Chocolate Cone, regular	230	7	27	115
Chocolate Sundae, regular	300	7	21	140
DQ Sandwich	140	4	26	135
Grilled Chicken Fillet Sandwich	300	8	24	800
Hamburger, single	310	13	38	580
Mr. Misty, regular	250	0	0	0
Side Salad, no dressing	25	0	0	15
Strawberry Breeze, small	290	<1	2	115
Strawberry Yogurt Sundae, regular	230	<1	2	80
Vanilla Cone, regular	230	7	27	95
Yogurt Cone, regular	180	<1	3	80
Yogurt Cup, regular	170	<1	3	70

(continued)

Slimmer Selections from Fast-Food Restaurants—Continued

Food	Calories	Fat (g.)	% Calories from Fat	Sodium (mg.)
DUNKIN' DONUTS				
Apple N'Spice Muffin	300	8	24	360
Banana Nut Muffin	310	10	29	410
Blueberry Muffin	280	8	26	340
Bran Muffin with Raisins	310	9	26	560
Cinnamon N'Raisin Bagel	230	2	8	330
Cranberry Nut Muffin	290	9	28	360
Oat Bran Muffin	330	11	30	450
Onion Bagel	210	1	4	410
Plain Bagel	210	2	9	330
HARDEE'S				
Chocolate Cool Twist Cone	180	4	20	85
Chocolate Shake	390	10	23	220
Grilled Chicken Salad	120	4	30	520
Hamburger	260	9	31	460
Hot Fudge Cool Twist Sundae	320	10	28	260
Mashed Potatoes (4 oz.)	70	<1	13	330
Pancakes, plain (3)	280	2	6	890
Roast Beef, regular	270	11	36	780
Strawberry Cool Twist Sundae	260	6	21	100
Strawberry Shake	390	8	18	200
Vanilla/Chocolate Cool Twist Cone	170	4	21	85
Vanilla Cool Twist Cone	180	4	20	80
Vanilla Shake	370	9	22	210

Food	Calories	Fat (g.)	% Calories from Fat	Sodium (mg.)
JACK IN THE BOX				
Beef Teriyaki Bowl	640	3	4	930
Chicken Fajita Pita	290	8	25	700
Chicken Teriyaki Bowl	580	1.5	2	1,220
Chocolate Shake	330	7	19	270
Double Fudge Cake	290	9	28	260
Hamburger	270	11	37	560
Sesame Breadsticks	70	2	26	110
Side Salad	50	3.4	61	85
Strawberry Shake	320	7	20	240
Vanilla Shake	320	6	17	230
KFC				
BBQ Baked Beans	132	2	14	535
Breadstick (1)	110	3	25	15
Garden Rice	75	1	12	576
Garden Salad	16	0	0	10
Green Beans	36	1	25	563
Mashed Potatoes with Gravy	70	1	13	370
Red Beans and Rice	114	3	24	315
Rotisserie Gold Chicken, White Quarter, skin and wing removed	199	5.9	27	667
Sourdough Roll (1)	128	2	14	236
Vegetable Medley Salad	126	4	29	240
LONG JOHN SILVER'S				
Baked Apples	123	2	15	20
Baked Potato	119	<1	4	0
Green Beans	20	<1	23	320
Honey Wheat Roll	110	<1	4	171
Lemon Crumb Fish	150	1	6	370
Light Herb Chicken	120	4	30	570
Parsley Potatoes	135	4	27	75

(continued)

Slimmer Selections from Fast-Food Restaurants—Continued

Food	Calories	Fat (g.)	% Calories from Fat	Sodium (mg.)
LONG JOHN SILVER'S—CONTINUED				
Rice	160	3	17	340
Side Salad	25	<1	18	20
McDONALD'S				
Apple Bran Muffin, fat-free	180	0	0	220
Cereal	85	1	11	215
Chicken Fajita	185	8	39	310
Chocolate Milk Shake, low-fat	320	1.7	5	240
Chunky Chicken Salad, no dressing	150	4	24	230
English Muffin with spread	170	4	21	285
Garden Salad, no dressing	50	2	36	70
Hamburger	225	9	36	490
Hot Caramel Frozen Yogurt Sundae	270	3	10	180
Hot Fudge Frozen Yogurt Sundae	240	3	11	170
McLean Deluxe	320	10	28	670
McLean Deluxe with Cheese	370	14	34	890
Scrambled Eggs (2)	140	10	64	290
Side Salad, no dressing	30	1	30	35
Strawberry Frozen Yogurt Sundae	210	1	4	95
Strawberry Milk Shake	320	1.3	4	170
Vanilla Frozen Yogurt Cone	105	1	9	80
Vanilla Milk Shake	290	1.3	4	170

Food	Calories	Fat (g.)	% Calories from Fat	Sodium (mg.)
Pizza Hut*				
Bigfoot Cheese Pizza	179	5	25	959
Cheese Hand-Tossed Pizza	253	9	32	593
Cheese Thin 'N Crispy Pizza	223	10	40	503
Chunky Veggie Hand-Tossed Pizza	224	6	24	633
Chunky Veggie Thin 'N Crispy Pizza	193	8	37	546
Veggie Lovers Hand-Tossed Pizza	222	7	28	641
Veggie Lovers Thin 'N Crispy Pizza	192	8	38	551
Roy Rogers				
Baked Beans (5 oz.)	160	2	11	560
Baked Potato, plain	130	1	7	65
Cinnamon Raisin Bagel	300	1	3	490
Grilled Chicken Salad	120	4	30	520
Grilled Chicken Sandwich	340	11	29	910
Hamburger	260	9	31	460
Hot Fudge Sundae	320	10	28	260
Mashed Potatoes (5 oz.)	92	<1	5	320
Pancakes, plain (3)	280	2	6	890
Plain Bagel	300	2	6	520
Roast Beef Sandwich	260	4	14	700
Roy's Roaster (¼, white meat, no skin)	190	6	28	700
Side Salad	20	<1	23	20
Strawberry Sundae	260	6	21	95
Vanilla Frozen Yogurt Cone	180	4	20	80

(continued)

Slimmer Selections from Fast-Food Restaurants—Continued

Food	Calories	Fat (g.)	% Calories from Fat	Sodium (mg.)
SUBWAY				
Roast Turkey Breast Sub† (6″, white bread)	312	7.8	23	1,190
Round Ham Sandwich‡ (4″)	317	2.8	8	670
Round Roast Beef Sandwich‡ (4″)	326	2.4	7	820
Veggies and Cheese Sub† (6″, wheat bread)	258	6.3	22	530
TACO BELL				
Chicken Soft Taco	213	10	42	615
Pintos 'N Cheese	190	9	43	642

Food	Calories	Fat (g.)	% Calories from Fat	Sodium (mg.)
WENDY'S				
Baked Potato, plain	310	0	0	25
Breadstick, soft	130	3	21	250
Chili, small	190	6	28	670
Frosty Dairy Dessert, small	340	10	26	200
Grilled Chicken Sandwich	290	7	22	720
Hamburger, Jr.	270	9	30	600

NOTE: All figures are based on nutritional analysis from each restaurant. If you would like nutritional information for other menu items, check with the individual restaurants.

*Bigfoot pizza values are for 1 slice. All other values are for 1 slice of a medium pizza.

†Subs include cheese, onions, lettuce, tomatoes, pickles, peppers and olives.

‡Rounds include lettuce, tomato and pickle.

Surprise! Foods Can Fool You

You could be in for some real surprises! Wait until you find out how many calories are in a piña colada or how much fat is in eggplant parmigiana. There are a lot of foods that have more calories or fat than they appear to have at first glance.

On the other hand, you may have a few pleasant surprises in store. Some of the foods you may have been avoiding aren't so bad after all.

Food	Portion	Calories	Fat (g.)	% Calories from Fat
FOODS SURPRISINGLY HIGH IN FAT				
Avocado	1 med.	306	30.0	88
Bean burritos	2	448	13.5	27
Bérnaise sauce, from mix	¼ cup	170	17.0	90
Cappuccino	1 cup	123	4.7	34
Chicken leg	3 oz.	181	8.0	40
Cream of chicken soup	1 cup	116	7.4	57
Chicken potpie, homemade	1 piece	545	31.3	52
Chicken sandwich, fried	1	515	29.5	52
Chicken sandwich spread	2 oz.	110	7.4	61
Chop suey	1 cup	300	17.0	51
Chow mein	1 cup	255	10.0	35
Coconut, dried, toasted	1 oz.	168	13.4	72
Coffee, instant Irish creme	1 cup	55	2.4	39
Coffee, instant Suisse mocha	1 cup	53	2.5	42
Cottage cheese, creamed	4 oz.	117	5.1	39
Cream, half-and-half	2 Tbsp.	40	3.4	77
Cream, light	2 Tbsp.	58	5.8	90

Food	Portion	Calories	Fat (g.)	% Calories from Fat
Creamer, nondairy, powdered	1 tsp.	11	0.7	57
Duck, no skin, roasted	3.5 oz.	201	11.1	50
Egg, scrambled	1	101	7.5	67
Eggplant parmigiana, frozen	5.5 oz.	293	18.2	56
Enchiladas, cheese	2	638	37.6	53
Fish sandwich, fried	3.2 oz. fillet	211	11.2	48
Granola bar, regular	1 (0.75 oz.)	134	4.2	28
Herring, pickled	1 oz.	39	2.7	62
Hollandaise sauce, from mix	¼ cup	170	18.0	95
Hummus	½ cup	210	10.4	45
Olives, green	10	45	5.8	100
Mackerel, Atlantic, cooked, dry heat	3 oz.	223	15.1	61
Parmesan cheese, grated	1 Tbsp.	23	1.5	59
Piña colada, canned	6.8 oz.	525	16.9	29
Pork egg roll	3 oz.	165	5.5	30
Potato, baked with cheese sauce and broccoli	1	402	21.4	48
Potato salad, homemade	½ cup	179	10.3	52
Pumpkin seeds, roasted	1 oz.	148	12.0	73
Seafood Newburg	10 oz.	350	12.0	31
Soft-shell crab, fried	4.5 oz.	334	17.9	48
Taco salad	1.5 cups	279	14.8	48
Tartar sauce	1 Tbsp.	74	8.0	97
Tofu, raw, firm	½ cup	183	11.0	54
Turkey, ground	3 oz. patty	188	11.4	55
Turkey bologna	1 slice	70	6.0	77
Turkey frank	1	90	6.0	60

(continued)

Surprise! Foods Can Fool You—Continued

Food	Portion	Calories	Fat (g.)	% Calories from Fat
FOODS SURPRISINGLY HIGH IN FAT—CONTINUED				
Whipped topping, nondairy	2 Tbsp.	22	1.8	74
White sauce, from mix	¼ packet	151	8.4	50
Yellow mustard	1 tsp.	4	0.2	45
FOODS SURPRISINGLY LOW IN FAT				
Angel food cake, from mix	¹⁄₁₂ cake (2 oz.)	126	0.1	<1
Apple butter	1 Tbsp.	33	0.1	3
Barbecue sauce	1 Tbsp.	12	0.3	23
Chestnuts, roasted	3–4 (1 oz.)	70	0.6	8
Chocolate fudge	0.6 oz.	65	1.4	19
Cocktail sauce	1 Tbsp.	12	0	0
Cod, cooked, dry heat	3 oz.	89	0.7	7
Fortune cookie	1	15	0	0
Fig bar	1	60	1.0	15
Gelatin, sugar-free	½ cup	8	0	0
Gingerbread, from mix	¹⁄₉ cake	174	4.3	22
Gingersnaps	5	100	3.0	27
Graham crackers	2	60	1.0	15
Haddock, cooked, dry heat	3 oz.	95	0.8	8
Hard candy	1 oz.	106	0	0
Honey	1 Tbsp.	64	0	0
Horseradish	1 Tbsp.	6	0	0
Hot chocolate, from mix, with water	6 oz.	103	1.1	10

Food	Portion	Calories	Fat (g.)	% Calories from Fat
Jam/preserves	1 Tbsp.	48	0	0
Jelly	1 Tbsp.	52	0	0
Jelly beans	10 large	104	0.1	<1
Ketchup	1 Tbsp.	16	0.1	6
Ladyfingers	2	79	1.7	19
Licorice	1 oz.	120	3.0	23
Lobster, cooked, moist heat	3 oz.	83	0.5	5
Lollipop	1	22	0	0
Maple syrup	1 Tbsp.	52	0	0
Pierogies, boiled	2	120	1.0	8
Popsicle	2 oz.	42	0	0
Pork tenderloin	3.5 oz.	166	4.8	26
Red wine	3.5 oz.	74	0	0
Rice pudding, with raisins	½ cup	193	4.1	19
Rose wine	3.5 oz.	73	0	0
Salsa	3 Tbsp.	25	0	0
Sapsago cheese	1 oz.	16	0.5	28
Shrimp, cooked, moist heat	3 oz.	84	0.9	10
Soy sauce	¼ cup	38	0	0
Steak sauce	1 Tbsp.	15	0	0
Sweet relish	1 Tbsp.	19	0.1	5
Tabasco sauce	½ tsp.	0	0	0
Teriyaki sauce	1 Tbsp.	15	0	0
Top round steak, select, broiled	3.5 oz.	169	3.7	20
Veal leg, roasted	3.5 oz.	150	3.4	20
Venison	3.5 oz.	158	3.2	18
Waffle/pancake syrup	1 Tbsp.	57	0	0
White wine	3.5 oz.	70	0	0
Worcestershire sauce	1 Tbsp.	11	0	0

One Hundred 100-Calorie Snacks

High-fat, high-calorie snacks can sabotage weight-loss efforts. Next time you can't resist those midmorning or late-night munchies, reach for one of the snacks listed below. The following list contains 100 low-fat, low-calorie snacks that will satisfy your hunger without sacrificing your figure.

The number of calories and fat grams are based on averages of the brands available. Please check individual labels because some products may be higher or lower than these averages.

Food	Portion	Calories	Fat (g.)	% Calories from Fat
Animal crackers	5	56	1.2	19
Apple	1 med.	81	0.5	6
Applesauce, unsweetened	½ cup	53	0.1	2
Apricots	3 med.	51	0.4	7
Bagel, plain	½	82	0.7	8
Banana	½ med.	53	0.3	5
Bean salad	½ cup	90	0.3	3
Beets, pickled, canned, sliced	½ cup	75	0.1	1
Blackberries	½ cup	37	0.3	7
Blueberries	1 cup	82	0.6	7
Bran cereal	½ cup	60	0.5	8
Breadsticks	2	77	0.6	7
Broccoli	½ cup	12	0.2	15
Candy corn	10 pieces	51	0.3	5
Cantaloupe, cubed	1 cup	57	0.4	6
Carambola (starfruit)	1 med.	42	0.4	9
Carrot	1 med.	31	0.1	3
Cauliflower	½ cup	12	0.1	8
Celery	1 stalk	6	0.1	15
Cheese, nonfat	1 oz.	40	0	0
Chestnuts, roasted	3–4 (1 oz.)	70	0.6	8
Chewing gum	1 stick	5	0	0
Chicken noodle soup, canned	1 cup	75	2.5	30

Food	Portion	Calories	Fat (g.)	% Calories from Fat
Chocolate pudding, instant, sugar-free	½ cup	92	2.7	26
Chocolate pudding pop	1	79	1.9	22
Cornflakes	1 cup	100	0.7	7
Cottage cheese	4 oz.	90	1.0	10
Couscous	½ cup	100	0.2	2
Cranberries	1 cup	46	0.2	4
Cucumber, sliced	½ cup	7	0.1	13
Currants	½ cup	34	0.2	5
Dill pickle	1 med.	12	0.1	8
English muffin	½	68	0.6	8
Fig	1 med.	37	0.2	5
Fig bar	1	53	1.0	17
Fortune cookie	1	15	0	0
Frozen yogurt, nonfat	½ cup	100	0	0
Fruit and juice bar, frozen	3 oz. bar	75	0.1	1
Fruit bar	0.8 oz. bar	81	1.2	13
Fruit cocktail, water-packed	½ cup	40	0.1	2
Fruit-filled cookie	0.75 oz. cookie	80	2.0	23
Fruit roll	0.75 oz.	73	0.6	7
Fruit salad	½ cup	67	0.1	1
Gelatin	½ cup	80	0	0
Gingersnaps	2	59	1.2	18
Graham crackers	2	66	2.6	35
Graham snacks	11 pieces	60	2.0	30
Grapefruit	½ med.	37	0.1	2
Grapes	1 cup	58	0.3	5
Guava	1 med.	45	0.5	10
Gummy bears	3	20	0	0
Hard candy	1 piece	25	0	0
Honeydew melon, cubed	1 cup	60	0.2	3
Ice pop	2 fl. oz. bar	42	0	0

(continued)

One Hundred 100-Calorie Snacks—Continued

Food	Portion	Calories	Fat (g.)	% Calories from Fat
Jellied candy	1 oz.	100	0	0
Jelly beans	10 large	104	0.1	<1
Kiwifruit	1 med.	46	0.3	6
Kumquat	1 med.	12	0	0
Licorice, red	6 bite-size pieces	75	0.3	4
Life Savers	1	9	0	0
Lollipop	1	22	0	0
Mandarin oranges, canned	½ cup	76	0.1	1
Mango	½ med.	68	0.3	4
Marshmallow	1 regular	23	0	0
Melba toast	2 pieces	25	0.1	4
Mints	¼ cup	100	0.6	5
Mulberries	1 cup	61	0.6	9
Nectarine	1 med.	67	0.6	8
Orange	1 med.	65	0.2	3
Oyster crackers	10	33	1.0	27
Papaya	½ med.	58	0.2	3
Peach	1 med.	37	0.1	2
Pear	1 med.	98	0.7	6
Persimmon	1 med.	32	0.1	3
Pineapple, chunked	1 cup	77	0.7	8
Plum	1 med.	36	0.4	10

Food	Portion	Calories	Fat (g.)	% Calories from Fat
Pomegranate	½ med.	52	0.3	5
Popcorn, plain	1 cup	23	0.3	12
Popcorn cake	2	77	0.6	7
Pretzels	0.5 oz.	54	0.5	8
Prunes, boxed	5	100	0.2	2
Puffed rice cereal	1 cup	54	0.1	2
Puffed wheat cereal	1 cup	52	0.1	2
Radishes	10	7	0.2	26
Raspberries	1 cup	61	0.7	10
Rice cakes	2	70	0.5	6
Rye crackers	2	45	0.2	4
Saltine crackers	2	26	0.6	21
Shredded wheat cereal	1 biscuit	81	0.3	3
Strawberries	1 cup	45	0.6	12
Sweet cherries	10	49	0.7	13
Sweet peppers, sliced	½ cup	13	0.1	7
Sweet potato, baked	1 med.	59	0.1	2
Tangerine	1 med.	37	0.2	5
Vanilla ice milk	½ cup	92	2.8	27
Vanilla wafers	3½	60	3.2	48
Vegetable soup	1 cup	81	1.9	21
Watermelon, cubed	1 cup	50	0.7	13
Whole-wheat toast, with 2 tsp. jam	1 slice	91	1.1	11
Yogurt, nonfat	3 oz.	75	0	0

TERMS FOR PERFECT WEIGHT

There's plenty of confusion in the world of dieting, nutrition and exercise. But these simple explanations should help make it easier for you to understand what you're eating and how you're working out, and the ways these things may or may not contribute to your weight-loss efforts.

Aerobic. Exercise that makes you breathe faster than normal for an extended period of time, such as hiking or swimming.

Anorexia. An eating disorder characterized by self-starvation due to an intense fear of becoming overweight.

Appetite. A strong desire or craving for food, not to be confused with *hunger,* which is a physiological response to a lack of food.

Basal metabolic rate. The rate at which the body burns calories while at rest.

Bench press. An exercise used in resistance training that builds and strengthens muscles in the chest, upper arms and back.

Biceps. A set of muscles located in the front of the upper arms.

Bingeing (binge eating). Periods of uncontrolled eating in which large quantities of food are consumed within a short period of time.

BMI (body-mass index). A measure used to determine a person's level of obesity, based on height and weight. (Multiply your weight in pounds by 700, divide that number by your height in inches, then divide again by your height.) A BMI of between 20 and 25 is considered good for most middle-aged adults.

Bulimia. An eating disorder characterized by recurrent episodes of bingeing, followed by attempts to lose weight through self-induced vomiting, diuretics or severely restrictive diets.

Calipers. An instrument that measures the percentage of body fat by "pinching" the skin.

Calorie. The amount of heat necessary to raise the temperature of one gram of water 1°C. Expressed another way, it is a measure of the energy-producing value of food—the more energy food produces, the greater its calorie count. One pound of body weight is produced by 3,500 calories.

Carbohydrate. One of the basic food categories, carbohydrates are organic compounds containing carbon, hydrogen and oxygen. When broken down, carbs are the main energy source for muscular work.

Cellulite. A word coined in the 1970s referring to the puckered, cottage cheesy type of fat found around the hips, thighs and buttocks. However, this fat is no different from fat found anywhere else in the body and cannot be eliminated differently from any other body fat.

Cholesterol. A fatty substance found in the cells of humans and animals. (All foods of animal origin contain this substance.) Cholesterol helps form hormones, cell membranes and other life-enhancing substances, but the body is able to manufacture all it needs naturally, and too much can clog arteries and interfere with health. An acceptable cholesterol reading is between 150 and 200. That's equivalent to about 3.9 to 5.2 in the Canadian system.

Fat. A compound containing glycerol and fatty acids. Fats serve as a concentrated source of energy for muscular work. Fat is stored very efficiently by the body, so excess fat can cause obesity and interfere with health.

Fatty acids. Types of fat found in the body. They include nonessential fatty acids (manufactured by the body) and essential fatty acids (obtained through the foods we eat). Fatty acids may be saturated or unsaturated—all dietary fats are made up of mixtures of both. Fatty acids are necessary for healthy skin, blood, arteries, nerves and normal growth.

Fiber. Thick-walled cells found in plants and in such foods as whole-grain cereals and breads, raw fruits and vegetables. Eating fiber promotes satiety and aids digestion, and soluble fiber (which dissolves in water) has been found to lower cholesterol levels.

Food Guide Pyramid. The U.S. Department of Agriculture (USDA) diagram indicating types and quantities of foods that comprise a healthy daily diet.

Hamstrings. The muscles located on the back of the thighs.

High-density lipoproteins (HDLs). A type of cholesterol—actually, proteins that carry unused fat to the liver for disposal. A lipid (fat) must be attached to a protein in order to be carried in the body. HDLs are considered "good" because they're able to remove harmful LDLs (low-density lipoproteins) and, in so doing, lower the cholesterol level. Aerobic exercise helps boost the body's HDLs.

Hydrogenated oil. Liquid oil, such as vegetable oil, that's been turned into a semisolid state, such as margarine, giving it cholesterol-elevating properties.

"Lat" (latissimus dorsi). A back muscle.

Light or lite. According to the newest USDA regulations, a product containing one-third fewer calories or 50 percent less fat than the same serving size of the regular product.

Lipid. Fat.

Low-calorie. According to the newest USDA regulations, a product containing 40 or fewer calories per serving.

Low-density lipoproteins (LDLs). The "bad" form of cholesterol. These proteins get deposited on artery walls. This deposit then forms plaque, which contributes to coronary artery disease and high blood pressure.

Low-fat. According to the newest USDA regulations, a product containing three or fewer grams of fat per serving.

Maximum heart rate. Theoretically, the maximum rate at which your heart can beat per minute at your age. The formula for your maximum heart rate is 220 minus your age.

Metabolic rate. The rate at which the body burns calories.

Monounsaturated fats. Fatty acids found in both plant and animal fat, appearing mainly in vegetable and nut oils. Foods high in monounsaturated fatty acids include olive oil, peanut oil and vegetable shortening. Substituting monounsaturated fats for saturated fats reduces blood cholesterol levels.

Polyunsaturated fats. Fatty acids found in most foods, mainly in the fat from plants, including safflower, sunflower, corn and soybean oils. Polyunsaturated fats are liquid at room temperature and contain the essential nutrient linoleic acid.

Protein. One of the basic food categories, it is essential for building and repairing muscles, red blood cells, hair and other tissues.

"Quads" (quadriceps). Muscles on the front of the thighs.

RDAs (Recommended Dietary Allowances). The amounts of vitamins and minerals that should be included in the daily diet, according to the USDA.

Recovery heart rate. Your heart rate measured at the end of your workout after cooling down. It is used to determine when the heart rate has returned to its normal, pre-exercise pulse.

Resistance training. The process of increasing muscle strength (the ability to lift heavy objects) and muscular endurance (the ability to repeat a movement requiring strength). It involves repetitive sets of exercises aimed at strengthening specific areas of the body.

Saturated fats. Fatty acids, which are solid at room temperature, that tend to raise blood cholesterol to dangerously high levels. Saturated fat is found in all foods from animal sources, including meat and dairy products, but also in such oils as coconut oil and palm-kernel oil.

Sodium. A mineral used by the body to help maintain fluid balance in and around the cells. However, an excess of sodium (which comprises 40 percent of table salt) can lead to high blood pressure, as well as to water retention, which can slow weight loss.

Spot reducing. A popular myth that fat can be "burned" only in desired areas of the body.

Strength. The maximum force or tension that a muscle or muscle group can produce against resistance.

Strength training. (See resistance training.)

Triceps. A set of muscles located at the back of the upper arms.

Triglycerides. One of the major fats carried in the blood. Triglyceride levels above 100 are considered high and may interfere with health.

Unsaturated fats. Fatty acids, either polyunsaturated or monounsaturated, that lower blood cholesterol levels.

Weight cycling. Repeatedly gaining and losing weight, usually caused by an inconsistent pattern of dieting and overeating.

Weight training. (See resistance training.)

WHR (waist-to-hip circumference ratio). A measurement used to compare the size of your waist to your hips that helps determine heart disease risk. (Divide the number of inches in your waist by the number of inches in your hips.) A number above 0.8 for women and above 1.0 for men indicates a higher-than-normal level of risk.

Yo-yo dieting. (See weight cycling.)

INDEX

Note: Underscored page references indicate boxed text. **Boldface** references indicate illustrations.

A

Abdominal crunches, 117
Abdominal curl, 77, 220, 262–63
Additives, food, 43
Aerobic exercise, 351
   in circuit training, 70
   for weight loss promotion, 63, 122–23, 126
Affirmations, 94
Afterburn from exercise, 238
Aging
   easing process of
      body fat, decreasing, 9
      resistance training, 72, 73
      weight loss, 8–9
   effects of, on
      cholesterol levels, 6
      energy level, 118, 155
      exercise, 8–9
      metabolism, 15–16, 72
      muscles, 72
Alcohol
   cordials, 143
   dieting and, 151
   mixed drinks, 143
   at parties, avoiding, 269
   selections when dining out, 143
   weight gain by men and, 110, 112
   in weight loss failure, 156–57
   wine, 143, 151, 232
Anorexia, 351
Appetite, 351
   body temperature and, 156
   fiber and, 105
   water intake in controlling, 198
Appetizers, low-fat, 311–14
Applesauce, to replace cooking fat, 48
Apple-shaped body, 15
Arm curl, 77, 78
Arteries, 5, 24
Assertiveness, 79–81

B

Back problems, weight loss in preventing, 9
Basal metabolic rate, 351
Basil, 245
Beans
   Black Bean Soup, 298–99
   Butterflies and Beans, 310
   Kidney Bean and Chick-Pea Salad,
      300
   Shortcut Chili, 298
Beef
   dietary fat in, 124
   hamburgers, low-fat, 48
   substitutes for, low-fat, 124
Beer belly, 107
Behavior modification
   alternatives to eating and, 93
   for cravings, 91
   goals for, sample, 178–79
   need for, 89–90
   social support for, 98
   triple-A program for
      action, 95–98
      attitude, 92, 94–95
      awareness, 90, 92
Bench press, 77–78, 77, 246, 351
Biceps, 351
Biceps curl, 220, 262
Bingeing/binge eating, 351
   coping with, 97–98
   exercise after, 241
   giving into, **325**
   responding to, 240–41
   reward systems for avoiding, 241
   water intake after, 241
Blender, 39
Blood flow, 5
Blood pressure, 4–5, 15, 121
Blood sugar levels, 6, 15, 105, 121, 190
BMI, 351

Body fat. *See also* Obesity; Overweight
    aging and, 9
    cellulite, 352
    distribution, 62, 122
    gender and, 122
    of models/actresses, 16
    in stomach, 15, 107, 122, 263–64
    swimming and, 156
    of women, average, 16
Body image
    children's, 135
    gender and, 108, 120
    men's, 108, 120
    unrealistic, eliminating, 234
    women's, 108, 120, 121
Body-mass index (BMI), 351
Body makeovers, real-life stories of, 158–67
Body shape, 15
Body Shop, 130
Bone strengthening, 73, 136
Breakfasts
    for children, 131
    for cold-weather walking, 217–18
    fast-food, 138
    for football players, 25
    healthy, 187
    importance of, 95, 147, 187–88
    obesity and, 95
    recipes for low-fat, 293–96
Breast cancer, 6–7
Breast-feeding, 115, 116
Bulimia, 351
Butter, 39, 142

C
Caesar salads, 142
Caffeine drinks, avoiding, 199
Cakes
    Angel Food Cake with Blueberries and
        Strawberry Sauce, 318–19
    Lemon Glazed Coffee Cake, 317
Calcium, 44, 56
Calf raise, 77
Calipers, 351
Calorie-free food, 44
Calories, 351–52
    activities for losing 500, 221–23
    burning
        body fat and, 72
        exercises for, 65, 156, 221–23
        gender and, 123

    metabolism and, 20–21, 154, 177
    muscles and, 72
    in butter, 39
    in carbohydrates, 19, 182, 190
    deficit, for weight loss, 103, 177
    in dietary fat, 19, 182
    in food
        80-calorie, 27
        100-calorie, **346–49**
        specific, **328–33**
    intake of
        for breast-feeding mothers, 116
        for men, average, 17
        reducing, 49, 103–4
        for women, average, 17
    in oil, 39
    in proteins, 19, 182
Cancer
    breast, 6–7
    prevention
        low-fat diet, 7
        weight loss, 6–7
    prostate, 7
    risks for developing
        obesity, 7
        saturated fat, 24
Carbohydrates, 352
    calories in, 19, 182, 190
    complex, 52, 187, 189–90
    diet rich in, 25
    in football players' diets, 25
Cellulite, 352
Cereals
    for children's breakfasts, 131
    Maple-Almond Oatmeal, 293
Chair push-ups, 220
Cheeses
    Cheese-Topped Mushroom Caps with
        Spinach, 313
    Herbed Cheese Spread, 314
    Mozzarella and Asparagus Canapés, 312
Chef's salads, 108
Chest pull, 197
Chicken
    lean, 52
    recipes using
        California Chicken Salad Sandwiches,
            316
        Chicken and Garden Vegetable Stir-Fry,
            309
        Minted Chicken Salad, 301
    skin removal, 48

Childbirth, ideal weight in easing, 9
Children
    activities for, 228–29
    body image of, 135
    breakfasts for, 131
    exercise for, 130, 133–34, 136
    fast food and, 132
    including vegetables in diet of, 133
    lunches for, brown-bag, 131–32
    metabolism of, while watching TV,
        227–28
    nutrition for, 129–31
    overweight
        exercise for, 130, 133–34, 136
        factors causing, 128
        motivation to lose weight for,
            134–36
        statistics on, 128–29
        strategies for preventing, 129–36
        weight-loss programs for, 130
    resistance training for, 136
    snacking and, 129, 132
    supermarket shopping with, 42, 129
    walking with, 228, 242–43
Chili
    Shortcut Chili, 227, 298
Chocolate cravings, 124
Cholesterol, 352
    aging and, 6
    dietary fat and, 156
    exercise and, 6
    stomach fat and, 15
    levels
        acceptable, 352
        desired, 121
    vegetable oil in lowering levels of, 57
    weight loss in increasing good, 6
Chopsticks, speed of eating and, 143
Circuit training, 70
Clothing, 151, 217, 238–40
Club soda, 199
Commitment
    to exercise as weight maintenance strategy,
        272
    to exercise program, 192–93
    to lifestyle changes, 178
    public, 257–58
    to weight-loss plan, 178
    as weight maintenance strategy, 170
Condiments, 245–46
Contracts
    eating, 96

exercise, 192–93
    for motivation, 100
Cooking
    with herbs, 50
    for later eating, 261
    low-fat, 46–50
    meal planning and, low-fat, 226–27
    men's views of, 109–10
    utensils, 38–40, 260
    with vegetables, 204–5
Cooking fat, 48. *See also* Oil
Cool-down, 75
Cordials, after-dinner, 143
Cortisol, 263
Cost-benefit analysis of weight-loss program,
    99–100
Cravings
    for chocolate, 124
    curing, 91
    dietary fat and, 26–27
    gender and, 124
    satisfying, 154
    stress and, 82
    taste/texture and, 152
Cream, milk vs., 143
Cross-training, 70
Crunches, abdominal, 117
Curls
    abdominal, 77, 220, 262–63
    arm, 77, 78
    biceps, 220, 262
    hamstring, 77, 247

D

Dairy products, 52, 201–2. *See also specific types*
Dancing, 270–71
Deficiencies, nutritional, 56
Dehydration, 57
Denial, 171
Depression, weight gain by women and,
    118
Desserts
    fruit, 49–50, 131, 317–19
    recipes for low-fat, 317–19
    selections when dining out, 143
Diabetes, 6, 9
Diary, success, 275–90
Diet. *See also* Low-fat diet
    arteries and, 5
    breast-feeding and, 116
    carbohydrate-rich, low-fat, 25

Diet *(continued)*
  changes to
    gradual, 148
    seasonal, 155
    for variety, 101, 148, 211, 245–46, 272
  for football players, 25
  smoking cessation and, 4
  weight maintenance strategies and, 103–5,
    170, 272
Dietary fat, 352
  animal, 149
  in beef, 124
  in butter, 39
  calories in, 19, 182
  cholesterol and, 156
  counting, 20–21, 22
  cravings, 26–27
  essential fatty acid deficiency and, 56
  excess, health problems caused by, 10
  in food
    high content of, **342–44**
    low content of, **344–45**
    specific, **28–34, 325–27, 328–33**
  hydrogenated, 24
  insulin's effects on, 218
  intake of
    for breast-feeding mothers, 116
    for ideal weight, **23**
    recommended, 22
    safe, 22–23, **23**
  monosaturated, 24, 353
  in oil, 39
  polyunsaturated, 24, 353
  reducing
    "Fat Budget" table and, 22–24, **23**
    food plan for, 182–85
    gradual approach to, 24–26
    labels (food) in helping, 103–4
    recommended amount, 22
  saturated, 24, 353
  substitutes for foods high in
    for calorie reduction, 49
    eating on run and, 110
    80-calorie foods, 27
    in low-fat kitchen, 36–38
    mayonnaise, low-fat, 149
    treats, 236–37
    as weight loss strategy, 104
  sugar and, 157
  taste for, losing, 26–27
  in turkey, 124
  types of, 24

unsaturated, 354
  in weight loss failure, 156
Diet-induced thermogenesis (DIT), 97
Dieting
  alcohol and, 151
  dining out and, 137, 214
  gender and, 108
  for lifestyle change, 157
  limitations of, 102–3
  mantras for, 173–74
  men's view of, 108, 111
  mentality about, 92, 94, 151
  repeated, 154
  reversibility and, law of, 211
  rigidity in, avoiding, 153–54
  saboteurs, responding to, 266–67,
    323–24
  social support for, 98
  work and, 112
  yo-yo, 169, 354
Diet plan, 52-week, 177–273
Dining out
  dieting and, 137, 214
  at ethnic restaurants, 138
  fast food
    breakfasts, 138
    children and, 132
    low-fat selections of, **334–41**
  low-fat diet and, 137–38
  "playing" with food and, 151
  selections
    alcohol, 143
    to avoid, 138
    desserts, 143
    low-fat, 140–41, **334–41**
    phrases to watch for, 139
    from restaurants, specific, **334–41**
    salads, 142
    soups, 142
    substitutes for high-fat foods, 140–41
    water, 143
  survival guide for, 214–15
  tips for healthy, 139–43
Dinners
  fruits for, 120
  leftover, for brown-bag lunches, 209
  recipes for low-fat
    Almond-Baked Halibut, 302
    Angel Hair Pasta with Carrots and Basil,
      306
    Black Bean Soup, 298–99
    Butterflies and Beans, 310

Chicken and Garden Vegetable Stir-Fry, 309
Creamy Carrot Soup, 299
Flounder with Lemon Broccoli, 305
Kidney Bean and Chick-Pea Salad, 300
Mexican Meatballs, 304
Minted Chicken Salad, 301
Pork Chops with Apricots, 297
Ratatouille, 300–301
Scallops Véronique with Linguine, 307
Shortcut Chili, 227, 298
Stuffed Peppers, 303
Thyme Turkey Scallops, 310–11
Turkey Cutlets with Herbed Mushroom Stuffing, 308
DIT, 97
Dumbbell row, 77

E

Eating disorders, 351
Eating habits. *See also* Bingeing/binge eating; Cravings
action modifications about, 95–98
alternatives to eating and, 93
attitude modifications about, 92, 94–95
awareness of, 90, 92
breakfasts and, importance of, 95
cleaning one's plate, 157, 260
contracts in controlling, 96
emotions and, 82, 106, 155
gender and, 82, 125
high-risk situations for bad, 96–97, 101
"invisible" eating and, 155
log of, 92
mealtimes and, 261
after menopause, 118
pleasing other people and, 157
servings and, 155–56, 200
small meals vs. big meals and, 150
speed of eating and, 142, 143
stress and, 81, 83, 84
understanding, 148
variety and, 245–46
in warm weather, 265
water intake and, 199
Eggs, 52
Electrolytes, 57
Emotions
eating habits and, 82, 106, 155
log for recording, 188–89
massage and, 254

overeating and, 90
as triggers for eating, 230
Endurance, 76, 80
Energy level
aging's effects on, 118, 155
increasing
complex carbohydrates, 189–90
exercise, 80
weight loss, 11
ERT, 117
Essential fatty acid deficiency, 56
Estrogen, 122
Estrogen replacement therapy (ERT), 117
Estrone, 7
Evaporation, during warm-weather exercise, 265
Exercise. *See also* Aerobic exercise; *specific types*
afterburn from, 238
aging's effects on, 8–9
after bingeing, 241
calorie-burning, **65**, 156, 221–23
for children, 130, 133–34, 136
commitment to program of, 192–93
contracts, 192–93
deficiency, men's, 110
effects of, on
cholesterol, increasing good, 6
energy level, increasing, 80
high-density lipoprotein, increasing, 6
self-esteem, improving, 74
stress, reducing, 195
enjoying, 64, 65, 67
firming, 116–17
gender and, 126
health benefits of, 64
house-cleaning, 188
interval training and, 156, 237–38, 268
lite, 66
mat, 206
mentality about, 151
overweight caused by deficiency of, 58
in past, 58–59
after pregnancy, 116–17
in present, 59–61
program, 67–70, 192–93
quotas, 67, **68–69**
seasonal changes and, 154–55
selecting, 68–70, 180–81
smoking cessation and, 5
during social gatherings, 67
for stress reduction, 195
supermarket shopping, 63
time for, 62–63, 182, 206

Exercise *(continued)*
  varying, 67, 101, 211
  videos, 250–51
  in warm weather, 265
  weight loss promotion and, 60–61, 61–62
  as weight maintenance strategy
    commitment to, 272
    for men, 112–13
    importance of, 62–63
    moderate, 63–64
    options for, 105–6
    for relapse prevention, 170–71
    for women, 116–17
Extensions
  leg, 197–98
  quadriceps, 77
    seated, 247
  triceps, 262

F
Fast food
  breakfasts, 138
  children and, 132
  low-fat selections of, **334–41**
Fat. *See* Body fat; Dietary fat
"Fat Budget" table, 22–24, **23**
Fatty acids, 352
FDA, 44
Feelings. *See* Emotions
Fiber, 105, 187, 352
52-week diet plan, 177–273
Fish
  omega-3 and omega-6 acids in, 56
  poaching vs. frying, 47
  recipes
    Almond-Baked Halibut, 302
    Catalina Shrimp in Pita Pockets, 209, 316
    Flounder with Lemon Broccoli, 305
    Prawns with Peach Dipping Sauce, 311
    Scallops Véronique with Linguine, 307
    Tuna Shell Salad, 314–15
  servings of, 201–2
Fitness, 67, 71, 75
Food. *See also* Fast food; *specific types*
  additives, 43
  calorie-free, 44
  calories in specific, **328–33**
  dietary fat in
    high content of, **342–44**
    low content of, **344–45**
    specific, **28–34, 325–27, 328–33**

80-calorie, 27
elimination of one favorite, 260
enjoying, 148, 261
fat-free, 44
"grazing," 139, 218–19
high-fat, **342–45**
high-fiber, 105
high-sodium, 261
interest in, sparking, 245–46
labels
  changes in, recent, 243–44
  dietary fat reductions and, 103–4
  for milk, 44
  "no cholesterol," 261
  studying, 194
  supermarket shopping and, 44
light/lite, 44, **328–33**, 352
low-calorie, 353
low-fat, 44, 353
metabolism boosts by, 97
100-calorie, **346–49**
organic, 232
quality, 45, 231–32
in season, 43, 45, 194
sodium in specific, **328–33**
substitutes for high-fat
  for calorie reduction, 49
  eating on run and, 110
  in 80-calorie foods, 27
  in low-fat kitchen, 36–38
  mayonnaise, low-fat, 149
  treats, **236–37**
  as weight loss strategy, 104
sugar-free, 44, 52
trading off, 141–42, 248–49
water content in, 198
Food and Drug Administration (FDA), 44
Food cravings. *See* Cravings
Food diary, 5
Food Guide Pyramid, 352
  nutrition and, 51–52, **54–55**
Food shopping. *See* Supermarket shopping
Fracture threshold, 136
Freezer bags, plastic, 40
French toast
  Fruited French Toast, 294
Frittata
  Potato and Onion Frittata, 294–95
Fruit pizza, 120
Fruit
  complex carbohydrates in, 189, 190
  desserts made with, 49–50, 131, 317–19

for dinners, 120
juices, 132
for lunches, children's brown-bag, 131–32
recipes using
   Angel Food Cake with Blueberries and
     Strawberry Sauce, 318–19
   Breakfast Melon Bowl, 295
   Frozen Peach Pops, 318
   Fruited French Toast, 294
   fruit pizza, 120
   Lemon-Glazed Coffee Cake, 317
   Microwave Streusel Apples, 319
   Pork Chops with Apricots, 297
   Prawns with Peach Dipping Sauce,
     311
servings of, 52, 201
water content in, 198
Frying fish, 47

G

Gender. *See also* Men; Women
body fat and, 122
body image and, 108, 120
calorie burning and, 123
cravings and, 124
dieting and, 108
eating habits and, 82, 125
exercise and, 126
food preferences and, 119
stress reactions and, 82
weight loss and, 119
   approaches to, 127
   body fat reduction and, 122–23
   calorie burning and, 123
   cravings and, 124–25
   eating habits and, 125–26
   exercise and, 126–27
   food selection and, 120
   health/fitness strategies and, 121
Genetics, obesity and, 109
Girl Scout cookies, avoiding, 260
Glucose, 139
Goal weight
false ideals and, avoiding, 15–16
ideal weight vs., 16
importance of knowing, 178
individuality in determining, 12, 18
natural weight and, 17
physician in helping to determine, 18
realistic determination of, 16–17, 169–70
resistance training in reaching, 18

tables in determining, standard, 13–15, **13**
   in weight maintenance, 169–70
Grains, whole, 189, 200–201
"Grazing" food, 139, 218–19
Grocery shopping. *See* Supermarket shopping
Gum, sugarless, 4

H

Habits, 229
Half-and-half, milk vs., 143
Hamburgers, low-fat, 48
Hamstring curl, 247
Hamstrings, 352
HDL, 6, 121, 352
Health benefits
of exercise, 64
of resistance training, 77
of weight loss
   back problem prevention, 9
   cancer prevention, 6–7
   cholesterol, increased good, 6
   diabetes prevention, 6
   energy level, increased, 11
   heart problem prevention, 4–5
   high blood pressure prevention, 4–5
   immune system improvement, 10
   joint problem prevention, 9
   longevity, 8–9
   osteoarthritis prevention, 9
   sex drive, increased, 8
   sleep apnea prevention, 11
   ten-pound loss, 3
Heart attack, 4
Heart disease, 4, 6, 24, 121
Heart problems, weight loss in preventing, 4–5
Heart rate, 353
Height-weight charts, 13–15, **13**
Herbs. *See also specific types*
cooking with, 50
fresh, 43
recipes using
   Angel Hair Pasta with Carrots and Basil,
     306
   Baby Potatoes Filled with Dill Sour
     Cream, 312
   Herbed Cheese Spread, 314
   Herbed Sausage Muffins, 296
   Thyme Turkey Scallops, 310–11
   Turkey Cutlets with Herbed M
     Stuffing, 308
Heredity, obesity and, 109

High blood pressure, weight loss in prevent-
    ing, 4–5, _15_
High-density lipoprotein (HDL), 6, 121, 352
Hip flexor, _77_
Home gyms, 205–7
Hunger, _42_, 43, 260
Hydration, for warm-weather exercise, 265
Hydrogenated dietary fat, _24_
Hydrogenated oil, 352
Hypertension, weight loss in preventing, 4–5,
    _15_

I

Ideal weight
    dietary fat intake for maintaining, **23**
    goal weight vs., 16
    healthy life and, 3
    healthy weight vs., 121
    pregnancy and, 9
    terms in discussing, 351–54
Imaging, 233–34
Immune system, weight loss in improving, 10
Impulses, controlling, 92
Insulin, _4_, 218
Interval training, 156, 237–38, 268
"Invisible" eating, 155
Iron, 53, 56

J

Jelly beans, for snacking, 260
Job. *See* Work
Joint problems, weight loss in preventing, 9
Juices
    fruit, 132
    vegetable, 204
Jump rope, 205

K

Kitchen, low-fat
    cooking utensils in, 38–40
    high-fat food removal from, 182–83
    low-fat food substitutes in, 35, _36–38_, 38
    typical American kitchen vs., 35

L

Labels, food
    changes in, recent, 243–44
    dietary fat reductions and, 103–4

for milk, _44_
"no cholesterol," 261
studying, 194
supermarket shopping and, _44_
Lateral raises, _77_, 220
Latissimus dorsi muscle, 352
"Lat" muscle, 352
Lat pull-down, 78
LDL, 6, 353
Lean-body mass, 126
Leg extensions, 197–98
Leg press, 246
Legumes, 189, 200
Life expectancy, weight loss in increasing, 8–9
Lifestyle
    awareness of, 157
    commitment to changing, 178
    dieting for healthy, 157
    goals, as weight maintenance strategy,
        174
    in past, 58–59
    in present, 59–61
    varying, for motivation boost, 211
    weight maintenance and, 106, 256–57
Lifts, thigh, 197
Light/lite food, _44_, **328–33**, 352
Lipid, 353
Lite exercise, _66_
Log
    diary, 275–90
    eating habits, 92
    for emotions, recording, 188–89
    fitness goal, 149
    resistance training, 76, 220–21
    for stress reduction, 264
    walking, _61_
    for weight maintenance, 171–73
Longevity, weight loss in increasing, 8–9
Low-calorie food, 353
Low-density lipoprotein (LDL), 6, 353
Lower back exercise, 262
Low-fat diet. *See also* Recipes, low-fat
    dining out and, 137–38
    effects of, on
        blood flow, 5
        cancer, 7
    personalizing, 183–85
    rewards of, 19, 21–22
    weight loss promotion and, 19–21, 122–23
    as weight maintenance strategy, 170
Low-fat food, _44_, 353. *See also* Low-fat diet;
    specific types

Lunches, brown-bag
   for children, 131–32
   creative, 209–10
   dinner leftovers for, 209
   recipes for low-fat, 314–16

M
Massage, 253–54
Mat, exercise, 206
Maximum heart rate, 353
Mayonnaise, low-fat, 149
Meal planning, low-fat, 226–27
Mealtimes, 261
Meat loaf pan, double, 39
Meat. *See also* Chicken; Turkey
   lean, 52, 194
   recipe using
      Pork Chops with Apricots, 297
   reducing intake of, 104–5, 156
   servings of, 52, 201–2
   trimming fat from, 48, 124
Medications, weight gain from, 155, 188
Meditation, 90, 195–96, 264
Men. *See also* Gender
   body image of, 108, 120
   calorie intake for average, 17
   cancer risks of, 7
   dietary fat intake of, safe, **23**
   dieting and, view of, 108, 111
   height-weight chart for, **13**
   overweight, 107–8, 110, 112, 120
   social support for, 111–12
   weight gain by
      alcohol and, 110, 112
      casualness about, 108–9
      cooking views and, 109–10
      dieting views and, 108, 111
      exercise deficiency and, 110
      ignorance of nutrition and, 108
   weight maintenance strategies for,
      111–13
Menopause
   calcium supplements and, 56
   eating habits after, 118
   estrogen replacement therapy and, 117
   weight gain by women after, 114, 117–18
Metabolic rate, 353
Metabolism
   aging's effects on, 15–16, 72
   basal metabolic rate and, 351
   calorie burning and, 20–21, 154, 177

   children's, while watching TV, 227–28
   food-boosted, <u>97</u>
   metabolic rate and, 353
   nicotine's effects on, <u>4</u>
Microwave oven, 39
Military press, 78
Milk
   chocolate, 131
   cream vs., 143
   half-and-half vs., 143
   labels on, <u>44</u>
   skim, 48, 131, 191–92
   whole vs. low-fat, 48, 131
Minerals
   Reference Daily Intake of, **53**
   supplements, 52–53, 56
Mineral water, 199
Minigoals, 100, 101, 178
Mixed drinks, 143
Monosaturated fats, <u>24</u>, 353
Moods. *See* Emotions
Motivation
   boosting, 171–73, 211–12
   contracts for, 100
   maximizing, 99–101
   for overweight children to lose weight,
      134–36
   pretending to have, 97
   for resistance training, continued,
      220–21
   self-esteem as, 95
Muffins
   Herbed Sausage Muffins, 296
Muscles
   aging's effects on, 72
   calories burned by, 72
   "lat," 352
   lean-body mass and, 126
   "quad," 353
   tension and, 195
   toning, 76
   triceps, 221, 262, 354
Music
   for stationary bike riding, 268
   for stress reduction, 84

N
Natural weight, 17
Neck exercise, <u>77</u>
Nicotine, metabolism and, <u>4</u>
Non-insulin-dependent diabe

Nutrients
   deficiencies of, 56
   nutrition and, 52–53, **53**, 56–57
   Percent Daily Values and, 244
   Reference Daily Intake of, **53**, 56
Nutrition
   for children, 129–31
   Food Guide Pyramid and, 51–52,
      54–55
   learning about, 111
   men's ignorance of, 108
   nutrients and, 52–53, **53**, 56–57
   in past, 51
   in present, 51
Nutrition Facts, 194, 243–44. *See also*
      Labels, food

O

Oatmeal
   Maple-Almond Oatmeal, 293
Obesity
   breakfasts and, <u>95</u>
   effects of, on
      cancer, 7
      diabetes, 6
      health, general, 3, <u>10</u>
   genetics and, <u>109</u>
   heredity and, <u>109</u>
Oil. *See also* Cooking fat
   calories in, 39
   dietary fat in, 39
   extra-virgin, 47
   vegetable, 57
Omega-3 acids, 56
Omega-6 acids, 56
One-pot meals, shopping for, 43
Onions
   Potato and Onion Frittata, 294–95
Organic food, 232
Organization, for stress reduction,
      84–85
Osteoarthritis, 9
Osteoporosis, <u>44</u>, 73, 126, <u>136</u>
Overeaters Anonymous, 98
Overeating. *See also* Bingeing/binge
         eating
   emotions and, 90
   responses to, 261
   stress causing, 81, <u>82</u>, 84
   water intake in preventing, 198
Overhead press, 262

Overweight. *See also* Weight gain
   children
      exercise for, <u>130</u>, 133–34
      factors causing, 128
      motivation to lose weight for, 134–36
      statistics on, 128–29
      strategies for preventing, 129–36
      weight-loss programs for, <u>130</u>
   effects of, on
      back, 9
      breast cancer, 7
      health, general, 3
      pregnancy, 9
      sleep apnea, 11
      surgery, 10
   exercise deficiency causing, 58
   men, 107–8, 110, 112, 120
   physicians in U.S., <u>7</u>
   women, 109

P

"Pain words," 216
Parties
   alcohol at, avoiding, 269
   recipes for low-fat food at, 311–14
   tips for healthy enjoyment of, 269–70
Pasta
   Angel Hair Pasta with Carrots and Basil,
      306
   Butterflies and Beans, 310
   primavera, 48
   Scallops Véronique with Linguine, 307
Pear-shaped body, <u>15</u>
Peppers
   Stuffed Peppers, 303
Percent Daily Values, 244
Perfectionism, avoiding, 98
Pets, walking with, 242
Physical activity. *See* Aerobic exercise;
         Exercise
Pizza
   fruit, 120
   low-fat, 47
Plateau
   resistance training, 75
   weight-loss, 223–24
Poaching fish, 47
Polyunsaturated fats, <u>24</u>, 353
Popcorn popper, 39
Pork chops
   Pork Chops with Apricots, 297

Portions. *See* Servings
Positive messages, 94, 214–17, <u>216</u>
Posture, <u>61</u>
Potassium deficiency, 56
Potatoes
  complex carbohydrates in, 189
  potato salad, 48
  recipes using
    Baby Potatoes Filled with Dill Sour
      Cream, 312
    Potato and Onion Frittata, 294–95
  toppings for, 120
  vegetables with, 204–5
  yam or sweet potato "fries," 47
Potbelly, <u>15</u>, 107, 122, 263–64
Poultry. *See* Chicken; Turkey
"Power words," 216
Prawns
  Prawns with Peach Dipping Sauce, 311
Prayer, before meals, 260
Pregnancy
  diabetes during, 9
  exercise after, 116–17
  ideal weight in easing, 9
  overweight effects on, 9
  weight gain after, 114–17
Prescription drugs, weight gain from, 155, 188
Presses
  bench, 77–78, <u>77</u>, 246, 351
  leg, 246
  military, 78
  overhead, 262
  thigh, 197
  triceps, 220
Progressive muscular relaxation, for stress
    reduction, 84
Prostate cancer, 7
Proteins, 353
  animal, 149
  calories in, 19, 182
  deficiency of, 56
Pulling exercises
  chest pull, 197
  pull-down lat, 78
Pureeing, 124–25
Push-ups, chair, 220

Q
Quadriceps, 353
Quadriceps extension, <u>77</u>
"Quads," 353

R
Raises
  calf, <u>77</u>
  lateral, <u>77</u>, 220
RDAs, 353
RDI, **53**, 56
Recipes, low-fat
  adapting old recipe into, 261
  breakfasts, 293–96
  desserts, 317–19
  dinners
    Almond-Baked Halibut, 302
    Angel Hair Pasta with Carrots and Basil,
      306
    Black Bean Soup, 298–99
    Butterflies and Beans, 310
    Chicken and Garden Vegetable Stir-Fry,
      309
    Creamy Carrot Soup, 299
    Flounder with Lemon Broccoli, 305
    Kidney Bean and Chick-Pea Salad, 300
    Mexican Meatballs, 304
    Minted Chicken Salad, 301
    Pork Chops with Apricots, 297
    Ratotouille, 300–301
    Scallops Véronique with Linguine, 307
    Shortcut Chili, 227, 298
    Stuffed Peppers, 303
    Thyme Turkey Scallops, 310–11
    Turkey Cutlets with Herbed Mushroom
      Stuffing, 308
  lunches, brown-bag, 314–16
  new, finding, 243
  party food, 311–14
Recommended Dietary Allowances (RDAs),
    353
Recovery heart rate, 353
Reference Daily Intake (RDI), **53**, 56
Resistance training, 353
  aging and, 72, <u>73</u>
  amount of, to reap benefits, 197
  beginner work-out, 76–78
  benefits of, 196
  cautions in starting, 72–73, 197
  for children, <u>136</u>
  circuit training and, 70
  cool-down after, 75
  for endurance, 76
  equipment, 75, 206
  exercises
    slowing down, 220
    specific, 77–78, <u>77</u>, 197–9

Resistance training (*continued*)
  fitness and, 71, 75
  goal weight attainment and, 18
  gradual approach to, 76
  gratification of, immediate, 71–72
  habit of, 219
  health benefits of, 77
  log, 76, 220–21
  motivation for continued, 220–21
  in past, 71
  personalizing program of, 75–76
  plateau reached in, 75
  in present, 71
  questions about, 74–75
  realistic goals of, 76
  repetitions in, 74, 76, 77
  reward systems for, 76
  self-esteem improvement and, 74
  social support for, 76
  strategies for successful, 75–76
  strength training and, 127, 246–47, 262–63
  stretching before, 197
  time allotted for, 74
  for toning, muscle, 76
  varying, 76, 220
  warm-up before, 75
  weight loss promotion and, 72
  women and, benefits of, 73, 126–27
Resolutions, new week, 247–48
Restaurants. *See* Dining out
Reversibility, law of, 211
Reward systems
  for bingeing avoidance, 241
  for resistance training, 76
  "reward jar" vs. "cookie jar," 100–101
  setting up, 202–4
  as weight maintenance strategy, 272
  for women, 117
Rice, quick-cooking, 47
Role model, for children, 129–30, 135
Rows
  dumbbell, 77
  seated pulley, 246–47
  standing arm, 198

S
Salad bars, 142
Salads
  Caesar, 142
  chef's, 108
  dressings for, 124–25, 149
  before meals, 151
  potato, 48
  recipes for low-fat
    Kidney Bean and Chick-Pea Salad, 300
    Minted Chicken Salad, 301
    Tuna Shell Salad, 314–15
  selections when dining out, 142
  tuna, 47–48
  vinegar for tasty, 50
Salad spinner, 39
Salt. *See* Sodium
Sandwiches
  California Chicken Salad Sandwiches, 316
  Catalina Shrimp in Pita Pockets, 209, 316
  Turkey and Cucumber Sandwiches, 315
Saturated fats, 24, 353
Sausage
  Herbed Sausage Muffins, 296
Sautéing, without oil, 47
Scale, bathroom, 17
Scallops
  Scallops Véronique with Linguine, 307
Seafood. *See* Fish
Seasonings, 245. *See also specific types*
Seated pulley row, 246–47
Seated quadriceps extension, 247
Self-esteem
  exercise in improving, 74
  as motivation, 95
  resistance training in improving, 74
  weight loss and, 106
Self-image, 233–34
Self-massage, 254
Self-talk, 94, 172, 214–17, 216
Seltzer water, 199
Servings
  classic portion, 155, 156
  of dairy products, 201–2
  determining sizes of, 200–202
  eating habits and, 155–56, 200
  of fish, 201–2
  of fruits, 52, 201
  of grains, 200–201
  of legumes, 200
  of meats, 52, 201–2
  recommended daily, 52
  standard sizes of, 44
  traditional portion, 155–56
  underestimating, 155–56
  of vegetables, 52, 200–201
Sex drive, weight loss in increasing, 8
Shapedown, 130

Shoes
　alternating, 265
　athletic, 206
　hiking, 217
　walking, <u>60</u>, 185–86
Shopping list, 43, 194
Shrimp
　Catalina Shrimp in Pita Pockets, 209, 316
　Prawns with Peach Dipping Sauce, 311
Sit-ups, 122
Skillet, no-stick, 39, 47
Skin protection, 217, 228, 265
Sleep apnea, weight loss in preventing, 11
Smoking, quitting, <u>4–5</u>
Smoking-cessation clinics, <u>5</u>
Snacking
　children and, 129, 132
　distractions to avoid, 207–8
　jelly beans for, 260
　low-calorie, 190
　nighttime vs. daytime, <u>97</u>
　100-calorie foods for, **346–49**
　plans to avoid, 230–31
　smoking cessation and, <u>4</u>
　supermarket shopping with children and,
　　<u>42</u>
　triggers for, 230
　vegetables for, 204
Social support
　for behavior modification, 98
　for dieting, 98
　for men, 111–12
　for motivation
　　of children, 135
　　of self, 101
　for resistance training, 76
　walking and, 242–43
　for weight maintenance, 257–58
　for women, 127
Socks, for walking, 186, 217
Sodium, 353
　in foods, specific, **328–33**
　foods high in, 261
　reducing intake of, 27
　requirements, 261
Soups
　broths for, 46
　recipes for low-fat
　　Black Bean Soup, 298–99
　　Creamy Carrot Soup, 299
　selections when dining out, 142
　supermarket shopping for, 43

Spas
　Canyon Ranch in the Berkshires, 148
　The Greenhouse, 151
　Green Valley Spa and Tennis Resort, 151
　La Costa Hotel and Spa, 150–51
　Le Pli Health Spa and Salon at the Charles
　　Hotel, 150
　The New Age Spa, 147
　Norwich Inn and Spa, 148
　The Oaks, 149
　The Palms, 149
　The Phoenix Spa, 151–52
　Safety Harbor Spa and Fitness Center,
　　148–49
Special occasions, 144–46, 173, 269–70
SPF, 217, 228, 265
Spices, 43, 50
Sports drinks, 57
Spot reducing, 353
Sprays, no-stick, 47
Squats, 78
Stamina, 76, 80
Standing arm row, 198
Stationary bike, riding
　alternatives to, 101
　benefits of, 267
　bone strengthening from, <u>73</u>
　fun while, 268
　in home gym, 205–6
　interval training and, 268
　music while, 268
　reading while, <u>63</u>, 268
Steamer, 39
Steaming vegetables, 48
Stereotypes, 109–10, 111
Stock, fat-free, 46–47
Stomach crunches, 117
Stomach curls, <u>77</u>, 220, 262–63
Stomach fat, <u>15</u>, 107, 122, 263–64
Strainer, plastic/metal, 39
Strength, 354
Strength training. *See* Resistance training
Stress
　cravings and, <u>82</u>
　eating habits and, 81, <u>83</u>, 84
　gender differences in reacting to, <u>82</u>
　muscle tension and, 195
　overeating caused by, 81, <u>82</u>, 84
　reducing
　　assertiveness, 79–81
　　exercise, 195
　　ideas for, general, <u>83</u>

Stress (*continued*)
  reducing (*continued*)
    log for, 264
    meditation, 195–96
    music, 84
    organization, 84–85
    progressive muscular relaxation, 84
    walking, 79, 80–81, 264
    as weight maintenance strategy, 173
    yoga, 195–96
  stomach fat and, 263–64
  symptoms of, personal, 195
  understanding, 264
  weight gain and, 262–63
  work-induced, 81
Stretching, 61, 197
Stroke, 4
Sugar, 157
Sugar-free food, 44, 52
Sun protection factor (SPF), 217, 228, 265
Sunscreen, 217, 228, 265
Supermarket shopping
  with children, 42, 129
  dangers for weight watchers and, 41
  as exercise, 63
  food labels and, 44
  hunger during, avoiding, 42, 43
  low-fat food purchase and, 260
  samples while, free, 43, 193
  shopping list for, 43, 194
  smaller amounts and, buying, 148–49
  for soups, 43
  tips for, 43, 45, 194
  trends in, 41
Suppers. *See* Dinners
Supplements, vitamin/mineral, 52–53, 56
Support groups, weight loss, 98, 258
Surgery, effects of overweight on, 10
Sweets, avoiding during smoking cessation, 4.
    See also Desserts
Swimming, 156

T

Target weight. *See* Goal weight
Thigh exercises, 197
Three-pound alarm, 170, 272
Time management, for stress control, 84–85
Toning muscles, 76
Trading off, 141–42, 248–49
Triceps, 221, 262, 354
Triceps extension, 262

Triceps presses, 221
Triglycerides, 121, 354
Triple-A program for behavior modification
  action, 95–98
  attitude, 92, 94–95
  awareness, 90, 92
Tuna
  in low-fat cooking, 47–48
  Tuna Shell Salad, 314–15
Turkey
  dietary fat in, 124
  lean, 52
  recipes using
    Herbed Sausage Muffins, 296
    Mexican Meatballs, 305
    Thyme Turkey Scallops, 310–11
    Turkey and Cucumber Sandwiches,
        315
    Turkey Cutlets with Mushroom
        Stuffing, 308
Type II diabetes, 6, 9

U

Unsaturated fats, 354

V

Vacations, 145, 228–29, 261
Vegetables. *See also specific types*
  in children's diet, encouraging, 133
  cooking with, 204–5
  fresh, 245
  intake of, increasing, 204–5
  juices, 204
  with potatoes, 204–5
  recipes using
    Angel Hair Pasta with Carrots and
        Basil, 306
    Cheese-Topped Mushroom Caps with
        Spinach, 313
    Chicken and Garden Vegetable Stir-Fry,
        309
    Creamy Carrot Soup, 299
    Flounder with Lemon Broccoli, 305
    Mozzarella and Asparagus Canapes, 312
    Ratatouille, 300–301
    Stuffed Peppers, 303
    Turkey and Cucumber Sandwiches,
        315
    Turkey Cutlets with Herbed Mushroom
        Stuffing, 308

sautéing, 47
servings of, 52, 200–201
for snacking, 204
starch, 200
steaming, 48
water content in, 47, 198
Vending machines, avoiding, 261
Videos, exercise, 250–51
Vinegar, for tasty salads, 50
Visualization, 233–34
Vitamins
Reference Daily Intake of, **53**
supplements, 52–53, 56
vitamin E, 57

W

Waffles, 131
Waist-to-hip ratio (WHR), 15, 15, 122, 354
Walking
with children, 228, 242–43
in cold weather, 216–18
enjoying, 180, 181
indoors, 217
interval training and, 237–38
log, 61
with pets, 242
posture during, 61
Prevention Club, 159
program, 60–61, 192
fine-tuning, 225–26
shoes for, 60, 185–86
social support and, 242–43
speed vs. distance and, 259
for stress reduction, 79, 80–81, 264
tips, 60–61
for weight loss promotion, 60–61
at work, 243
Warm-up, 75, 271
Water intake
in appetite control, 198
after bingeing, 241
caffeine drinks, avoiding, 199
dehydration and, 57
when dining out, 143
eating habits and, 199
from food, 198
hydration and, 265
overeating prevention and, 198
requirements, 57
smoking cessation and, helping, 5
tap water vs. bottled and, 199

tips for ensuring adequate amount of, 199
water loss vs., 198
weight loss promotion and, 105
at work, 261
Weigh-ins, 5, 17, 179, 191
Weight, suggested adult, 13–15, **13**
Weight control. *See* Weight maintenance
Weight cycling, 169, 354
Weight gain. *See also* Overweight
from medications, 188
by men
alcohol and, 110, 112
casualness about, 108–9
cooking views and, 109–10
dieting views and, 108, 111
exercise deficiency and, 110
ignorance of nutrition and, 108
with smoking cessation, 4–5
during special occasions, 144–45
stress and, 262–63
by women
depression and, 118
after menopause, 114, 117–18
after pregnancy, 114–17
Weight loss
aging and, 8–9
calorie deficit for, 103, 177
commitment to program of, 178
cost-benefit analysis of, 99–100
expectations about, 251–53
failure, 153–57, 183
fantasy vs. reality of, 155, 251–53
gender and, 119, 127
body fat reduction and, 122–23
calorie burning and, 123
cravings and, 124–25
eating habits and, 125–26
exercise and, 126–27
food selection and, 120
health/fitness strategies and, 121
health benefits of
back problem prevention, 9
cancer prevention, 6–7
cholesterol, increasing good, 6
diabetes prevention, 6
energy level, increased, 11
heart problem prevention, 4–5
high blood pressure prevention, 4–5
immune system, improved, 10
joint problem prevention, 9
longevity, 8–9
osteoarthritis prevention, 9

Weight loss *(continued)*
    health benefits of *(continued)*
        sex drive, increased, 8
        sleep apnea prevention, 11
        ten-pound loss, 3
    personalizing plan for, 150–51
    plateau in, 223–24
    promotion
        aerobic exercise, 63, 122–23, 126
        breast feeding, 115
        diet, 103–5
        exercise, 60–61, 61–62, 105–6
        goal-setting, 178–79
        low-fat diet, 19–21, 122–23
        resistance training, 72
        self-esteem, 106
        strategies, top 20, 103, 104
        walking, 60–61
        water intake, 105
    scale use in, 17
    self-esteem and, 106
    social support in, 98, 101, 111–12, 257–58
    spa tips for
        Canyon Ranch in the Berkshires, 148
        The Greenhouse, 151
        Green Valley Spa and Tennis Resort,
            151
        La Costa Hotel and Spa, 150–51
        Le Pli Health Spa and Salon at the
            Charles Hotel, 150
        The New Age Spa, 147
        Norwich Inn and Spa, 148
        The Oaks, 149
        The Palms, 149
        The Phoenix Spa, 151–52
        Safety Harbor Spa and Fitness Center,
            148–49
    terms in discussing, 351–54
    tricks, 221–23, 260–61
Weight maintenance
    challenges of, 168–69, 271–72
    goal weight in, 169–70
    gradual steps toward, 102
    lifestyles and, 106, 256–57
    log for, 171–73
    social support for, 257–58
    strategies
        commitment, 170, 272
        diet, 103–5, 170, 272
        diet mantra, 173–74
        exercise *(see* Exercise, as weight mainte-
            nance strategy)

forgiveness for lapses, 174
goal weight, realistic, 169–70
lifestyle changes, 106
lifestyle goals, 174
log, 171–73
low-fat diet, 170
men's, 111–13
motivation, 171–73
refresher courses, 174
reward systems, 272
self-praise, 173
self-talk, 172
special occasion preparation, 171
stress management, 173
three-pound alarm, 170, 272
top 20, 103, 104
women's, 114–18
successful, 169–74, 171, 256
yo-yo syndrome and, avoiding, 169
Weight training. *See* Resistance training
Weight Watchers, 98
WHR, 15, 15, 122, 354
Wine, 143, 151, 232
Women. *See also* Gender
body fat of average, 16
body image of, 108, 121
calorie intake for average, 17
cancer risks of, 6–7
dietary fat intake for, safe, 22–23, **23**
height-weight chart for, **13**
overweight, 109
resistance training and, benefits of, 73,
    126–27
reward systems for, 117
social support for, 127
weight gain by
    depression and, 118
    after menopause, 114, 117–18
    after pregnancy, 114–17
weight maintenance strategies for, 114–18
Work
dieting and, 112
stress caused by, 81
walking at, 243
water intake at, 261
Workouts. *See* Exercise; Resistance training

Y
Yoga, 149, 195–96
Yogurt, 48
Yo-yo dieting, 169, 354